Lecture Notes on General Surgery

TO OUR WIVES

Lecture Notes on General Surgery

HAROLD ELLIS
CBE, MA, DM, MCh, FRCS
Emeritus Professor of Surgery
University of London

SIR ROY CALNE
MA, MS, FRCS, FRS
Professor of Surgery
Addenbrooke's Hospital, Cambridge

EIGHTH EDITION

Blackwell
Science

© 1965, 1968, 1970, 1972, 1977, 1983,
1987, 1993 by
Blackwell Science Ltd
Editorial Offices:
Osney Mead, Oxford OX2 0EL
25 John Street, London WC1N 2BL
23 Ainslie Place, Edinburgh EH3 6AJ
238 Main Street, Cambridge
  MA 02142, USA
54 University Street, Carlton
  Victoria 3053, Australia

Other Editorial Offices:

Arnette Blackwell SA
1, rue de Lille, 75007 Paris
France

Blackwell Wissenschafts-Verlag GmbH
Kurfürstendamm 57
10707 Berlin, Germany

Blackwell MZV
Feldgasse 13, A-1238 Wien
Austria

First published 1965
Revised edition 1966
Second edition 1968
Greek edition 1968
Third edition 1970
Fourth edition 1972
Reprinted 1974
Revised reprint 1976
Fifth edition 1977
Portugese edition 1979
Reprinted 1979, 1980
Sixth edition 1983
Reprinted 1984, 1985, 1986
Seventh edition, 1987
Reprinted 1989 (twice)
Eighth edition 1993
Reprinted 1994, 1995

DISTRIBUTORS

  Marston Book Services Ltd
  PO Box 87
  Oxford OX2 0DT
  (Orders: Tel: 01865 791155
          Fax: 01865 791927
          Telex: 837515)

North America
  Blackwell Science, Inc.
  238 Main Street
  Cambridge, MA 02142
  (Orders: Tel: 800 215-1000
          617 876-7000
          Fax: 617 492-5263)

Australia
  Blackwell Science Pty Ltd
  54 University Street
  Carlton, Victoria 3053
  (Orders: Tel: 03 347–5552)

A catalogue record for this title
is available from the British Library

ISBN 0-632–03335–5
     0-632-03667-2 Four Dragons

Set by Semantic Graphics Services
Singapore
Printed and bound
in Great Britain by
Hartnolls of Bodmin, Cornwall

Contents

Introduction

The ideal medical student at the end of his clinical course will have written his own textbook — a digest of the lectures and tutorials he has assiduously attended and of the textbooks he has meticulously read. Unfortunately few students are perfect, and most approach the qualifying examinations depressed by the thought of the thousands of pages of excellent and exhaustive textbooks wherein lies the wisdom required of them by the examiners.

We believe that there is a serious need in these days of widening knowledge and expanding syllabus for a book which will set out briefly the important facts in general surgery which are classified, analysed and as far as possible rationalized for the revision student. These lecture notes represent our own final year teaching; they are in no way a substitute for the standard textbooks but are our attempts to draw together in some sort of logical way the fundamentals of general surgery.

Because this book is written at student level, principles of treatment only are presented, not details of surgical technique.

We recommend the companion volume *Spot Diagnosis in General Surgery*, which provides colour illustrations and questions and answers based on the text of *Lecture Notes*.

The need for an eighth edition has enabled us to update and carry out a detailed revision of the whole text.

HAROLD ELLIS
SIR ROY CALNE

Acknowledgements

We are grateful to our colleagues — registrars, housemen and dressers — who have read and criticized this text during its production and to many readers and reviewers for their constructive criticisms.

Finally, we should like to acknowledge the continued help given by the staff at Blackwell Scientific Publications.

H.E.
R.C.

Chapter 1
Acute Infections

There is an important general principle in treating acute infection anywhere in the body: antibiotics are invaluable when the infection is spreading through the tissues (e.g. cellulitis, peritonitis, pneumonia), but drainage is essential when abscess formation has occurred.

CELLULITIS

Cellulitis is a spreading inflammation of connective tissues. It is generally subcutaneous, but the term may also be applied to pelvic, perinephric, pharyngeal and other connective tissue infections. The common causative agent is the β-haemolytic streptococcus.

The invasiveness of this organism is due to the production of hyaluronidase and streptokinase, which respectively dissolve the intercellular matrix and the fibrin inflammatory barrier.

Characteristically the skin is dark red with local oedema and heat. There may be vesicles and, in severe cases, cutaneous gangrene. Cellulitis is often accompanied by lymphangitis and lymphadenitis, and there may be an associated septicaemia.

Treatment

Immobilization, elevation and antibiotics. If a local abscess forms, this must be drained.

ABSCESS

An abscess is a localized collection of pus, usually, but not invariably, produced by pyogenic organisms; occasionally a sterile abscess results from the injection of irritants into soft tissues (for example, thiopentone).

An abscess commences as a hard, red, painful swelling which then softens and becomes fluctuant. If not drained, it may discharge spontaneously onto the surface or into an adjacent viscus or body cavity. There are the associated features of bacterial infection; a swinging fever, malaise, anorexia and sweating with a polymorph leucocytosis.

Treatment

An established abscess in any situation requires drainage. Chemotherapeutic agents cannot diffuse in sufficient quantity to sterilize an abscess completely. Pus left undrained continues to act as a source of toxaemia and becomes surrounded by dense fibrous tissue.

The technique of abscess drainage depends on the site. The classical method, which is applicable to a superficial abscess, is to wait until there is fluctuation and

1

to insert the tip of a scalpel blade at this point. The track is widened by means of sinus forceps, which can be inserted without fear of damaging adjacent structures. If there is room, the surgeon's finger can be used to explore the abscess cavity and break down undrained loculi. Drainage is then maintained until the abscess cavity heals from below upwards, otherwise the superficial layers can close over, with recurrence of the abscess. The cavity is therefore kept open by means of a gauze wick, a corrugated drain or a tube; the drain is gradually withdrawn until complete healing is achieved.

Deep abscesses are usually localized and drained using ultrasound or CT scanning.

BOILS

A boil (furuncle) is an abscess, usually due to the pyogenic staphylococcus, which involves a hair follicle and its associated glands. It is therefore not found on the hairless palm or sole, but is usually encountered where the skin is hairy, injured by friction, or dirty and macerated by sweat; thus it occurs particularly on the neck, axilla and the perianal region. Occasionally a furuncle may be the primary source of a staphylococcal septicaemia and be responsible for osteomyelitis, perinephric abscess or empyema, particularly in debilitated patients. On the face it may be complicated by a cavernous sinus thrombosis, via the facial veins.

Differential diagnosis

Multiple infected foci in the axillae or groins due to infection of the apocrine sweat glands of these regions (Hydradenitis suppurativa) are usually misdiagnosed as boils. They do not respond to antibiotic therapy and can only be treated effectively by excision of the affected skin area; if this is extensive, the defect may require grafting.

Treatment

When pus is visible the boil should be incised. Recurrent crops of boils should be treated by improving the general hygiene of the patient, and by the use of ultraviolet light and hexachlorophene baths, but systemic antibiotic therapy is not indicated.

CARBUNCLES

A carbuncle is an area of subcutaneous necrosis which discharges onto the surface through multiple sinuses. It is usually staphylococcal in origin. The subcutaneous tissues become honeycombed by small abscesses separated by fibrous strands. The condition is often associated with general debility and particularly with diabetes. The urine should always be tested for sugar in this or any other septic condition.

Treatment

Surgery is rarely indicated initially. Antibiotic therapy is given and the carbuncle merely protected with sterile dressings. Occasionally a large sloughing area eventually requires excision and a skin graft. Diabetes, if present, should be controlled.

Chapter 2
Specific Infections

TETANUS

Tetanus is now a rare disease in the United Kingdom, thanks to a comprehensive immunization policy. In the developing world it remains prevalent with a mortality of up to 60 per cent.

Pathology

Tetanus is caused by the clostridium tetani; an anaerobic, flagellated, exotoxin-secreting and Gram-positive bacillus, which forms a characteristic terminal spore ('drumstick'), and which is a normal inhabitant of soil and faeces. The bacillus remains at the site of inoculation and produces a powerful exotoxin. This is a protein with a high molecular weight that prevents renal excretion. This results in its having a long half life in the blood stream and allows time for penetration into nervous tissue. The toxin enters peripheral nerve axons and travels proximally to the spinal cord, where it blocks inhibiting spinal reflex mechanisms and gives rise to the characteristic features of the disease.

Tetanus follows the implantations of spores into a deep, devitalized wound where anaerobic conditions occur. Infection is related less to the severity of the wound than to its nature; thus an extensive injury which has received early and adequate wound toilet is far less at risk than a contaminated puncture wound which has been neglected. Occasionally, dressings or catgut which have been contaminated with tetanus spores are the source of infection of surgical wounds. In primitive communities, where dung is used to dress the umbilical cord in newborn, *tetanus neonatorum* may occur.

Clinical features

The incubation time is 24 hours to 24 days. Muscle spasm first develops at the site of inoculation and then involves the facial muscles and the muscles of the neck and spine. As a rule it is the trismus of the facial spasm (producing the typical 'risus sardonicus', or 'lock-jaw' to the layman) which is the first reliable indication of developing tetanus. This may be so severe that it becomes impossible for the patient to open his mouth. The period of spasm is followed, except in mild cases, by violent and extremely painful convulsions, which occur within 24–72 hours of the onset of symptoms and may be precipitated by some trivial stimulus, such as a sudden noise. The convulsions, like the muscle spasm, affect the muscles of the neck, face and trunk. Characteristically, the muslces remain in spasm between the convulsions. The temperature is a little elevated but the pulse is rapid and weak.

In favourable cases the convulsions, if present at all, become less frequent and then cease and the tonic spasm gradually lessens. It may however, be some weeks before muslce tone returns to normal and the risus sardonicus disappears. In fatal cases paroxysms become more severe and frequent; death occurs from asphyxia due to involvement of the respiratory muscles or from exhaustion, inhalation of vomit, or pneumonia.

The prognosis is serious when the incubation period from the time of injury to the onset of spasm is under 5 days and when convulsions occur within 48 hours of the onset of muscle spasm.

Differential diagnosis

1   Tetany: characteristically affects the limbs, producing carpopedal spasm.
2   Strychnine poisoning: flaccidity occurs between convulsions whereas in tetanus the spasm permits.
3   Meningitis: because of the neck stiffness.
4   Epilepsy.
5   Hysteria.

Treatment

Prophylaxis

Active immunization comprises two initial injections of tetanus toxoid (formalin treated exotoxin) at an interval of 6 weeks. Booster doses are given at intervals of not more than 7 years, or at the time of any injury. Toxoid should be given to any population at risk of injury, for example, service personnel.

The risk of tetanus can be reduced almost to zero if penetrating and contaminated wounds are adequately excised to remove all dead tissue and a course of prophylactic penicillin (or tetracycline in sensitive patients) is given. Patients who have previously received toxoid should be given a booster dose. If toxoid has not been given in the past, human antitetanus immunoglobulin, prepared from fully immunized subjects, should be given if the wound is heavily contaminated.

There is no justification for the use of anti-tetanus serum as a passive immunization agent. There has never been a controlled trial of the value of ATS; severe reactions may occur, particularly if serum therapy has been given in the past, and skin sensitivity tests to a small subcutaneous dose give no reliable guide to subsequent severe reactions. Tetanus may occur after ATS has been given and, at present, it seems that the risk of mortality from serum is of the same order as that of an unimmunized subject acquiring tetanus after injury.

Curative treatment

1. Control convulsions.
The patient is nursed in isolation, quiet and darkness and is heavily sedated with phenobarbitone or chlorpromazine. In severe cases curarization with tracheostomy and intermittent positive pressure artificial respiration is required and this may have to be continued for up to 4 weeks. It is terminated when the spasms and rigidity are absent during a trial period without relaxants. These serious cases are best transferred to a special respiratory unit.

2. Control the local infection.
Excision and drainage of any wound is carried out under a general anaesthetic. Penicillin or erythromycin are administered and these will also act as a prophylactic against pulmonary infection.

3. Maintain the general condition and electrolyte balance
Feed the patient by naso-gastric tube to maintain the general condition and electrolyte balance.

4. Administer human antitetanus immunoglobulin.
Tetanus does not confer immunity and therefore, if the patient has not previously been immunized, the first dose of tetanus toxoid should be given. If previous active immunization has been carried out, then a booster dose of toxoid is administered.

GAS GANGRENE

Pathology

Results from infection by *Clostridia welchii (perfringens), oedematiens, septicum* and *sporogenes*; anaerobic, encapsulated, spore forming, gas-producing, Gram-positive organisms which produce an exotoxin. This group includes both proteolytic and saccharolytic organisms. The characteristic gas formation in the tissues is produced by the liberation of CO_2, H_2S and NH_3 by protein destruction. The organisms are found in soil and in faeces.

Typically gas gangrene is an infection of deep penetrating wounds, particularly of war, but sometimes involvement of the abdominal wall or cavity may follow operations upon the alimentary system. Occasionally gas gangrene complicates amputation of an ischaemic lower limb, or follows abortion or puerperal infection.

Clinical features

The incubation period is about 24 hours. Toxaemia is severe with tachycardia, shock and vomiting. The temperature is first somewhat elevated and then becomes sub-normal. The affected tissues are swollen and crepitate due to gas. The skin becomes gangrenous and the infection spreads along the muscle planes, producing at first dark red swollen muscle and then frank gangrene.

Treatment

Prophylaxis
Consists of adequate excision of wounds, which removes both the organisms and the dead tissues which are essential for their anaerobic growth. Seriously contused wounds (such as those produced by a gunshot wound) or contaminated wounds are left open and lightly packed with gauze. Delayed primary suture can then safely be performed after 5 or 6 days, by which time the wound is usually healthy and granulating. Penicillin is given in all heavily contaminated wounds and to patients with atherosclerosis undergoing amputation of the leg.

Curative

In the established case, all involved tissue must be excised. Implication of all muscle groups in a limb is an indication for amputation. Penicillin and blood transfusion are given. Hyperbaric oxygen therapy, to eliminate the anaerobic environment, is theoretically sound but as it is combined with all the other modalities of treatment, its efficacy cannot be judged. If a hyperbaric chamber is available, it should certainly be employed.

The value of anti-gas gangrene serum, both as a prophylactic and curative measure, is not established.

ACTINOMYCOSIS

Pathology

Actinomycosis is an infection produced by the *Actinomyces israelii* or ray fungus, so called because the mycelial threads may be seen radiating from the main fungal mass in culture. The fungus is micro-aerophilic and exists as a saprophyte in the mouth (especially where there is dental caries) and in the alimentary canal. Infection may occur via a breach in the mucous membrane, for example following dental extraction, and produces a dense fibrous tissue reaction within which pockets of pus develop. The pus contains typical 'sulphur granules', which are yellow specks of mycelium. The infection spreads along the fascial planes and occasionally by the blood-stream, but not via the lymphatics.

Clinical features

Actinomycosis can be classified into three main groups: cervico-facial, abdominal and pulmonary.

Cervico-facial

This form occurs typically after dental extraction or tonsillitis. Although actino-myces do grow on grasses and decayed vegetable matter, these varieties are not pathogenic in man and the infection does not occur, as was once taught, by chewing contaminated straw. Nor is the disease transmitted from cattle or horses to man. Swelling occurs over the angle of the jaw and the adjacent tissues become greatly indurated. The skin develops a typical bluish discoloration, then sinuses appear, which discharge thin pus. Pain may or may not be a feature, but there is usually marked trismus. Spread may occur by direct infiltration to the orbit, base of skull, jaw, or mediastinum.

Abdominal actinomycosis

Usually located in the ileo-caecal region and follows upon an attack of perforative appendicitis, a perforated peptic ulcer or an abrasion of the alimentary mucosa by some foreign body. A hard fibrous mass, honey-combed with abscess cavities, develops in the right iliac fossa and multiple sinuses may appear on the abdominal wall. Spread may occur via the portal vein producing a portal pyaemia, the liver being riddled with abscess cavities.

Pulmonary actinomycosis

May follow inhalation of fungus from the infected mouth. Spread occurs through the lung to the pleura and eventually the chest wall. Pulmonary disease may also occur secondary to spread from the neck via the mediastinum, or from the abdominal cavity through the diaphragm.

Treatment

Comprises a 12-week course of daily injections of penicillin. Obvious collections of pus should be drained. The actinomyces should be tested for sensitivity and occasionally other antibiotics, e.g. tetracycline, may be required.

Chapter 3
Shock

Shock is the term used to describe a clinical state comprising pallor, sweating, coldness and peripheral cyanosis. The pulse is usually rapid and the blood pressure low. In severe cases there may be dyspnoea, thirst, nausea or vomiting. The patient may be confused and restless or semi-conscious.

Aetiology

Shock is produced by a wide variety of circumstances, the common factor being a *reduction in the effective circulating blood volume*, with resultant decreased tissue perfusion, particularly of vital organs. This clinical picture may be seen in:

1 *Severe haemorrhage*, an actual reduction of blood volume.

2 *Extensive fluid loss* as a result of exudation of plasma from burns, or loss of extra-cellular fluid in severe vomiting or diarrhoea.

3 *The vasovagal syndrome*, produced by severe pain or emotional disturbance. The mechanism of this is reflex vasolidation in muscle together with vagal cardiac slowing. This syndrome can be recognized because the shock picture is accompanied by slowing of the heart and responds to the simple measure of lying the patient flat with elevation of the legs.

4 *Severe toxaemia*, as in peritonitis, septicaemia (particularly Gram-negative organisms) or pancreatitis. Here there is a combination of fluid loss into the extravascular space, pain and the effect of chemical or bacterial toxins on the heart; once again the shock picture is produced by circulatory failure. However, in contrast to the other types of shock, bacterial endotoxins produce peripheral vasodilatation so that the patient's skin is usually hot and flushed.

5 *Heart failure* from myocardial infarction or pulmonary embolus.

6 *Adrenal cortical failure* following adrenalectomy, Addison's disease or lack of cortico-steroid replacement in patients who have been on long-term corticoids, who develop infection or undergo surgery. This last cause of unexplained shock is very important to remember since treatment is straightforward whilst failure to recognize the cause usually leads to death.

7 *Sympathetic interruption*, which reduces the effective blood volume by widespread vasodilatation; for example, the spinal shock following transection of the spinal cord, or after a high spinal anaesthetic.

The physiological basis of haemorrhagic shock

Severe haemorrhage produces the following chain of events: reduction in blood volume — diminution in the venous return to the heart — fall in cardiac output (Starling's law: the output depends on the degree of stretch of the heart muscle in diastole) — fall in blood pressure — this is counteracted by the carotid sinus and aortic arch reflexes, which increase the heart rate, and by sympathetic vasocon-striction of the splanchnic bed and of the peripheral cutaneous vessels.

This mechanism maintains essential coronary, renal, cerebral and lung blood flow. The blood pressure remains at first relatively normal, but continued haemor-rhage eventually reaches a stage which can no longer be compensated and the blood pressure then falls.

The clinical features of shock which have already been described are thus easily explicable on this physiological basis. The intense peripheral vasoconstric-tion produces the cold, pale skin. The rapid pulse and low blood pressure are typical features of the impaired cardiac output. The sweating results from sym-pathetic overactivity. The cerebral disturbances follow inadequate perfusion of the brain.

A continued low blood pressure produces a series of irreversible changes so that the patient may die in spite of later blood replacement. The oxygen lack affects all the vital organs; there may be tubular necrosis of the kidney resulting in renal failure, the adrenals may lose their normal reaction to stress, the heart may fail due to inadequate coronary perfusion and there may be damage to the cardiac and vasomotor centres in the medulla. In the tissues themselves anoxia produces capillary paralysis and dilatation so that a copious fluid loss occurs into the interstitial spaces.

With intensive treatment, life may be preserved despite continuing disease. In such instances, the condition of 'shock lung' may develop. There is progressive impairment of pulmonary gaseous perfusion with interstitial oedema due to 'leaky' capillaries which may result from multiple blood transfusions causing platelet and fibrin pulmonary microemboli, toxicity from prolonged oxygen ther-apy and opportunist lung infection.

Eventually the build up of 'sick cells' and tissue necrosis results in death — *irreversible shock.*

Septic shock

Shock may be produced as the result of severe infection from either Gram-positive or, more commonly, Gram-negative organisms. The latter is particularly seen after colonic, biliary and urological surgery and with infected severe burns. Endotoxin release damages the myocardium with resultant congestive cardiac failure so that, in contrast to the patient with haemorrhagic shock, the neck veins may be congested and the central venous pressure increased. Damage to capillary endothelium produces *disseminated intra-vascular coagulation* (DIC) with block-age of the arterial microcirculation. Fibrin and platelets are consumed excessively with resultant haemorrhages into the skin, the gastro-intestinal tract, the lungs, mouth and nose. Post-partum bleeding from the uterus may be a severe problem.

Treatment

This depends on diagnosis. A vasovagal attack, or faint, rapidly responds to lowering the head and elevating the legs; if the patient does not improve after this, it is suggestive that some complicating factor such as internal haemorrhage coexists with the vasovagal syndrome. It is important to know that considerable loss of blood into the tissues occurs with major fractures of the limbs even if these are not compound.

Where haemorrhage is the cause of the shock
Take the following steps:
1   Further haemorrhage is arrested; this may require direct pressure to a wound or surgical exploration where continued bleeding is the result of a peptic ulcer haemorrhage, ruptured spleen or ruptured ectopic pregnancy.
2   Blood transfusion to replace the blood loss.
3   Relief of pain by means of an injection of morphia where pain is a marked feature.
4   Elevation of the foot of the bed is a quick and effective temporary means of raising the blood pressure and is a useful emergency measure.

Excessive warmth should be avoided; this produces vasodilatation of the skin vessels thereby diverting available blood from the vital tissues.

Oxygen is seldom required since the blood is usually fully oxygenated unless there is an associated chest injury, pulmonary oedema or respiratory depression due to a head injury.

Shock from other causes
This may require appropriate fluid replacement; plasma or plasma substitute in the case of burns, or saline in severe vomiting or diarrhoea.

In septic shock, treatment comprises intravenous fluid replacement with plasma expanders, broad spectrum antibiotics and the tracing and elimination of the source of infection. This may be simply a matter of removing an infected central venous catheter or may involve major surgery for a leaking bowel anastomosis.

Treatment of DIC comprises intravenous heparin to arrest the coagulation process and transfusion of fresh frozen plasma to replace the necessary clotting factors.

In all these situations, regular and frequent monitoring of the central venous pressure is an aid in the correct replacement of fluid and the prevention of fluid overload.

The management and monitoring of the critically-ill patient
The severely-shocked patient should be admitted to an intensive care ward where his continuous supervision by specially-trained nursing staff is available. As well as careful clinical surveillance, the following need to be monitored:
1   Rectal temperature, pulse, respiration rate and blood pressure.
2   Central venous pressure.
3   Urine output (via catheter).
4   ECG.
5   Serum electrolytes, haemoglobin and white blood count.
6   Arterial Po_2, Pco_2, pH.

7 The cardiac output, left atrial and pulmonary arterial pressures can be monitored using a Swann Ganz cathether which is 'floated' into the pulmonary artery
via a systemic vein.

The frequency of these measurements depends on the patients condition and
response to treatment. It is particularly important to remember that, in this
environment of recording machinery and scientific nursing, the patient remains a
human being, who deserves to be treated with dignity and tenderness. If he is
conscious he may well be terrified, in pain and acutely aware of all that is going on
around him.

Chapter 4
Burns

Pathology

A burn may be partial or full thickness, depending on whether or not the germinal layer of the skin is intact or destroyed. (Fig. 4.1).

A *partial thickness* burn may be quite superficial, with erythema due to capillary dilatation and with or without areas of blistering produced by exudation

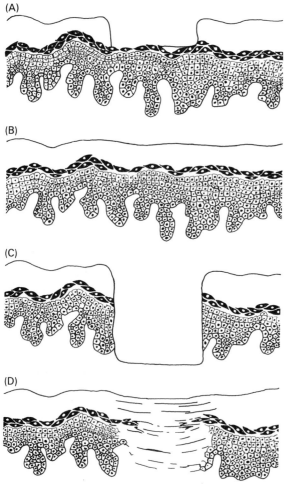

(A)

(B)

(C)

(D)

Fig. 4.1. A partial thickness burn (A) leaves part or the whole of the germinal epithelium intact. Complete healing takes place (B). A full thickness burn (C) destroys the germinal layer and, unless very small, can only heal by dense scar tissue (D).

of plasma beneath coagulated epidermis. The underlying germinal layer is intact and complete healing takes place within a few days. Deeper partial thickness burns extend down to the germinal layer and may partially destroy it. There is intense blistering followed by the formation of a slough. This separates after about 10 days, leaving healthy newly formed pink epithelium beneath.

Full thickness burns completely destroy the skin. There may be initial blistering but this is soon replaced by a coagulum or slough; more often this is present from the onset in an intense deep burn. Unlike the more superficial burns, this slough separates only slowly over three or four weeks, leaving an underlying surface of granulation tissue. Very small deep burns may heal from an ingrowth of epithelium from adjacent healthy skin; more extensive burns, unless grafted, heal by dense scar tissue with consequent contracture and deformity.

General effects of burns

Pain

This is due to the stimulation of numerous nerve endings in the damaged skin. It is more severe in superficial burns and, indeed, deep burns may be relatively painless due to extensive destruction of nerve endings.

Plasma loss

There is intense exudation of plasma through the damaged capillaries, especially during the first 24 hours after burning; by the time a coagulum has formed (about 48 hours) this plasma loss ceases.

Airway

Smoke inhalation or thermal injury of the respiratory tract may rapidly result in respiratory obstruction from pharyngeal or laryngeal oedema.

Oligaemic shock

Shock is a direct result of plasma loss, partly into blisters and partly as leakage into the interstitial spaces. It is therefore proportional to the surface area of the body which is burnt.

Anaemia

This results partly from destruction of red cells within involved skin capillaries and partly from toxic inhibition of the bone marrow if infection of the burnt area occurs.

Stress reaction

The adrenocortical response of sodium and water retention, potassium loss and protein catabolism occurs as in any severe injury.

Toxaemia

This is a combination of factors, which include biochemical disturbances, plasma loss and infection. It has also been postulated that a toxin is produced by the burnt tissues. But no specific toxic substance has so far been isolated. It is less often seen now that burns are treated adequately.

Treatment

The principles of the treatment of burns are: first the management of the local condition, to prevent infection and to promote healing, and second, the general treatment to mitigate the more widespread effects of burns listed above.

Local treatment

If smoke has been inhaled, humidified oxygen is given through a face mask. Early endotracheal intubation may be required for thermal injury of the upper respiratory tract or urgent tracheostomy may be necessary if intubation is unsuccessful.

Minor partial thickness burns are cleaned with a detergent and protected by a sterile dressing. A small full thickness burn is best treated by immediate excision and split skin grafting.

The treatment of major burns may either be by the open or the closed method; sometimes a combination of the two is required. The open (or exposure) method is based on the principle that bacteria will not grow on the dry coagulum which rapidly forms over the exposed burn surface. The closed treatment aims at excluding bacteria from the burnt area by means of sterile dressings.

In the *open treatment* the burn is exposed in a warm, isolated room. Elevation is used where possible to reduce oedema. It is excellent for the face, the limbs or where only the front or the back of the trunk is involved. It is obviously impossible to apply to circumferential burns of the trunk and is best avoided for burns of the fingers.

In the *closed treatment* the burn is cleaned with detergent, covered with silver-sulphadiazine, vaseline gauze and thick layers of sterile dressings. If these dressings become soaked with plasma they are changed immediately, otherwise they are left for approximately a week.

At the end of 10 days, in both methods of treatment, the slough will separate from superficial burns leaving a healthy healed epithelium beneath. No further local treatment is required. In contrast, the slough over a full thickness burn is still densely adherent. Attempts to remove it reveal an underlying bleeding granulation tissue; healing can only occur naturally by a process of dense fibrous scar tissue formation, therefore full thickness burns at this stage are excised and covered with split skin grafts.

Replacement of skin is carried out immediately if the eyelids are involved, in order to prevent ectropion with the risk of corneal ulceration. The face, hands and the joint flexures are next in priority for skin grafting procedures, since scarring at these sites will obviously produce considerable deformity and disability.

General treatment

1. Pain

Relieve pain with morphia, which is best given intravenously.

2. Oligaemic shock

Treat by replacing fluid with plasma or plasma substitute (for example, 5 per cent albumin or Dextran 70). The amount of plasma to be given depends on careful clinical assessment of the patient, including urinary output, general condition of shock, central venous pressure monitoring, together with 4-hourly haematocrit estimations.

As a guide to the amount of fluid replacement the 'rule of nine' is helpful. The body is divided into zones of percentage of surface area as follows (Fig. 4.2):

	Per cent surface area
Head and neck	9
Each arm	9
Each leg	9×2
Front of the trunk	9×2
Back of the trunk	9×2
Perineum	1

As a rough rule the patient's hand is approximately 1 per cent of his surface area.

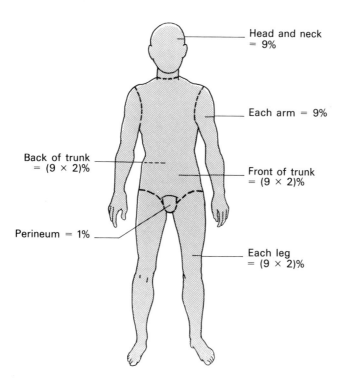

Fig. 4.2. The 'rule of nine' — a useful guide to the estimation of the area of a burned surface. (Note also that a patient's hand represents 1 per cent of his body surface.)

In adults, as a guide, 1 litre of fluid is required for each 9 per cent of the body affected. The maximum loss of fluid occurs during the first 12 hours and half of the estimated replacement should be given in this period. The rest is given over the subsequent 24 to 36 hours.

Another useful rule is the Mount Vernon Burns Unit formula:

$$\text{Weight in kg} \times \frac{\% \text{ burn area}}{2}$$

This gives a figure for fluid in ml; for example, a 70 kg patient with a 40 per cent burn would, on this formula, give a figure of 1400 ml. This amount is given every 4 hours for the first 12 hours, every 6 hours for the next 12 hours and then 12-hourly over the next day.

If the burns are full thickness, approximately 50 per cent of the fluid replacement should be given as blood in order to replace the extensive red cell destruction within the affected area.

3. Systemic chemotherapy

Antibiotics are given to cover both Gram positive and Gram negative organisms. Secondary infection of the burns may require local application of antibiotics, the choice of which will depend on culture of the burnt area.

Antibiotics seldom eliminate infection and there is the risk that resistant organisms will eventually proliferate. The best protection against infection is to obtain skin cover. Unfortunately, this is difficult to achieve rapidly in extensive burns; temporary biological dressings of cadaver homografts or porcine xenografts may help to prevent infection until autografting can be carried out. The use of sheets of skin epithelium produced by autologous skin culture is producing encouraging early results.

Prognosis

Depends on the extent and depth of the burns, and whether or not infection occurs. Young infants and the elderly carry a higher mortality than young adults. No matter which methods of treatment are used, few patients survive more than a 70 per cent full thickness body area burn. As a very rough guide, if the patient's age + percentage body area of full thickness burn exceeds 100, then the chances of survival are low.

Chapter 5
Post-operative Complications

Classification

Any operation carries with it the risk of complications. These should be considered as:

1 *Local:* involving the operation site itself.

2 *General:* affecting any of the other systems of the body, e.g. respiratory, urological or cardiovascular complications.

In addition post-operative complications should be classified into:

3 *Immediate:* within the first 24 hours.

4 *Early:* the first 2 to 3 weeks post-operatively.

5 *Late:* any subsequent period, often long after the patient has left hospital.

A useful table of post-operative complications following abdominal surgery is presented in Table 5.1. This scheme can be modified for operations concerning any other system.

Table 5.1. Post-operative complications — abdominal surgery.

Time	Local	General
0 hours to 24 hours	Reactionary haemorrhage	Asphyxia — Obstructed airway / Inhaled vomit
2nd day to 3 weeks	Paralytic ileus	
	Infection — Wound / Peritonitis / Pelvic / Subphrenic	Pulmonary — Collapse / Broncho-pneumonia / Embolus
	Secondary haemorrhage	Urinary — Retention / Suppression (Tubular necrosis)
	Dehiscence — Wound / Anastomosis	Deep venous thrombosis
	Obstruction due to fibrinous adhesions	Enterocolitis
		Bed sores
Late	Obstruction due to fibrous adhesions	After extensive resections or gastrectomy:
	Incisional hernia	Anaemia
	Persistent sinus	Vitamin deficiency
	Recurrence of original lesion (e.g. stomal ulcer or malignancy)	Steatorrhoea and/or diarrhoea
		Osteoporosis
		Dumping syndrome

WOUND INFECTION

The incidence of wound infection after surgical operations is still in the region of 10 per cent. It is especially high, of course, where pre-operative sepsis already exists. In pre-antibiotic days it was particularly the haemolytic streptococcus which was feared, but now, since this remains penicillin-sensitive, the principal causes of wound infection are the penicillin resistant or much feared methicillin resistant *Staphylococcus aureus*, together with *Streptococcus faecalis, pyocyaneus,* coliform bacilli and other bowel bacteria including bacteriodes.

Aetiology

In considering the aetiology of any post-operative complication the following classification should be used:

1   *Pre-operative*: factors already existing before the operation is carried out.
2   *Operative*: factors which come into play during the operation itself.
3   *Post-operative*: factors introduced after the patient's return to the ward.

Pre-operative factors

There may be pre-existing infection, e.g. a perforated appendix or an infected compound fracture. The patient may be a nasal carrier of staphylococci or have a skin infection, e.g. a crop of boils.

Operative factors

These are lapses in theatre technique; failure of adequate sterilization of instruments, the surgeon's hands or dressings. There may be nasal or skin carriers of staphylococci among the nursing and surgical staff. Wound infections are especially common when the alimentary, biliary or urinary tract is opened during surgery, allowing bacterial contamination to occur.

Post-operative factors

Cross infection may occur from infected cases in the ward during dressing, or there may be contamination of the wound from the nose or hands of the surgical or nursing staff.

Clinical features

The onset of wound infection is usually a few days after operation; this may be delayed still further, even up to weeks, if chemotherapy has been employed. The patient complains of pain and swelling in the wound, of the general effect of infection (malaise, anorexia, vomiting) and runs a swinging pyrexia. The wound is red, swollen, hot and tender. Removal of sutures or probing of the wound releases the contained pus.

Treatment

Prophylaxis comprises scrupulous theatre and dressing technique, the isolation of infected cases and the elimination of carriers with colds or septic lesions among the medical and nursing staff.

Established infection is treated by drainage; antibiotics are given if there is, in addition, a spreading cellulitis.

Prophylactic antibiotics

In the early days of antibiotic therapy, it was hoped that the problem of surgical infection would be overcome merely by the prescription of prophylactic chemotherapy. Unfortunately, this soon proved to be a false hope, and the widespread use of these drugs simply saw the emergence of resistant strains of bacteria and of many examples of diarrhoea, skin rashes and other unpleasant side-effects.

However, there are instances where prophylactic antibiotics are indicated:

1   Where a foreign body is to be implanted: prosthetic heart valves, joints etc.
2   In patients with mitral valve disease, as prophylaxis against subacute bacterial endocarditis.
3   In vascular and organ transplant surgery.
4   In amputation of the leg for ischaemic disease. Here the risk of gas gangrene is high and penicillin is the antibiotic of choice.
5   In penetrating wounds and compound fractures, again principally as prophylaxis against clostridial infections.
6   Because of the high risk of bacterial contamination in operations which involve opening the biliary or alimentary tract, (especially the large bowel) prophylactic systemic or local broad spectrum antibiotics are indicated.

Antibiotic associated enterocolitis

Shortly after the introduction of antibiotics, there were reports of post-operative severe watery diarrhoea due to extensive enterocolitis. The bowel shows mucosal inflammation with pseudo-membrane formation.

The probable mechanism is the destruction of normal bowel commensals allowing overgrowth of resistant bacteria. While *Staphylococcus pyogenes* was implicated in early epidemics, more recent evidence strongly supports a pathogenic role for toxin-producing strains of *Clostridium difficile* which may be demonstrated in the stools of patients with pseudomembranous colitis (PMC). Although this condition may follow administration of any of a range of antibiotics, there is a strong association with preceding lincomycin or clindamycin therapy.

Clinical features

Antibiotic associated enterocolitis usually occurs in the first post-operative week in patients who have received broad-spectrum antibiotics. The condition is particularly likely to occur after large bowel surgery. Mild cases present simply with watery diarrhoea. Severe cases have a cholera-like picture; a sudden onset of profuse watery diarrhoea with excess mucus, abdominal distension and shock due to the profound fluid loss.

Sigmoidoscopy reveals a red friable mucosa with whitish yellow plaques which may run together to form a pseudomembrane.

Treatment

Intravenous fluid and electrolyte replacement is essential; blood and hydrocortisone are given if shock is severe. Other antibiotics are stopped and oral vanco-mycin, which rapidly eliminates *Clostridium difficile*, is prescribed.

PULMONARY COLLAPSE

This is an extremely common post-operative complication; indeed, some degree of pulmonary collapse occurs after almost every abdominal or trans-thoracic procedure.

Mucus is retained in the bronchial tree, blocking the smaller bronchi; the alveolar air is then absorbed, with collapse of the supplied lung segments (usually the basal lobes). The collapsed lung may become secondarily infected by inhaled organisms.

Aetiology

1. Pre-operative factors
Pre-existing acute or chronic pulmonary infection increase the amount of bron-chial secretion and add the extra factor of pathogenic bacteria; heavy smokers are at particular risk and every effort must be made to dissuade patients from smoking for as long a period as possible before elective surgery. Emphysema, ankylosing spondylitis or any other condition which will make coughing difficult in the post-operative period predispose to mucus retention.

2. Operative factors
Irritant anaesthetic drugs, which increase mucus secretion and depress the action of the bronchial cilia. Atropine in addition increases the viscidity of the mucus.

3. Post-operative factors
The pain of the thoracic or abdominal incision which inhibits expectoration of the accumulated bronchial secretions is the most important cause of mucus retention.

Clinical features

Pulmonary collapse occurs within the first 48 hours post-operatively. The patient is dyspnoeic with a rapid pulse and elevated temperature. There may be cyanosis. He attempts to cough, but this is painful and unless he is encouraged, he may fail to expectorate. The sputum is at first frothy and clear, but later may become purulent.

Examination reveals that the patient is distressed with a typical painful 'fruity cough'; this results from the sound of the bronchial secretions rattling within the chest and a good clinician should be able to make the diagnosis while still several yards away from his patient. The chest movements are diminished, particularly on the affected side; there is basal dullness and air entry is depressed with the addition of râles.

X-ray of the chest may reveal an opacity of the involved segment (usually basal or mid-zone) and there may be mediastinal shift to the affected side.

Treatment

Pre-operatively, breathing exercises are given, smoking is forbidden and antibiotics prescribed if any chronic respiratory infection is present. Post-operatively, the patient is encouraged to cough and breathing exercises instituted. Small repeated doses of opiates diminish the pain of coughing but are insufficient to dull the cough reflex. Antibiotics are only prescribed if the sputum is infected; their selection is based on the sensitivity of the cultured organisms.

DEEP VEIN THROMBOSIS IN THE LOWER LIMB

In the post-operative period the patient has an increased predisposition to venous thrombosis in the veins of the calf muscles, the main deep venous channels of the leg and in the pelvic veins, due to:

1 *Increased thrombotic and clotting tendency* (increase in platelets and their adhesiveness and increase in fibrinogen).

2 *Increased stagnation* within the veins (immobilization in bed and depression of respiration).

3 *Damage to the vein wall* produced by pressure of the mattress against the calf or direct damage at operation (particularly the pelvic veins during pelvic procedures).

Platelets deposit on the damaged intima, the vein is occluded by thrombus and a propagated fibrin clot then develops, which may detach and form a pulmonary embolus (see below).

This complication is particularly likely to occur in elderly patients, the obese, those with malignant disease, patients who have varicose veins or a history of previous deep vein thrombosis, those undergoing abdominal, pelvic and particularly hip surgery and women who are taking steroid contraceptives.

Clinical features

Deep vein thrombosis can be 'silent' but typically the symptoms and signs usually occur during the second post-operative week, but it may be earlier or later; earlier thrombosis particularly occurs when the patient has already been in hospital for some time pre-operatively. Studies using radioiodine labelled fibrinogen, which is deposited as fibrin in the developing thrombus and which can be detected by scanning the leg, suggest that the thrombotic process usually commences at, or soon after, the operation.

The patient complains of pain in the calf, and on examination there is tenderness of the calf and swelling of the foot, often with oedema, raised skin temperature and with dilatation of the superficial veins of the leg. This is accompanied by a mild pyrexia. If the pelvic veins or the femoral vein are affected then there is massive swelling of the whole lower limb — a 'white leg'.

Special investigations

1. Venography
This is the definitive investigation but cannot be repeated frequently nor employed for routine screening.

2. I^{125} labelled fibrinogen
This is a highly sensitive test and enables the legs to be scanned at daily intervals. It

demonstrates the presence of deep vein thrombosis in approximately one-third of all post-operative patients, with a particularly high incidence in those groups of high risk subjects listed above. Only approximately 50 per cent of thrombi picked up on scanning can be detected on careful clinical examination. Due to scatter from the radioactive iodine excreted in the urine and held in the bladder, the test is unreliable in the pelvic and thigh region and is only significant from the knee downwards.

3. Doppler ultrasound
This depends on the loss of the Doppler effect over the femoral vein if this is totally or partially occluded. It is simple, non-invasive and has the advantage that it picks up occlusion of major veins which are the potentially dangerous ones.

Treatment
Prophylaxis consists of active mobilization and breathing exercises in the immediate post-operative period. An elective major operation on a patient taking contraceptive tablets should be delayed for several weeks after stopping the pill. Elevation of the legs increases the venous return and elastic graded compression stockings are effective, particularly if there are pre-existing varicose veins or the patient has a history of previous thrombosis.

The use of intermittent calf compression using inflatable bags have been shown to reduce the incidence of thrombosis as detected by the iodine-labelled fibrinogen scanning test. Intravenous infusion of low molecular weight dextran during, and for 48 hours after, operation is also effective.

The most widely-used prophylactic technique is the use of small doses of subcutaneous heparin, 5000 units twice or three times a day, commenced at the time of operation and continued while the patient remains at risk, in order to reduce the post-operative hypercoagulable state. Controlled trials have shown reduction in the incidence of venous thrombosis and a less certain reduction in pulmonary embolism in the treated group.

In the established case anticoagulant therapy with intravenous heparin is commenced to prevent formation of further propagated clot; this is best given by continuous pump infusion. Once anti-coagulated, the patient can be mobilized with the lower limbs supported in elastic stockings to prevent oedema. If thrombosis occurs in the immediate post-operative period a very difficult decision must be made whether or not to anticoagulate the patient, since the former carries with it the serious risk of haemorrhage at the operation site. If bleeding occurs, the heparin is immediately discontinued and protamine sulphate given intravenously on the basis of 1 ml of 1 per cent solution per 1000 units of heparin.

Ligation, plication or insertion of a sieve into the inferior vena cava are seldom performed but may be indicated when recurrent episodes of pulmonary embolization occur in spite of adequate anticoagulant therapy.

PULMONARY EMBOLUS
This occurs when a clot from a vein, originating in the calf muscles or especially

the femoral vein or the pelvis, detaches and becomes lodged in the pulmonary arterial tree. A massive embolus obstructs the right heart output and causes rapid death from right heart circulatory failure, probably with additional reflex cardiac arrhythmia, while the less severe cases present with shock, breathlessness and cyanosis, accompanied often by marked retrosternal pain or discomfort. Still milder cases present with pleural pain, dyspnoea and, in 50 per cent of cases, haemoptysis. If the patient survives the embolus, complete clearing of the clot occurs quite rapidly. Infarction of the lung only takes place in patients with cardiac failure where there is pre-existing pulmonary congestion.

Diagnosis of massive embolus in the acute phase is often difficult although there may be helpful signs in the chest — a pleural rub with diminished air entry and crepitations. Chest X-ray in the early stages is also often normal, although within a few hours patchy shadowing of the affected segment takes place. The jugular venous pressure will be raised.

Obviously the differential diagnosis is from a post-operative coronary infarction. An ECG may help in differentiating between these two conditions. In the case of pulmonary embolus there will be the electrocardiographic changes of right heart strain.

A perfusion lung scan will show uneven circulation through the lungs, with multiple perfusion defects, but a simultaneous ventilation scan is normal in the absence of pre-existing pulmonary disease.

Definitive diagnosis can be made by pulmonary arteriography which will demonstrate the filling defect in the pulmonary artery. This may be indicated in the critically ill patient if the diagnosis is in doubt and is also performed if pulmonary embolectomy is planned.

It is important to know that pulmonary embolus may occur without any preceding warning signs of thrombosis in the leg. Indeed, once there are obvious clinical features of deep vein thrombosis, detachment of an organized and adherent clot from this limb is rather unlikely, especially if anticoagulant therapy has been commenced so that fresh clot formation is inhibited. The great majority of fatal pulmonary emboli are unheralded.

Treatment

Morphia is given for pain, oxygen administered and heparin commenced if the patient is not already on anticoagulants. Lysis of a massive embolus may be effected with an intravenous infusion of streptokinase. In the critically ill patient, pulmonary embolectomy carried out with cardio-pulmonary bypass may be successful.

BURST ABDOMEN

Dehiscence of the abdominal wound may result from a number of factors:

1. Pre-operative

Uraemia, cachexia with protein deficiency, vitamin C deficiency, jaundice, obesity, steroids, distension and chronic cough (the latter two because of the strain put upon the abdominal incision).

2. Operative

Poor technique in closing the abdominal wound or the use of suture material of low tensile strength which ruptures postoperatively. Badly tied knots may come undone and sutures too near the edge of the incision may cut through the tissues like a cheese wire through cheese.

3. Post-operative

Cough or abdominal distension which put a strain on the suture line; infection or haematoma of the wound which weaken it.

Clinical features

The abdomen usually dehisces on about the tenth day. There may be a warning of this if pink fluid discharges through the abdominal incision. This represents the serous effusion, (which is always present during the first week or two within the abdominal cavity after operation), which is tinged with blood and which seeps through the breaking-down wound. If this 'pink fluid sign' is ignored the patient finds a loop of intestine or the omentum protruding through the wound, usually after a cough or strain — a most alarming finding both for the patient and staff.

Sometimes the deep layer of the abdominal incision give way but the skin sutures hold; such cases result in a massive incisional hernia.

Treatment

The patient with a burst abdomen is usually in mortal fear. He should be reassured and the reassurance supplemented by an injection of morphia. The abdominal contents are covered with sterile towels soaked in saline and the patient prepared for operation. The abdominal wound is resutured under a general anaesthetic using strong nylon stitches passed through all the layers of the abdominal wall. The prognosis after this procedure is good unless the patient succumbs to his underlying disease. The wound usually heals rapidly, but there is a high incidence of subsequent incisional herniation.

POST-OPERATIVE FISTULA

A serious complication following abdominal surgery is the development of a fistula involving the alimentary canal or its biliary or pancreatic adnexae.

This may result from:

1 Poor surgical technique.

2 Poor blood supply at the anastomotic line, particularly in operations on the oesophagus and rectum.

3 Sepsis incurred before or during the operation leading to suture line breakdown. (Sepsis is, of course, inevitable once leakage has occurred.)

4 Poor condition of the patient: uraemia, anaemia, jaundice, protein deficiency or cachexia from malignant disease.

5 Presence of distal obstruction. Thus, a biliary fistula is likely to occur if stones are left behind in the common bile duct after cholecystectomy. Moreover, a fistula will not heal spontaneously under these circumstances.

6 Local malignant or inflammatory disease, e.g. Crohn's.

Clinical features

Diagnosis is usually all too obvious, with the escape of bowel contents or bile through the wound or drainage site. If there is any doubt, methylene blue given by mouth will appear in the effluent of an alimentary fistula, the fluid can be tested for bile and the fluid from a pancreatic leak is rich in amylase. An injection of radio-opaque fluid will outline the fistulous tract and give valuable information about its size and whether or not distal obstruction exists.

The enzyme-rich fluid of the upper alimentary tract and of a pancreatic fistula produces rapid excoriation of the surrounding skin. This is much less marked in a faecal fistula since the contents of the colon are relatively poor in proteolytic enzymes. The patient is toxic and passes into a severe catabolic state compounded by infection and starvation due to loss of intestinal fluid. Rapid wasting occurs from fluid loss and protein depletion.

Treatment

The early management has three aims:

1 To protect the skin around the fistula from ulceration. The edges of the wound are covered by Stomahesive (which adheres even to moist surfaces), or aluminium paint or silicone barrier cream. It may be possible to collect the effluent by means of a colostomy appliance and thus reduce skin soilage but if the mouth of the fistula is too large, then continuous suction may be necessary.

2 To replace the loss of fluid, electrolytes, nutriments and vitamins. In a high alimentary fistula this will require intravenous feeding via a central line. Calories are given in the form of glucose and fat emulsion and protein depletion is countered by amino-acids. Vitamins and electrolytes are also required. Such prolonged intravenous feeding must be carefully monitored by serial biochemical studies. If the fistula is low in the alimentary tract, the so-called space diet can be given by mouth. This is rapidly absorbed in the upper intestine and is thus not lost through the fistula.

3 To reduce sepsis by judicious drainage of pus collections and by antibiotic therapy.

On this conservative regime a side-fistula without distal obstruction may well heal spontaneously. However, if the fistula is large or complete or if there is a distal obstruction then subsequent surgery is required to close the leak and to deal with the obstruction. This can only be successful if carried out at the stage when the patient's condition has improved and when a positive nitrogen balance has been achieved.

POST-OPERATIVE PYREXIA

The following drill is valuable in elucidating the cause of fever following operation:

1 Inspect the wound: superficial wound infection or haematoma.

2 Rectal examination: pelvic abscess.

3 Examine the legs: deep vein thrombosis.

4 Examine the chest clinically and if necessary order a chest X-ray, screening and ultrasound: pulmonary collapse, bronchopneumonia, infarct, subphrenic abscess.

5 Laboratory examination of the urine: urinary infection.

6 Laboratory examination of the stools: enterocolitis.

7 Finally, consider the possibility of drug sensitivity.

Chapter 6
Post-operative Fluid and Electrolyte Balance and Peri-operative Nutrition

The relative volumes of fluid in the different body compartments and their ionic concentration remain remarkably constant, so that for a healthy individual there is a well balanced intake of fluid and electrolytes to compensate for the loss that occurs in perspiration, respiration, defaecation and the urine (Table 6.1). The internal milieu is maintained chiefly by the selective control of excretion of water and minerals by the kidneys. Changes in temperature and humidity of the external environment will result in appropriately modified intake and excretion of fluid and electrolytes with the internal environment remaining constant.

If a patient is injured or subjected to an anaesthetic and surgery he may be unable to adapt his intake and loss, and the desirable compensatory renal response may not be possible. Under these circumstances the patient's general condition can rapidly deteriorate. Artificial administration of fluid and electrolytes by the intravenous route can protect the patient from serious disturbances of fluid and electrolyte change. A simple plan to provide sufficient fluid and electrolytes is usually successful without the need for precise calculations because of the enormous reserve of renal function that can cope with most minor insults. If, however, renal function is impaired, either by pre-existing disease or additional damage from hypotension, haemorrhage, septicaemia or nephrotoxic drugs, then minor errors of fluid and electrolyte balance can result in the rapid development of fatal complications. Just as the patient under an anaesthetic is not able to control his ventilation and this becomes the prime responsibility of the anaesthetist, so a patient unable to take fluid and electrolytes by the normal oral route must have his fluid balance controlled by the surgeon.

It is necessary to assess renal function, and to measure the plasma electrolytes and fluid and electrolyte input and output. The balance is determined and future requirements planned. If the patient develops persistent abnormal loss of fluid and electrolytes, for example from an intestinal fistula, balance can be difficult to

Table 6.1. Fluid and electrolyte loss — approximate values for 70 kg adult per 24 hours.

	Average loss		
	H_2O ml	Na mmol/l	K mmol/l
Insensible (lungs and skin)	700		
Urine	1300		
Total	2000	100	60

achieve. Similarly, an inbalance may develop between energy expenditure and calorie replacement, and, after a few days, malnutrition may lead to protein catabolism, reduced resistance of the body to infection, and impairment of healing ability. Prolonged intravenous feeding may be necessary to allow the patient to be restored towards nitrogen balance, so that his tissues will heal and the fistula will either close spontaneously or can be closed by surgery.

Impairment of kidney function makes the control and balance an extremely difficult task and the help of a nephrologist will be needed since the patient may require dialysis.

Once the patient has returned to normal oral intake of fluid and electrolytes, provided his renal function is satisfactory, balance will be restored to normal without external aid. With these principles in mind the following empirical management of a patient with normal renal function in the perioperative phase will usually be satisfactory.

A patient admitted for elective surgery, for example, an anterior resection of the rectum, will have been in fluid balance until the period of starvation before the operation. Following surgery, the response to the trauma is secretion of anti-diuretic hormone and corticosteroids, resulting in oliguria in the first 24 hours. An intravenous infusion is usually set up during the induction of anaesthesia and infusion of three litres per day of the solution containing sodium chloride, dextrose and potassium is usually continued until the patient's bowel sounds return and oral fluid intake and nutrition can begin.

Table 6.2(a) represents a suitable fluid and electrolyte replacement regime for a previously fit 70 kg patient requiring post-operative intravenous fluid replacement therapy for 2 to 3 days. Table 6.2(b) represents a slightly more complex scheme where more prolonged replacement is required.

Although 3 litres of fluid for a 70 kg subject is a good guide, note that fluid replacement can be calculated on the basis of 40 ml per kg body weight per day.

It must be stressed that excessive alimentary losses (nasogastric aspiration, fistulae, diarrhoea) are replaced ml per ml by additional normal saline.

The patient who has suffered severe trauma or repeated vomiting from, for example, a strangulated inguinal hernia causing intestinal obstruction, may require rehydration prior to surgery depending on the estimated state of the fluid loss. Patients with severe burns are a special case (see Chapter 4). The regimen outlined is suitable for patients with good renal function and additional nutrition is not generally required unless there is a delay in intestinal function.

Whilst the patient is receiving parenteral fluids, daily estimations of the plasma urea and electrolytes should be performed. Any deviations from the normal limits will require urgent assessment and arterial blood gases and pH may indicate disturbances of acid-base balance. Abnormalities of lung function rapidly occur following excessive fluid administration when excretion is impaired. Also, tissue destruction, for instance from infarcted bowel, may caused metabolic acidosis and a rise in serum potassium, findings which should lead to urgent therapy to remove the infarcted tissue and prevent further damage occurring.

Common disturbances of the plasma electrolytes include hyponatraemia, which usually responds to a reduction in water intake, and hypokalaemia, which

Table 6.2. Alternative replacement regimens.

	H_2O	Total Na mmol	Total K mmol	Calories
(a) 3 × 1 litre (1 every 8 hours) of 0.15% KCl 0.18% NaCl 4.0% Dextrose	3000	90	60	450
(Prolonged use of this may lead to water retention and hyponatraemia)				
(b) 2 × 500 ml of 0.15% KCl 0.9% NaCl	1000	150	20	0
4 × 500 ml of 0.15% KCl 5.0% Dextrose Each 500 ml bag in 4 hours One of solution A alternating with 2 of solution B	2000	0	40	380
Total in 24 hours	3000	150	60	380

Any additional losses should be replaced: for example, excessive drainage from a nasogastric tube or intestinal fistula should be replaced intravenously by a similar amount of normal saline, or hyponatraemia and metabolic alkalosis are likely to develop.

often accompanies a metabolic alkalosis or malnutrition.

Careful observation of the patient and his fluid and electrolyte balance and renal function will in most cases be rewarded by an uneventful hospital course and full recovery.

NUTRITION

Most patients coming to both elective and emergency surgery are reasonably well nourished and do not require special supplementation, since they will have recovered from the operation sufficiently to resume ordinary eating before they have become seriously malnourished. There are, however, certain categories of patients where nutrition prior to surgery is poor and may be a critical factor in determining the outcome of an operation, for example, patients with chronic intestinal fistulae, malabsorption, chronic liver disease, neoplasia, starvation and after chemo- and radiotherapy.

Enteral feeding

If the gastro-intestinal tract is functioning satisfactorily, it is best to supplement feeding by a basic diet introduced through a fine nasogastric tube directly into the stomach. The constituents of the diet are designed to be readily absorbable protein, fat and carbohydrate, which can provide in a total nutritional volume of 2 litres/day, 8400 kJ with 70 g protein. The commonest complication is diarrhoea which is usually self limiting.

Parenteral feeding

For patients with intestinal fistulae, ileus or malabsorption, nutrition cannot be supplemented through the gastro-intestinal tract and therefore parenteral feeding is necessary, usually introduced through a central venous line, although peripheral venous feeding can supplement nutrition up to 4000 kJ per day. Total parenteral nutrition (TPN) must be administered into a major vein because of the high osmolarity of the solutions used. The exact management is best directed by an expert in nutrition, but in principle is to provide the patient with 15g of nitrogen and 10 000 kJ, as amino-acids, dextrose and intralipid in 2.5 litres over 24 hours with added vitamin and essential elements. The ability of a patient to benefit from intravenous feeding depends on the general state of metabolism and residual liver function. It may be necessary to continue nutritional support in the post-operative period until gastro-intestinal function returns and the patient is restored to positive nitrogen balance from the perioperative catabolic state; often apparent to the nurses and doctors as a sudden occurrence, when the patient starts smiling and asks for food. In chronic malnutrition with intestinal fistulae or in patients who have lost most of the small bowel, parenteral feeding may be necessary on a long-term basis, similar to haemodialysis patients with renal failure. Complications of TPN include sepsis, hyponataemia and hyperglycaemia.

Chapter 7
Tumours

A particularly bad student was asked on a ward round 'What would you think of if a patient had central abdominal pain, vomited and then the pain shifted to the right iliac fossa?' He replied 'Cancer, Sir.' In this answer there existed a grain of truth. New growths are so common and widespread that their consideration must at least pass through the mind in most clinical situations. It therefore behoves the student, both for examinations and, still more important, for future practical doctoring, to have a standard scheme with which to tabulate the pathology, diagnosis, treatment and prognosis of neoplastic disease.

PATHOLOGY

When considering the tumours affecting any organ this simple classification should be used:

Benign

Malignant

    1. Primary

    2. Secondary

It is surprising how often failure to remember this basic scheme leads one to omit such an elementary fact that common tumours of brain and bone are secondary deposits.

For each particular tumour, the following headings should be used:
1 Incidence
2 Age distribution.
3 Sex distribution.
4 Geographical distribution (where relevant).
5 Predisposing factors.
6 Macroscopic appearances.
7 Microscopic appearances.
8 Pathways of spread of the tumour.
9 Prognosis.

Reference to page 164 (stomach) and page 210 (rectum) will show how this scheme functions in practice.

Clinical features and diagnosis

A malignant tumour may manifest itself in three ways:

1   The effects of the primary tumour itself.
2   The effects produced by secondary deposits.
3   The general effects of malignant disease.
(The only common exceptions are tumours of the CNS, which do not produce secondary deposits.)

Diagnosis is always made by history, clinical examination and, where necessary, special investigations. Let us now, as an example, apply this scheme to carcinoma of the lung, the commonest killing cancer in this country.

History

1   *The primary lesion* may present with cough, haemoptysis, dyspnoea.
2   *Secondary deposits* in bone may produce pathological fracture or bone pains, cerebral metastases may produce headaches or drowsiness, liver deposits may result in jaundice.
3   *General effects of malignant disease*: the patient may present with malaise, lassitude or loss of weight.

Examination

1   *The primary tumour* may produce signs in the chest.
2   *Secondary deposits* may produce cervical lymph node enlargement, hepatomegaly or obvious bony deposits.
3   *The general effects of malignancy* may be suggested by pallor or weight loss.

Special Investigations

1   *For the primary lesion:* chest X-ray, bronchoscopy, cytology of sputum.
2   *For secondary deposits:* X-ray skeletal survey, ultrasound liver.
3   *For general manifestation of malignancy:* a blood count may reveal anaemia. The ESR may be raised.

This simple scheme applied to any of the principal malignant tumours will enable the student to present a very full clinical picture of the disease with little mental effort.

Treatment

The treatment of malignant disease should be considered under two headings:
1   *Curative:* an attempt is made to ablate the disease completely.
2   *Palliative:* although the disease is incurable or has recurred after treatment, measures can still be taken to ease the symptoms of the patient.

In this section we shall summarize the possible lines of treatment for malignant disease in general; in subsequent chapters the management of specific tumours will be considered in more detail.

Curative

1   *Surgery.*
2   *Radiotherapy* alone (e.g. tumours of the mouth and pharynx).
3   *A combination* of surgery and radiotherapy (e.g. carcinoma of cervix).

Palliative

1 *Surgery:* the palliative excision of a primary lesion may be indicated although secondary deposits may be present; for example, a carcinoma of the rectum may be excised to prevent pain, bleeding and mucous discharge although secondary deposits may already be present in the liver. Irremovable obstructing growths in the bowel may be shortcircuited. Inoperable obstructing tumours of the oesophagus or cardiac end of the stomach may be intubated by means of a plastic tube so that dysphagia can be relieved. Surgery may also be used to interrupt nerve pathways for pain relief, e.g. cordotomy in which the contralateral spinothalamic tract within the spinal cord is divided.

2 *Radiotherapy:* palliative treatment may be given to localized secondary deposits in bone, irremovable breast tumours, inoperable lymph node deposits, etc. It is particularly indicated for *localized irremovable disease.*

3 *Sex hormones and endocrine gland surgery:* these are only applicable to carcinoma of the breast and prostate.

4 *Cytotoxic therapy:* a wide range of drugs have anti-cancer action but this is not specific and all of them also damage normal dividing cells, especially those of the bone marrow, the gut, the skin and the gonads. They may be classified into:

(a) Alkylating agents (e.g. cyclophosphamide).
(b) Antimetabolites (e.g. 5-flurouracil).
(c) Plant alkyloids (e.g. vincristine).
(d) Antibiotics (e.g. adriamycin).

Multiple drugs are frequently used (combination chemotherapy).

A balance must be made between the chances of regression of the tumour in relatively fit patients with tumours likely to be sensitive (e.g. breast, ovary, testis) and the toxic effects of the drug regime.

5 *Drugs:* for pain relief (analgesics, opiates), hypnotics, tranquillizers and antiemetics, for example chlorpromazine.

6 *Nerve blocks* with phenol or alcohol for relief of pain.

7 *Maintenance of morale* by cheerful and kindly attitude of medical and nursing staff.

Prognosis

The prognosis of any tumour depends on four main features:

1 The extent of spread.
2 Microscopic appearance.
3 Anatomical situation.
4 General condition of the patient.

The extent of spread

The extent of the tumour (its *staging*) on clinical examination, at operation or on studying the excised surgical specimen is of great prognostic importance. Obviously the clinical findings of palpable distant secondaries or gross fixation of the primary tumour are serious. Similarly the local invasiveness of the tumour at operation or evidence of distant spread are of great significance. Finally, histological study may reveal involvement of the nodes which have not been detected clinically or of microscopic extension of the growth to the edges of the resected specimen with consequent worsening of the outlook for the patient.

Microscopic appearance

As a general principle, the prognosis of a tumour is related to its degree of histological differentiation (its *grading*).

These two factors, the spread of the tumour and this histological differentiation, should be taken in conjunction with each other; a small tumour with no apparent spread at the time of operation may still have poor prognostic significance if its highly anaplastic, whereas an extensive tumour is not incompatible with long survival of the patient after operation if the microscopic examination reveals a high degree of differentiation.

Anatomical situation

The site of the tumour may preclude its adequate removal and thus seriously affect the prognosis. For example, a tumour at the lower end of the oesophagus may be easily removable whereas an exactly similar tumour situated behind the arch of the aorta may be technically inoperable; a brain tumour located in the frontal lobe may be resected whereas a similar tumour in the brain stem will be completely hopeless as a surgical proposition.

The general condition of the patient

A patient apparently curable from the point of view of the local condition may be inoperable because of his poor general health. For example, gross congestive cardiac failure may render what is technically an operable carcinoma of the rectum a hopeless surgical risk.

Chapter 8
The Chest and Lungs

INJURIES OF THE CHEST

Ventilation of the lungs depends on a patent main airway and pulmonary alveoli, a rigid bony skeleton of the thorax, and on the integrity of the nerves and muscles that control the movements of the ribs and diaphragm. Traumatic disruption of the chest wall is likely to be lethal unless treatment is instituted rapidly. Dangerous complications of chest injury are: paradoxical respiration, pneumothorax, penetration of the lung, haemothorax, cardiac tamponade due to laceration of the heart, and large vessel damage. Serious harm can also result from crush injuries which do not penetrate the chest; thus a main bronchus or the aorta may be ruptured, the lung contused and papillary muscles of the heart or the coronary arteries may be damaged.

FRACTURES OF THE RIBS

Clinical features

The commonest injury to the chest is fracture of the ribs by a direct blow. The most commonly affected ribs are the 7th, 8th and 9th in which the fracture usually occurs in the region of the mid-axillary line. The patient complains of pain in the chest overlying the fracture and this pain is intensified by springing the ribs by gentle but sharp pressure on the sternum.

Special investigation

The diagnosis is confirmed by a chest X-ray which should always be taken, as there may be underlying lung damage or haemorrhage that would not have been suspected from the trivial nature of the patient's symptoms. However, an X-ray may not always demonstrate a fracture and if the patient has clinical signs of fractured ribs, he should be treated for this condition in spite of a negative X-ray.

Complications

Flail chest (Fig. 8.1)

Crush injuries of the chest, in which multiple ribs are fractured at both ends or the whole sternum loosened, result in the condition of flail chest. On inspiration the flail part of the chest wall becomes indrawn as it is no longer in structural continuity with the bony thoracic cage. Similarly, in expiration the flail part of the chest is pushed out whilst the rest of the bony cage becomes contracted. This is termed *paradoxical movement*. The patient becomes grossly anoxic due to failure of adequate expansion of the affected side and also because of shunting of deoxygenated air from the lung on the side of the fracture into the opposite side. The

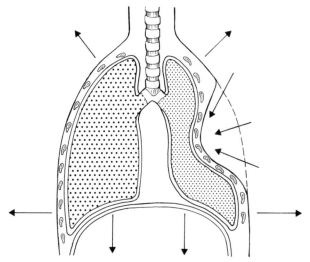

Fig. 8.1. Flail chest. On inspiration, the detached segment of the chest wall is sucked inwards, producing paradoxical movement.

pendulum movements of the mediastinum also produce cardiovascular embarrassment so that the patient becomes rapidly and progressively shocked.

Pneumothorax (Fig. 8.2)

If a bony spicule penetrates the lung then air escapes into the pleural cavity and will result in a pneumothorax. If the pleural tear is valvular a *tension pneumothorax*

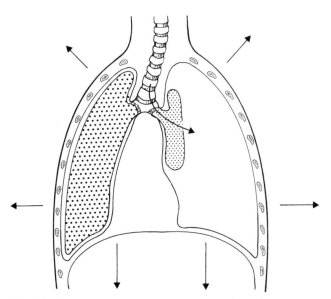

Fig. 8.2. Tension pneumothorax produced by a valvular tear in the lung. Air is sucked into the pleural cavity on inspiration and cannot escape on expiration.

results, since air is sucked into the pleural cavity at each inspiration but cannot return into the bronchi on expiration. A tension pneumothorax produces rapidly increasing dyspnoea; the apex beat is displaced away from the side of the pneumothorax and on the left side cardiac dullness may be absent. The chest on the affected side gives a tympanitic percussion note with bulging of the intercostal spaces. If, in addition, the torn rib allows air to enter the subcutaneous tissues, gross *surgical emphysema* will result. The skin over the trunk, neck and sometimes face gives a peculiar crepitating feel to the examining fingers and, in severe cases, the face and neck may become grossly swollen.

A pneumothorax will also result from a penetrating wound of the chest wall produced, for example, by a knife stab or gunshot wound. The lips of the wound may also have a valvular effect so that air is sucked into the cavity at each inspiration, but cannot escape on expiration, thus resulting in another variety of tension pneumothorax which has been vividly named a *sucking wound of the chest*.

It is important to remember that penetrating wounds of the chest may also injure the underlying diaphragm and thence the abdominal viscera. Thus it is not uncommon for a knife or bullet wound of the left chest to penetrate the spleen or, on the right side, to damage the liver.

Haemothorax

A haemothorax often accompanies a chest injury and may indeed be associated with a pneumothorax (*haemo-pneumothorax*). The bleeding usually comes from the lacerated chest wall or underlying contused lung, but on occasions may result from injury to the heart or great vessels. Retropleural bleeding may compress the thoracic viscera without breaching the pleural cavity.

Traumatic asphyxia

With severe crush injuries of the chest the sudden sharp rise in venous pressure produces extensive bruising and petechial haemorrhages over the head, neck and trunk. There is often subconjunctival haemorrhages and nasal bleeding. Any area of the skin which has been subjected to compression at the time of injury, e.g. from a tight collar, braces or spectacles, is protected and these areas remain mapped out on the body as strips of normal skin, giving a completely characteristic appearance to the patient.

Treatment

For any serious chest injury, the first important principle is to control the airway. It may be necessary to pass an endotracheal tube, particularly where a head injury coexists with chest trauma. Aspiration of vomit is prevented by passing a nasogastric tube to empty the stomach. Underwater drainage is essential for a pneumothorax and/or haemothorax. Continued observations are required and these include repeated X-rays of the chest and estimation of the blood gases. If the patient continues to bleed then thoracotomy is indicated. If the P_{CO_2} is above 7.3 kPa (50 mmHg) and the airway clear, then this is an indication for positive pressure ventilation. If recovery does not occur in a few days, management may be facilitated by performing a tracheostomy.

Simple rib fracture

Pain is relieved by analgesics or by the injection of local anaesthetic in the para-vertebral region to block the intercostal nerves or by a thoracic epidural block, which can be repeated by means of an indwelling plastic catheter. The patient is given vigorous physiotherapy to encourage deep breathing. Strapping of the chest wall inhibits thoracic movement and encourages pulmonary collapse so that most surgeons have abandoned this practice.

A flail chest

Treat as an emergency by supporting the flail segment by means of a firm pad held by strapping. On admission to hospital endotracheal intubation is performed, followed if necessary by tracheostomy, and positive pressure respiration instituted. This immediately stops the paradoxical ventilation, since the chest wall now moves as a single functional unit. The treatment is continued for about 10 days until fixation of the chest wall is effected. In cases of gross instability, wire fixation of the chest wall may be necessary.

Tension pneumothorax

Urgent emergency treatment is required. An intercostal tube drain is inserted by means of a trocar and cannula. The tube is then led to an underwater seal. When the pressure in the pleural space is increased on expiration, the air escapes through the water but air cannot enter the chest at inspiration since this is prevented by the water seal. This essential safety valve has been a most important step in the development of safe thoracic surgery (Fig. 8.3). If a pneumothorax persists, rupture of a bronchus should be suspected and bronchoscopy carried out, followed, if confirmed, by thoracotomy and repair.

Penetrating wounds of the chest

Immediate application of a dressing is required in order to prevent suction of air into the pleural space. Minor cases require only wound toilet with an underwater intercostal drain to allow escape of any accumulated blood or air in the pleural space. Large wounds demand formal exploration with excision or repair of damaged lung tissue, repair of any diaphragmatic tear and exclusion of injury of underlying abdominal viscera.

Cardiac tamponade

This may follow open or closed injuries to the chest or upper abdomen. It is characterized by a rise in venous pressure and a fall in the blood pressure. The heart sounds are distant and the cardiac shadow enlarged on X-ray. Treatment is emergency surgical exploration; the pericardium is opened, the blood is evacuated and the cardiac laceration sutured.

PULMONARY TUBERCULOSIS

In recent years the treatment of tuberculosis has been transformed by the successful introduction of specific antibiotic therapy. Progressive cavitating pulmonary tuberculosis is now uncommon in Great Britain except among immigrants from the developing countries and patients suffering from AIDS. Rarely, surgery is still

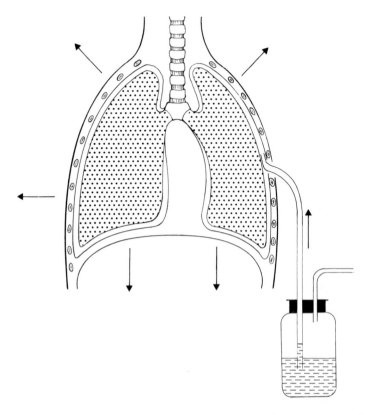

Fig. 8.3. Underwater seal chest drain in the treatment of a pneumothorax. Air escapes from the pleural cavity on expiration but cannot be sucked back through the water seal on inspiration (as shown here).

required for this condition especially in two situations — first, when an anatomical cavity has already occurred in the lung and this has become secondarily infected and second, when a tuberculous focus persists is spite of anti-tuberculous treatment.

Surgical treatment

The affected segment or lobe is resected under antibiotic cover. The operation of thoracoplasty, in which the cavity is obliterated by resection of portions of the ribs, is now hardly ever necessary.

BRONCHIECTASIS

Pathology

Bronchiectasis is the state of dilatation of the bronchi, commonly accompanied by sepsis. It is usually secondary to a combination of a bronchial obstruction and infection. In children it may follow measles or whooping cough, tuberculosis or inhalation of a foreign body, and there is often an associated sinusitis. In the adult it may be secondary to a tumour or stricture of the bronchial wall. Since the introduction of efficient antibiotic treatment of pulmonary infection in children the incidence of this condition has fallen.

The basal segments of one or both lungs are commonly affected, but the lingula on the left and the middle lobe on the right may also be involved, or, indeed, may be the only site of the lesion. The bronchi develop saccular or fusiform dilatations with inflamed walls and are distended with pus. The surrounding lung tissue may show collapse and consolidation and there may be an overlying pleurisy.

Clinical features

Typically there is a chronic productive cough with foul sputum. There may be associated pyrexia and toxaemia. The fingers may be clubbed and examination of the chest reveals moist sounds over the affected segments.

Complications

Haemoptysis.
Pleurisy, leading to empyema.
Haematogenous cerebral abscess.

Special investigations

1 *The chest X-ray*, surprisingly, may be normal although there may be some increased shadowing in the affected lung segments. Tuberculous mediastinal lymph nodes or the presence of an underlying lung carcinoma may be demonstrated.
2 *Bronchography* outlines the dilated bronchial tree.
3 *Bronchoscopy* may reveal a foreign body or malignant stricture.

Treatment

Conservative treatment comprises postural drainage and antibiotic therapy, and suffices in the milder cases.

Surgical treatment involves resection of the affected lung segments.

LUNG ABSCESS

Aetiology

1 Carcinoma of the lung.
2 Inhalation pneumonitis, e.g. inhaled vomit or pus.
3 Inhaled foreign body, e.g. at dental extraction.
4 Infected cyst.
5 Infected pulmonary infarct.
6 Blood-borne, secondary to staphylococcal septicaemia.
7 Secondary to pulmonary infection, e.g. pneumonia, bronchiectasis or tuberculosis.

Clinical features

The history may suggest the primary cause. There is usually acute fever and toxaemia, although the disease may sometimes run a more chronic course. If the abscess ruptures into the bronchus there is a foul productive cough.

Complications
1   Empyema.
2   Metastatic cerebral abscess (a feared complication of all pulmonary sepsis).

Special investigations
1   *The chest X-ray* shows a solid opacity or a fluid level if the abscess communicates with the bronchus.
2   *Bronchoscopy* may demonstrate the primary cause if this is a foreign body or carcinoma.

Treatment
The underlying cause may itself require treatment. The mainstay of therapy for lung abscess is postural drainage combined with antibiotics. On this the majority resolve and surgical excision is only required for the small percentage that fail to respond to this therapy, where some underlying cause needs to be treated, or where, in a late case, there is a complicating empyema that requires drainage.

EMPYEMA
An empyema (pyothorax) is a collection of pus in the pleural cavity.

Aetiology
1   Underlying lung disease: pneumonia, bronchiectasis or carcinoma of the lung; tuberculous empyema is now uncommon.
2   Penetrating wounds of the chest wall or infection following a transthoracic operation.
3   Perforation of the oesophagus.
4   Trans-diaphragmatic infection from a subphrenic abscess.
5   Haematogenous.

Complications
1   Rupture into a bronchus (broncho-pleural fistula).
2   Discharge through the chest wall (empyema necessitans).
3   Cerebral abscess.

Clinical features
There is usually a history of the underlying cause. The patient is febrile, toxic and may be anaemic. There are signs of fluid in the chest on the affected side. In chronic cases finger clubbing may be present.

Special investigations
1   *The white count* is raised.
2   *The chest X-ray* demonstrates an effusion and there may be evidence of the underlying lung disease.

3 *Bronchoscopy* is useful in determining the primary pathology.

4 *Aspiration* of the chest confirms the diagnosis and identifies the responsible bacteria. The infecting organisms are usually the pneumococcus, streptococcus or staphylococcus.

Treatment

An acute empyema may respond to repeated aspirations together with antibiotic therapy, based on the sensitivity of the responsible organism and given both systemically and into the pleural cavity. If the condition fails to respond to this treatment, drainage by means of excision of a rib overlying the empyema becomes necessary. An intercostal tube is inserted and progress followed by repeated sinograms to ensure adequate drainage and ultimate obliteration of the empyema cavity. In more chronic cases, the fibrous wall of the empyema cavity may require excision (decortication).

LUNG TUMOURS

Classification

Benign

(a) adenoma
(b) carcinoid (occasionally malignant)
(c) hamartoma
(d) haemangioma (rare)

Malignant

1 *Primary:* bronchogenic carcinoma, malignant carcinoid
2 *Secondary:*
(a) carcinoma (especially breast, kidney)
(b) sarcoma (especially bone)
(c) melanoma

ADENOMA

Pathology

Adenomas account for about 4 per cent of lung primary tumours. Two-thirds of the patients are female and the average age is 40 years.

The tumour arises from the mucosa usually of the main bronchus as a cherry-red swelling which ulcerates and bleeds (hence the common presenting symptom of haemoptysis). The growth may eventually block the bronchus with resulting pulmonary collapse and infection. Although slow growing, it cannot be considered benign since infiltration and metastases may eventually take place.

Occasionally serotonin is secreted, producing attacks of flushing and dyspnoea (carcinoid syndrome, see page 183).

Treatment
Removal by local resection, lobectomy or pneumonectomy.

CARCINOMA OF THE LUNG
This is the commonest growth affecting male adults and accounts for some 40 000 deaths a year in England and Wales.

Aetiology
Radioactive carcinogens in certain mines have been shown to be associated with development of carcinoma of the lung, but in Great Britain there are two main aetiological factors: smoking of cigarettes and pollution of the air with diesel, petrol and other fumes. The incidence is higher in urban than in rural populations.

There are many critics who complain of the lack of progress in cancer research that has been achieved by the medical profession and yet, when a dramatic advance is made and published in a well-known journal, many years pass before any steps are taken to try and remove this danger and then, for a variety of emotional and economic reasons, the steps are half-hearted. It requires a very stubborn, stupid man, or a smoker, to disregard the warning of the association of cigarette smoke with cancer of the lung, so clearly demonstrated in the report of Doll and Bradford Hill (*B.M.J.* 1952, 2, 1271).

Carcinoma of the lung has an extremely poor prognosis and the gravity of this condition should be impressed on all patients who are inveterate smokers. The decision whether or not to continue smoking depends on the patient, but there is no doubt that the doctor's advice should be against it. There is an increased incidence of carcinoma of the lung even in patients who smoke only a few cigarettes a day and this danger is greatly increased in patients smoking more than 20 cigarettes a day for a number of years.

Pathology
There is considerable predominance of males over females in this disease (six to one), but the ratio is decreasing as women tend to smoke more. It is uncommon before the fifth decade and peaks in the 60s.

Macroscopic appearance
About half the tumours arise in the main bronchi, and 75 per cent are visible at bronchoscopy. The growth may arise peripherally and some appear to be multi-focal.

The bronchial wall is narrowed and ulcerated. Surrounding lung tissue is invaded by a pale mass of tumour which may undergo necrosis, haemorrhage or abscess formation. The lung segments distal to the occlusion may show collapse, bronchiectasis or abscess formation.

Microscopic appearance
1 *Squamous cell* (40 per cent), mostly poorly differentiated and arising in an area of squamour metaplasia of bronchial epithelium.
2 *Adenocarcinoma* (15 per cent), very rapidly growing.

3 *Undifferentiated* (45 per cent), either large polygonal cells or small elongated cells, (the 'oat cell' or 'small cell' tumour). These have a most unfavourable prognosis.

SPREAD

1 *Local,* to pleura, recurrent laryngeal nerve, pericardium, oesophagus (broncho-oesophageal fistula) and brachial plexus (Pancoast's tumour).
2 *Lymphatic,* to mediastinal and cervical nodes. Compression of the superior vena cava by massive mediastinal node involvement produces gross oedema and cyanosis of the face and upper limbs (superior vena cava syndrome).
3 *Blood,* to bone, brain, liver and adrenals.
4 *Transcoelomic,* pleural seedlings and effusion.

Clinical features

Carcinoma of the lung may present with:
1 *Local features,* namely cough, dyspnoea, haemoptysis or lung infection.
2 *Secondaries,* which are especially likely to occur in the brain, adrenal, liver and bones; thus the patient may present with evidence of a space occupying lesion within the skull, pathological fracture, jaundice and hepatomegaly, or adrenal cortical failure.
3 *The general effects of neoplasm,* loss of weight, anaemia, cachexia and also peripheral neuropathies, myopathies and endocrine disturbances.

Unfortunately, by the time carcinoma of the lung is diagnosed, most cases are quite incurable. About half the patients will be found to have inoperable growths when they have had no symptoms at all, with a lesion discovered on routine chest X-ray. Certainly any middle-aged or elderly man presenting with a respiratory infection that has continued for more than 2 weeks should have a chest X-ray, and, if the symptoms persist and nothing shows on the chest X-ray, he should be bronchoscoped.

Patients may present with bizarre neuropathies and myopathies that can occur with cancer anywhere, but these are especially common in growths of the lung. Cancer of the lung is likely to lead to pulmonary infection and the patients often develop clubbing of the fingers, which are usually nicotine-stained.

On examination special attention should be paid to evidence of stridor or hoarseness of the voice due to recurrent laryngeal nerve involvement with growth. The heart may be invaded, resulting in atrial fibrillation or cardiac failure. There may be enlarged lymph nodes, especially at the root of the neck, and signs in the chest of consolidation, fluid or collapse.

Investigations

1 Chest X-ray and CT
2 Examination of the sputum for malignant cells.
3 Bronchoscopy and biopsy.

Chest X-ray and CT will usually show an opacity in the lung and quite often enlargement of the hilar lymph nodes. There may be paralysis of one side of the diaphragm due to involvement of the phrenic nerve.

The patient should be bronchoscoped, when histological diagnosis may be obtained by biopsy. Involved lymph nodes may widen the carina and an ulcerating or exuberant growth may be seen. Aspirated sputum should be sent for examination for malignant cells. Lymph nodes in the region of the carina may be removed for histological examination by mediastinoscopy performed through a small suprasternal incision.

Treatment

The surgeon has to determine which patients have an operable lesion. Generally, if there are secondary deposits in cervical lymph nodes or elsewhere, then removal of the primary tumour is valueless. Enlarged lymph nodes of the neck should be removed for biopsy and, if they contain growth, then surgery is not indicated. If the tumour appears to be confined to one lobe or one lung, without there being any evidence of secondary deposits and if the carina is free from growth on bronchoscopy, the patient should be submitted to a thoracotomy. In a favourable case it may be possible to remove all macroscopic growth by performing a lobectomy or a pneumonectomy. In these highly selected cases the 5-year survival rate of this disease is in the order of 20 to 30 per cent.

Radiotherapy may give useful palliation in the inoperable cases. Although it may not prolong life, it may stop distressing haemoptysis, cure the pain from bone secondaries and produce dramatic improvement in a patient with acute superior vena caval obstruction. It may also give some relief from the irritating cough and dyspnoea resulting from early bronchial obstruction.

Cyclical cytotoxic therapy combined with radiotherapy gives improved survival in small cell tumours but the other types of primary carcinoma of the lung are not responsive to chemotherapy.

SECONDARY TUMOURS

The lung is second only to the liver as the site of metastases, which may be from carcinoma (especially breast, kidney), sarcoma (especially bone) or melanoma. Spread may be either as a result of vascular deposits or retrograde lymphatic permeation from involved mediastinal nodes — lymphangitis carcinomatosa.

Pulmonary metastases are so common that it should be routine practice to X-ray the chest in every case of malignant disease.

Diagnosis of an abnormal shadow in the mediastinum

1 Retro-sternal thyroid.
2 Aneurysm of the thoracic aorta.
3 Thymic tumour and cysts.
4 Carcinoma of the lung with a mediastinal mass.
5 Pericardial effusion.
6 Enlarged lymph nodes.
   (a) sarcoid
   (b) Hodgkin's disease
   (c) leukaemia
   (d) non-Hodgkin's lymphoma
   (e) secondary deposits

7 The mega-oesophagus of achalasia of the cardia.
8 Paravertebral tuberculous abscess.
9 Scoliosis.
10 Dumb-bell tumour of neurofibroma.
11 Dermoid cyst or teratoma.

Chapter 9
The Heart and Great Vessels

Surgery has always been particularly successful in closing defects and relieving obstruction. However, it is only in recent years that the surgeon has been able to apply these techniques to the heart and great vessels. Not because the closure of defects or relieving of obstruction in these situations are particularly difficult to perform on their own, but because, in order to gain access, the circulation to the vital parts of the body is liable to be interfered with. Recent advances in anaesthesia and the development of methods of preservation of the vital organs of the body from anoxic damage have been responsible for the tremendous achievements in cardiovascular surgery.

In this chapter we shall first consider the congenital and acquired conditions of the heart and great vessels which can be treated surgically without interruption of the circulation, and then those cardiac conditions which require heart bypass or arrest.

PERSISTENT DUCTUS ARTERIOSUS (Fig. 9.1)

Pathology

If the channel between the aorta and pulmonary artery fails to close at the time of birth, the normal haemodynamics of the systemic and pulmonary circulations will be disordered. Blood will be shunted from the systemic circulation with its higher pressure into the pulmonary circulation and the result is pulmonary hypertension.

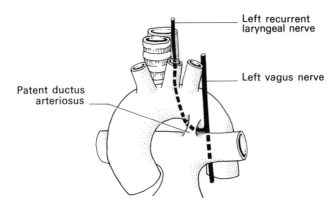

Left recurrent
laryngeal nerve

Left vagus nerve

Patent ductus
arteriosus

Fig. 9.1. A patent ductus arteriosus — note its close relationship to the left recurrent laryngeal nerve.

Clinical features

The patient is usually asymptomatic and the condition is most commonly diagnosed because of finding the characteristic machinery-like continuous murmur with systolic accentuation best heard over the second left space anteriorly. In infants the bruit may be purely systolic.

If this condition is not treated the abnormal strain on the heart may lead to cardiac failure and the pulmonary hypertension may be so great that there is a reversal of the direction of flow of blood so that deoxygenated blood from the pulmonary artery reaches the systemic circulation. Although usually subjects with persistent ductus arteriosus are acyanotic, patients with this complication will become cyanosed. Rarely, differential cyanosis may be noted in that flow from the aortic arch is of oxygenated blood and therefore the head and upper limbs are pink, whereas the lower half of the body, supplied via the distal aorta, is cyanosed.

Any congenital abnormality in the heart or the vessels is a potential source of infection. The most likely organism to produce this complication is the *Streptococcus viridans*; the resulting sub-acute bacterial endarteritis is treated by massive doses of penicillin — 10 million units a day for several weeks.

Special investigations

Chest X-ray will usually show left ventricular hypertrophy and increased pulmonary arterial markings. An angiocardiograph will demonstrate the patient ductus and indeed the cardiac catheter can often be manipulated through the ductus into the aorta.

Treatment

Treatment of a persistent ductus should be undertaken on diagnosis, and before irreversible pulmonary hypertension or cardiac failure have occurred. The channel is interrupted, preferably by ligation and division, but if this is technically difficult the duct is merely ligated. The disadvantage of simple ligation is that recanalization has occurred in a small proportion of cases. Transvascular insertion of an occlusive device into the ductus can lead to a cure without surgery.

COARCTATION OF THE AORTA

Pathology

This is a congenital narrowing of the aorta, which, in the majority of cases, occurs in the descending aorta just distal to the origin of the left subclavian artery. The stenosis is usually extreme, only a pinpoint lumen remaining. Coarctation can rarely occur in other sites up and down the aorta.

Blood reaches the intercostal arteries from collateral connections between branches of subclavian arteries and the intercostals by the anastomosis between the internal thoracic and inferior epigastric arteries. In this way there is a blood flow into the aorta distal to the stenosis. Although the blood supply to the lower part of the body is diminished, patients with coarctation seldom suffer from peripheral gangrene, although occasionally they complain of intermittent claudication. The danger of coarctation is due to the effects of hypertension, which is often severe and is likely to result in cerebral haemorrhage or left ventricular failure. Another hazard is the development of bacterial endarteritis.

Clinical features

The diagnosis is usually made on account of hypertension in a young adult or a child. The mechanism of the production of hypertension is not simple blockage of the aorta but is probably due in a large part to the relatively poor blood supply to the kidneys. The renal ischaemia causes a release of hypertensive agents, of which renin is probably an important component.

In addition to the hypertension, the most characteristic physical sign is absent, diminished or delayed femoral pulsations in relation to the radial pulse. A systolic murmur is sometimes present in the chest and large collateral blood vessels may be seen or felt in the subcutaneous tissues of the chest wall.

Special investigations

X-ray of the chest will show left ventricular hypertrophy and often the ribs are notched by the large intercostal collateral blood vessels bypassing the stenotic area. Angiocardiography will confirm the diagnosis.

Treatment

This is desirable before complications arise and consists of excision of the stenotic segment and either end-to-end anastomosis of the proximal and distal aorta, or, if the gap to bridge is too great, an arterial graft is used to join the two aortic ends.

AORTIC ANEURYSMS

Aneurysms can occur in any situation in the body (see pages 60 to 62) but the aorta is particularly liable to be affected. Aneurysms of the arch of the aorta are commonly syphilitic but may occur in Marfan's syndrome. Aneurysms of the descending thoracic aorta may be traumatic, syphilitic or atherosclerotic. With the exception of aneurysms with a very narrow neck, those involving the thoracic aorta require some form of vascular bypass in order to treat them surgically.

Abdominal aortic aneurysms are in the majority of cases due to atherosclerotic disease.

Clinical features

Aneurysms of the ascending aorta may present with chest pain, aortic regurgitation, obstruction of the superior vena cava, obstruction of the right main bronchus and eventually a pulsating mass in the front of the chest, which may even ulcerate the chest wall, resulting in exsanguination.

Aneurysms of the arch of the aorta may compress the trachea or ulcerate into it, they are liable to stretch the left recurrent laryngeal nerve leading to hoarseness and may obstruct the left lower lobe bronchus, producing an area of collapse.

Aneurysms of the descending thoracic aorta may produce pain in the back, erosion of vertebrae, or may press on the oesophagus producing dysphagia and even rupture into it. Not surprisingly, this is the most lethal cause of haematemesis.

Aneurysms of the abdominal aorta usually present with pain in the back, especially the lumbar region, and may cause sciatica. Many abdominal aneurysms, however, are diagnosed in symptomless patients who are found on abdominal examination to have a pulsatile mass. An aneurysm may not present clinically until it has ruptured, when the patient, if he does not die immediately, will manifest severe surgical shock. Haemorrhage from an abdominal aneurysm is usually first extraperitoneal and then, eventually, intraperitoneal. There may be a history of a pulsatile mass in the abdomen but on clinical examination no such mass may be found due to the hypotension and the shock. An elderly patient presenting with unrevealed internal haemorrhage should always be suspected of a ruptured aortic aneurysm. Rarely, abdominal aortic aneurysms may rupture into the inferior vena cava or duodenum.

Special investigations

An X-ray of the abdomen will probably show the extent of the aneurysm due to clacification in its walls. A lateral film is particularly valuable.

Ultrasound scanning is useful in delimiting the size and extent of the aneurysm, which can also be demonstrated on a CT scan.

Aortography may be dangerous and often does not help in establishing the diagnosis since the lumen of the aneurysm is narrowed by thrombus.

Treatment

Aneurysms of the ascending aorta and arch require total cardiopulmonary bypass for adequate surgical treatment, which consists of partial excision of the aneurysm and insertion of a prosthetic graft with appropriate junction limbs to the main aortic branches. Aneurysms of the descending thoracic aorta require a left heart bypass for their surgical treatment which is similar in principal to those of the arch.

Management of patients with abdominal aneurysms depends on the mode of presentation.

The patient with a symptomless pulsatile swelling in the abdomen should be carefully assessed as regards his general condition and the size of the aneurysm. If the aneurysm is small and symptomless, especially in the elderly patient, a conservative approach is adopted. The patient is kept under observation and surgery only adivsed if the aneurysm is enlarging or if it becomes painful.

In the relatively young, fit patient, especially if the aneurysm is large, elective surgical excision is advised as prophylaxis against future rupture.

If a patient presents with pain or the swelling has been observed to be enlarging over the past few weeks, then it is very likely that the aneurysm will soon rupture. Once rupture has occurred the mortality is close to 80 per cent, therefore the patient with an enlarging or painful aneurysm should be strongly advised to have surgery. A useful rule of thumb is that aneurysms larger than 5 cm in diameter measured on palpation, X-ray or ultrasound merit surgery.

The patient presenting in surgical shock with frank rupture of the aneurysm will certainly die if he is not operated on and is likely to die even if surgery is undertaken. It is essential to perform the operation as soon as possible after the diagnosis has been made and a large amount of blood should be available. The

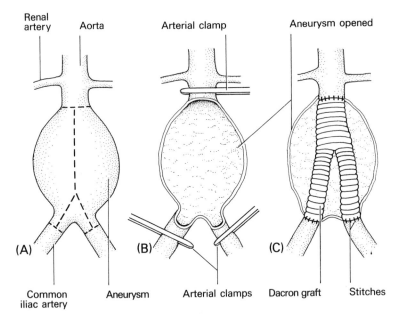

Fig. 9.2. Steps in the excision and grafting of an aortic aneurysm.

operation involves a long abdominal incision and control of the proximal and distal extremities of the aneurysm with clamps. The proximal point of the aneurysm is usually below the renal arteries. The distal point may well involve the iliacs. The sac is opened, clot evacuated and the aorta and iliac vessels divided above and below the aneurysm. The sac wall, especially where it is intimately adherent to the inferior vena cava and the common iliac veins, is left undisturbed (Fig. 9.2). If the iliac arteries are not involved, a straight Dacron tube graft restores continuity, otherwise a bifurcation graft is inserted and covered over snugly by the walls of the sac, which protect it from contact with, and possible fistulation into, the duodenum and intestines.

DISSECTING ANEURYSM

Pathology

A dissecting aneurysm consists of a tear in the wall of the aorta, usually in the region of its arch, which allows blood to dissect along a plane of cleavage in the media. The false aneurysm thus formed may rupture internally into the true lumen, thus decompressing itself and resulting in an aorta with a double lumen. Such a case may survive. However, more commonly, the aneurysm ruptures externally into the pericardium producing cardiac tamponade, or into the mediastinum or abdominal cavity with fatal haemorrhage.

The aetiology of this condition is a cystic medial necrosis of the wall of the aorta and its major branches which enables this splitting to occur. It is usually found in arteriosclerotic, hypertensive subjects.

Clinical features

The patient usually presents with sudden pain in the chest which may radiate to the arms, neck or abdomen. In addition there may be signs of surgical shock, either from cardiac tamponade or from external rupture of the aneurysm. Patients with dissecting aneurysm are therefore usually initially diagnosed as suffering from coronary thrombosis, and an electrocardiogram may not help differentiate between the two conditions. However, a chest X-ray may show widening of the mediastinum due to the aneurysm.

As the dissection in the wall of the aorta progresses the orifices of main arterial branches may become blocked, producing progression of symptoms and the disappearance of peripheral pulses. If the renal vessels are involved there may be haematuria or anuria.

Treatment

Initially this should be conservative; hypotensive drugs are used in order to try to prevent further extension of the dissection. The dissected portion may then thrombose. A chronic dissecting aneurysm may require treatment if it enlarges or produces pressure symptoms. In the acute stage, surgery is necessary if there is rapid development of aortic incompetence, if the aneurysm ruptures into the thorax or pericardium, if a major vessel becomes blocked or if the dissection continues despite hypotensive treatment. Surgery is difficult because of the problems in establishing the exact diagnosis, and the location of the distal and proximal tears as well as the technical difficulties of extensive arterial reconstruction. To excise the whole aneurysm in the arch of the aorta and replace the arch with a prosthetic graft is a major surgical procedure and requires cardiopulmonary bypass, but in recent years success has been achieved with this type of operation. If the dissection has proceeded into the descending thoracic aorta or the abdominal aorta without producing irreversible damage, then a satisfactory operation, which is less formidable, is to perform an artifical re-entry in which the dissection of the aortic wall is re-opened into the distal aorta by making a hole in the intima.

CONSTRICTIVE PERICARDITIS

This condition, which may be due to tuberculosis of the pericardium, virus pericarditis, an old haemopericardium or rheumatic pericarditis, results in the pericardium becoming fibrosed and often calcified; this impedes both the action of the heart and re-entry of blood into it. The impairment of return of blood to the heart may result in the liver becoming enlarged and the formation of ascites, the condition then mimics cirrhosis and, indeed, has been called 'pseudo-cirrhosis'.

Treatment

The treatment is to excise the pericardium and free the heart from its embarrassment.

PRINCIPLES OF CARDIAC OPERATIONS

The first assays at cardiac surgery comprised either operations on the main vessels emerging from the heart or on the pericardium. The early operations on the heart itself were carried out without interruption of the circulation and were performed without direct vision, mostly to relieve stenosis of the mitral, aortic or pulmonary valves and performed either with the finger or with special instruments introduced through the heart wall or the root of one or other of the main emerging vessels. Although these operations are still used, they have been increasingly displaced by surgery under direct vision with cardiopulmonary bypass. The difficulties and time limitation of performing surgery on the heart by blind methods led to the development of means of maintaining the circulation artificially so that the heart is operated on in a bloodless field. If the circulation is temporarily stopped at normal body temperature the different organs vary in their susceptibility to irreversible damage due to lack of oxygen. The brain is the most sensitive tissue in this respect and is liable to irreversible changes after 3 minutes of ischaemia. The spinal cord is next, followed by heart muscle, which will tolerate between 3 and 6 minutes of ischaemia at normal temperature. The liver can withstand 30 to 40 minutes of normothermic ischaemia. Renal tubular necrosis commences after 30–60 minutes cessation of circulation.

If the metabolic rate of the tissues is lowered by hypothermia, the period of permissible circulatory arrest will be prolonged. This depends on the the degree of hypothermia; at 28°C up to 10 minutes of arrest can be tolerated; in deep hypothermia, 10°C or lower, arrest can be carried out for periods of up to one hour. Hypothermia can be produced by surface cooling, but profound hypothermia requires circulation of the blood through a heat exchanger.

The second approach to this problem has been the development of cardiopulmonary bypass in which a machine is used to take over the pumping and oxygenation of the blood after full heparinization. Catheters are inserted into the venae cavae or the right atrium; the return of blood to the heart from the systemic circulation is thus syphoned off and pumped into a membrane oxygenator.

Once oxygenated, the blood is pumped through a heat exchanger via a catheter into the aorta, either through a femoral artery or directly into the ascending aorta. This form of bypass will perfuse the whole body with oxygenated blood at an adequate pressure while diverting it from the heart and lungs. If the aorta is cross clamped, it may be desirable to perfuse the coronary arteries separately and to drain the return of blood by means of a catheter in the coronary sinus; alternatively, the heart may be cooled locally, the myocardium being protected by infusion via the coronary arteries of cold 'cardioplegic' solution containing potassium, to produce cardiac arrest in diastole.

There have been a large variety of modifications of these techniques and a combination of hypothermia and cardiopulmonary bypass may be used.

MITRAL STENOSIS

Mitral stenosis commonly follows rheumatic carditis. The original attack of rheumatism may have been mild so that only half the patients give a previous history of rheumatic fever or chorea.

Clinical features

Patients usually present between the twentieth and fortieth year, females more commonly than males. The usual presenting feature is increasing dyspnoea due to progressive cardiac failure. There may be nocturnal dyspnoea and episodes of pulmonary oedema with recurrent lung infections.

On examination the patient may have the typical malar flush. There is a mid-diastolic murmur in the mitral area and the opening snap of the mitral valve may be audible. Atrial fibrillation is common and this is accompanied by the disappearance of the pre-systolic murmur as effective atrial contraction ceases.

Complications

1 Right heart failure.
2 Peripheral arterial embolism (particularly in atrial fibrillation).
3 Sub-acute bacterial endocarditis.

Treatment

In the absence of mitral regurgitation, evidence of valve calcification or history of emboli, and if the valve cusps are mobile on left ventricular angiography, then a closed operation gives excellent results. The original procedure was to insert the finger through the left atrium in order to split the mitral valve. This is now achieved more satisfactorily by means of a dilator inserted through the wall of the left ventricle at the same time as the finger is palpating the mitral valve through the left atrium. If a satisfactory split of the fused commissures can be achieved, then the prognosis is good.

With calcified and distorted valves, regurgitation may result from mitral valvotomy. In such cases open operation is preferable, with replacement by means of prosthetic, homograft, or xenograft valve.

PULMONARY STENOSIS

This is usually a congenital condition and may exist on its own or with stenosis of the infundibulum of the right ventricle as well. Sometimes the pulmonary outflow tract is the only abnormal part of the heart, but more frequently the pulmonary stenosis is part of *Fallot's tetralogy,* in which the other defects are: ventricular septal defect, over-riding of the root of the aorta to the right side of the heart, and right ventricular hypertrophy (Fig. 9.3).

Treatment

The first successful surgical approach to this condition was devised by Blalock, who performed an extra-cardiac operation and anastomosed the left subclavian artery to the pulmonary artery. Thus blood was shunted into the pulmonary circulation, which was previously deficient due to the pulmonary stenosis. Subsequently methods were devised to relieve the pulmonary stenosis directly by introducing a punch or a dilator into the right ventricle, excising the infundibular stenosis and dilating the stenotic pulmonary valve. These procedures were little more effective than Blalock's operation and now a far more satisfactory reconstructive operation of total correction is performed under direct vision using cardiopulmonary bypass. The Blalock procedure may still be used in an infant to tide him over until fit enough for definitive repair.

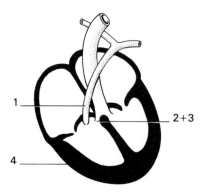

Fig. 9.3. The tetralogy of Fallot. **1** Pulmonary stenosis; **2** septal defect + **3** overriding aorta; **4** right ventricular hypertrophy.

AORTIC STENOSIS

Stenosis of the aortic valve may be congenital or acquired. In the acquired variety, rheumatic heart disease is the commonest cause. Unfortunately no matter what the cause, the aortic valve when stenosed is usually grossly distorted and is liable to be calcified.

Clinical features

The patient with aortic stenosis may suffer from angina pectoris. He has a slow rising pulse, a low blood pressure, and left ventricular hypertrophy, as shown on X-ray and electrocardiogram. If the disease progresses the patient is liable to develop left ventricular failure with attacks of dyspnoea, angina and syncope.

Treatment

Blind methods of dilation of the stenotic valve were introduced using similar procedures to those described for the pulmonary valve, namely instrumentation via the left ventricle to the aortic valve or, alternatively, retrograde dilatation was performed through the ascending aorta. However, the severe anatomical changes in the aortic valve made satisfactory results more difficult to achieve and modern treatment comprises valve replacement, either by prosthetic, homograft or xeno-graft valve, under cardiopulmonary bypass.

SEPTAL DEFECTS

Defects in the atrial or ventricular septal walls will allow blood to shunt between the pulmonary and systemic circulations. The direction in which the blood flows will depend on the pressures on the two sides of the defect. Very frequently there is a passage of blood in both directions. If there is an appreciable shunting of blood from the right side of the heart to the left, the patient is likely to be cyanosed, and this may be intense due to compensatory polycythaemia.

In a normal cardiac action, each side of the heart deals with exactly the same amount of blood, but when a shunt is present one part of the heart is likely to be overburdened with the amount of blood it has to cope with. In addition there may be abnormal stresses due to associated stenoses of valve outflow tracts. Patients with pure atrial or ventricular septal defects, with no other associated lesions, may not be cyanosed but they are liable to develop heart failure in the fourth decade.

Rarely, infants with a ventricular septal defect develop heart failure. This is treated by pulmonary artery banding to diminish the flow of blood into the pulmonary arterial tree.

Treatment

Open heart surgery can be performed by techniques described above and closures of the septal defects can be achieved under direct vision, either by suture of the margins of the defect, or, if the defect is too large, by sewing a patch of pericardium or synthetic material over the defect.

ISCHAEMIC HEART DISEASE

Severe angina due to myocardial ischaemia may be alleviated by increasing the arterial supply to the muscle. Procedures which were carried out in the past included attachment of the omentum to the heart, the induction of vascular adhesions from the pericardium by means of talc and implantation of the internal mammary artery into the heart muscle (Vineberg's operation). These have now been replaced by direct reconstructive surgery.

One of the most marked changes in surgical practice has been the introduction of internal mammary and aorto-coronary bypass surgery for the treatment of ischaemic heat disease. Now in the United Kingdom some 10 000 of these operations are performed each year and the figure is nearer 200 000 in the United States. This enormous effort is directed at rehabilitating patients and curing the angina. An accurate anatomical diagnosis is essential. Since the severity of symptoms does not directly relate to severity and extent of the coronary artery disease, all patients with angina should be given the benefit of selective coronary angiography and those with lesions suitable for surgery should be operated on. The procedure of choice is to join one or both of the internal mammary (internal thoracic) arteries to the diseased coronary artery distal to the blockage. If this is not possible then autogenous saphenous vein is used as a bypass from the aorta to the coronary artery (Fig. 9.4). In cases of stenosis, dilatation of the artery can be performed under angiographic radiological control (angioplasty). It may be necessary to perform more than one anastomosis to provide good revascularization of the heart, but the long term results of anastomosis to vessels less than one mm in diameter are poor. Many patients crippled by angina have been restored to a normal life and there is increasing evidence that not only are symptoms alleviated but also survival is prolonged.

Nevertheless, as with arterial surgery in any part of the body for atherosclerosis, there is a tendency for recurrent disease with the passage of time.

In young patients crippled by angina in whom direct bypass surgery is impossible or in those with gross myocardial disease, cardiac transplantation may be the only treatment that can give relief of symptoms and return to the normal life.

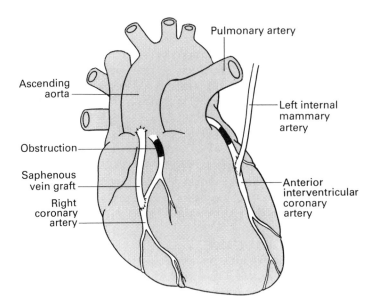

Fig. 9.4. A saphenous vein graft from the aorta to the right coronary artery and a direct left internal mammary (thoracic) artery graft to the anterior interventricular coronary artery.

HYPERTENSION

This section summarizes raised blood pressure in its surgical aspects.

Classification

1   *Primary* (cause unknown).
2   *Secondary* (causes at least partially understood).

Primary hypertension

Primary hypertension is a disease of middle-aged and elderly patients which tends to run in families. It is a very common condition and may be compatible with few symptoms and a long life. There is an increase in the peripheral resistance due to arteriolar thickening or spasm, but since arteriolar thickening is a consequence of hypertension the argument of which is the primary factor has not been resolved in this disease.

The kidney may be an important contributor to the hypertension when its blood supply is impaired due to arteriolar narrowing. There is a vicious circle of arteriolar spasm, arteriolar thickening, renal ischaemia and further hypertension, which leads to a progressive increase in the severity of this condition.

Secondary hypertension

Classification
1 Renal disease.
2 Coarctation of the aorta (page 47).
3 Endocrine causes:
   (a) Phaeochromocytoma (page 335)
   (b) Cushing's syndrome (page 337)
   (c) Conn's syndrome (page 339)
4 Raised intracranial pressure (page 92).
5 Toxaemia of pregnancy.

Renal causes

Aetiology
Ever since the experiments of Goldblatt, it has been known that impairment of blood perfusion to the kidneys can result in hypertension, which, if the renal perfusion remains impaired, may become permanent, due to the vicious circle that has already been mentioned. The mechanism of renal hypertension appears to be the release of a hormone, renin, from the juxta-glomerular cells in the renal cortex. Renin causes a serum protein, hypertensinogen (angiotensinogen) to give rise to a polypeptide, hypertensin (or angiotensin). This substance causes spasm of arterioles, an increase in peripheral resistance and release of aldosterone with sodium retention. Thus the features of hypertension are set in motion and renal perfusion is further impaired. It is likely that this renin mechanism is protective as far as the kidney is concerned and in a teleological manner can be considered as the method by which the kidney attempts to improve and maintain its circulation. How important renin is in the maintenance of normal blood pressure has not been established.

All forms of renal parenchymal disease are likely to produce hypertension. Especially common are chronic glomerulonephritis and chronic pyelonephritis. Chronic pyelonephritis may arise from lower urinary tract infections that have not been adequately treated.

The only surgical treatment for established bilateral renal disease producing severe hyperternsion is renal transplantation (see Chapter 50).

Unilateral renal disease producing hypertension
These are of especial surgical importance since they may sometimes be amenable to curative treatment either by nephrectomy or by reconstructive procedures on the kidney or on its blood supply.

Unilateral pyelonephritis
Rarely, pyelonephritis may affect one kidney only, especially if this kidney has been the site of previous trauma or of congenital malformation, if the ureter on that side has been blocked or if there is unilateral hydronephrosis. If the condition

is diagnosed early, before the hypertension has reached the chronic established stage and before hypertensive changes have taken place in the opposite kidney, then removal of the affected kidney may result in a return to normal blood pressure.

Renal artery stenosis

A fairly common cause of secondary hypertension. It occurs in two age groups: in the elderly, where the cause of the narrowing is atherosclerosis, and in young people, especially women, in whom the cause appears to be the thickening of the intima and media by hyperplasia of collagen and muscle — fibro-muscular hyperplasia.

An intravenous urogram may help the diagnosis of renal artery stenosis. There is usually delay in the excretion on the affected side, but the actual intensity of the shadow produced by the contrast medium when excretion occurs is greater than on the normal side. This is due to an impaired glomerular filtration, but relatively less impaired tubular function, so that reabsorption approaches normal; although the total amount of contrast medium excreted is less, its concentration is greater.

Arteriography should be performed in young patients with severe hypertension in such circumstances so that the stenosis of the renal artery may be demonstrated.

Treatment

If the stenosis is fairly proximal and the distal vessels relatively healthy, then it may be possible to remove the stenotic portion of the artery or bypass it; for instance, on the left side by joining the splenic artery to the renal artery distal to the blockage. Autotransplantation of the kidney may be performed after excising the stenosed portion of the artery. Alternatively, if the small ramifications of the renal artery are diseased, then a unilateral nephrectomy may result in relief of the hypertension. In suitable cases, a localized stenosis can be dilated by a balloon catheter passed under X-ray control (balloon angioplasty).

Other lesions of the renal arteries, for instance aneurysm and congenital bands, may also result in hypertension that can be cured by unilateral nephrectomy or direct arterial surgery.

It should be noted that since the introduction of effective anti-hypertensive drugs, enthusiasm for surgery in unilateral renal disease (apart from cases where the kidney's function is grossly impaired), has waned.

Other unilateral renal diseases can cause hypertension, including hydronephrosis, tuberculosis of the kidneys or tumours of the kidney; nephrectomy is indicated in these conditions.

Chapter 10
The Peripheral Arteries

TRAUMA
Peripheral arteries may be injured either by closed or open trauma.

Closed injuries
These include pressure from too tightly applied plaster of Paris splints, a tourniquet which has been left on for more than an hour, and damage to the artery, usually by spasm, but sometimes by penetration of a bone spicule, accompanying a closed fracture. The supracondylar fracture of the humerus is particularly prone to this complication.

Clinical features
A useful quintet by which to remember the clinical features of the acute ischaemia accompanying sudden arterial injury is: pain, pallor, pulselessness, paraesthesiae, paralysis. To this list a distinguished Professor of Surgery in Dublin has added 'perishing with cold'!

Treatment
When these features accompany a supracondylar fracture of the humerus in a child the fracture is gently reduced under a general anaesthetic, care being taken not to flex the elbow acutely. A cervical sympathetic block with local anaesthetic may help to relieve spasm. If the clinical features of the circulation in the arm do not rapidly improve within the next half hour the brachial artery is exposed. It may be found to be compressed by a haematoma beneath the deep fascia or to be caught against the fracture edge. The intense vascular spasm may respond to the local application of 2.5 per cent papaverine, which is the only effective local antispasmodic. More commonly, damage to the arterial wall requires direct repair with a vein graft.

If unrelieved, the continued muscle ischaemia results in necrosis of the muscles of the forearm. Subsequent fibrous replacement of the muscles produces the typical deformity of Volkmann's ischaemic contracture of the forearm muscles (see page 116).

Arteries may be injured as part of a compound fracture, from gunshot wounds or from penetrating stab injuries.

The following varieties of injury may occur:

1 *Spasm* from a 'near miss'.

2 *Thrombosis* of a vessel in spasm or which has been contused without actually being divided.

3 *Division* of the artery, which may be partial or complete. Partial division bleeds furiously whereas complete division of the artery, particularly if resulting from a

contused injury, may, suprisingly enough, bleed but little due to contraction and spasm of the divided vessel.

4   *Aneurysm — true and false.*

5   *Arterio-venous fistula.*

Clinical features

Arterial injury is suggested by severe bright red haemorrhage, often with signs of distal ischaemia. Another danger sign is a large haematoma developing beneath a puncture wound situated in the vicinity of a major artery. It is important to note that peripheral pulses may still be palpable distal to a completely divided artery in a young patient with a good collateral circulation.

Treatment

The bleeding can usually be controlled by direct pressure; the use of a tourniquet or proximal compression on a pressure point is seldom needed as a first aid measure. After a transfusion has been arranged the wound is explored in the theatre.

Partial laceration of an artery may be sutured or repaired with a vein patch. A complete division may be suitable for end to end suture or grafting by means of the patient's saphenous vein.

Small peripheral vessels, e.g. those below the brachial or popliteal arteries, can be sacrificed and ligated above and below the point of damage without jeopardy to the peripheral blood supply.

ANEURYSM

An aneurysm is defined as a sac which communicates with the lumen of an artery. The following types are recognized (Fig. 10.1): true (fusiform and saccular), false, arterio-venous and dissecting.

1   A *saccular aneurysm*: a dilated portion of the artery joins the main lumen by a small neck.

2   A *fusiform aneurysm*, in which there is a fusiform dilation of the artery.

This is the common type of aneurysm to affect the abdominal aorta.

3   A *false aneurysm*, in which the blood passes outside the torn wall of the blood vessel to produce a cavity containing blood and lined by laminated clot and fibrous tissue.

4   An *arterio-venous aneurysm*, in which there is a communication between an artery and the vein.

5   A *dissecting aneurysm*, where there has been a breach of the intima and blood dissects the wall of the blood vessel to form a second channel. This may either rupture back into the main lumen, or externally (see page 50).

Aortic aneurysms are considered in the section on the heart and great vessels (see page 48). In this section certain features of peripheral aneurysms will be considered.

Aetiology

1   *Congenital*: especially the berry aneurysm which occurs intracranially on the

ANEURYSMS

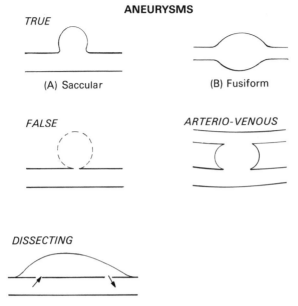

Fig. 10.1. The types of aneurysm.

circle of Willis and also the less common arteriovenous aneurysms and fistulae in the limbs.

2 *Traumatic*: the wall of an artery may be damaged by a penetrating wound, e.g. a bullet, and the weakened wall may subsequently distend into an aneurysm. Penetrating wounds may also produce a false aneurysm or an arteriovenous aneurysm.

3 *Inflammatory*: the mycotic aneurysms of subacute bacterial end-arteritis and the syphilitic aneurysm of the aorta which typically affects the thoracic course of the vessel.

4 *Degenerative*: in modern practice atheromatous degeneration of the vessel wall is the commonest cause of true aneurysm.

Clinical features

The clinical diagnosis of an aneurysm is usually obvious. There is a dilatation along the course of an artery which exhibits expansile pulsation. Direct compression may empty the sac or diminish its size, (the 'sign of emptying') and pressure on the artery proximal to the aneurysm again may reduce its pulsation. If the entering vessel has a narrow orifice there may be a thrill and bruit.

The commonest differential diagnosis is from a dilated, rather tortuous atheromatous artery which is not uncommon in elderly subjects.

Complications

1 Rupture.

2 Thrombosis, with impairment of the peripheral circulation.

3 Embolism, from contained thrombus.

4 Pressure, on adjacent structures.

5 Infection.

Treatment

Small peripheral aneurysms can be excised without endangering the peripheral circulation. More major aneurysms can be excised with a graft replacement. Occasionally the old-fashioned ligation of the artery proximal and/or distal to the sac may be carried out in order to induce thrombosis and hence obliteration of the sac. (The management of aortic atheromatous and dissecting aneurysms is considered on pages 49 and 51).

IMPAIRED CIRCULATION TO THE LIMBS

Causes of impaired circulation

1 Atherosclerosis.

2 Embolus.

3 Thrombosis.

4 Spasm: Raynaud's phenomenon.

5 Buerger's disease.

6 Diabetes.

7 Ergot poisoning.

8 Vessel injury due to trauma, cold or chemicals.

Although there are a large number of diseases that can cause impaired arterial blood flow to the limbs, three conditions are relatively common in Britain. First, and most important, atherosclerotic disease, second, embolism, and third, arteriolar spasm in Raynaud's phenomenon.

Buerger's disease is a rather poorly defined entity, confined to males, the salient features of which are similar to atherosclerosis but the age incidence is much younger and the association with heavy smoking is almost invariable. Peripheral vessels tend to be affected earlier in Buerger's disease and the veins may be inflamed together with the arteries.

Diagnosis

Surprisingly accurate pathological and anatomical diagnosis can be made by careful history taking and clinical examination.

History

In the history the points that will be sought particularly are as follows: the insidious progression of intermittent claudication of the calves over a period of months or years, will exclude embolus. A history of cold, painful hands since childhood, especially in the female, will be suggestive of Raynaud's disease. Sudden onset of pain in the leg with evidence of an impaired circulation is typical of an embolus and a history of cardiovascular disease, especially rheumatic carditis or coronary occlusion, should be sought.

The symptoms of atherosclerosis occurring in a young person, especially a heavy smoker and male, is typical of Buerger's disease.

Ergot poisoning is occasionally seen in patients with migraine who are consuming large doses of ergotamine.

It is important to determine the degree of disability produced by the symptoms, for on this will depend the selection of patients for reconstructive surgery. For example, a man with intermittent claudication which comes on after walking 500 metres, who is retired and seldom has need to walk this distance is obviously not a candidate for surgery. Similarly, if a patient suffers from angina pectoris as well as intermittent claudication, a fairly common combination, he may require coronary reconstruction (see page 55).

Atherosclerosis is usually a generalized disease and the cerebral circulation is quite often affected in addition to the circulation in the legs. Thus a history of intermittent loss of consciousness, blindness and hemiparesis is of importance and may indicate atherosclerosis of the arterial supply to the brain.

Examination

Careful clinical examination will usually provide a very clear indication of the severity and nature of the ischaemic disease. It is important that attention should be directed to other systems of the body, especially the heart and blood pressure.

The peripheral pulses throughout the body should be examined. Whereas normal pulsation can be appreciated easily, palpation of weak pulsations requires practice, care and, above all, time. The presence of a weak pulse that is definitely palpated is of considerable significance diagnostically and can be important prognostically, since even a weak pulse means that the vessel is patent. In addition to determination of the presence and intensity of pulsation, the regularity should be appreciated and atrial fibrillation or other cardiac arrhythmias noted.

The abdomen should be examined for any evidence of abnormal aortic pulsation and if distal pulses are absent then it is possible that no aortic pulsation will be felt due to thrombosis of the terminal aorta (*Leriche's syndrome*, absent femoral pulses, intermittent claudication of the buttock muscles, pale cold legs and impotence).

In all areas where pulses are felt auscultation should be performed. Partial blockage of arteries very often causes bruits which are usually systolic in timing. Arterio-venous communications will produce continuous bruits with systolic accentuations and pulsating dilated veins.

Attention is then directed to the legs. Inspection may reveal gangrene, marked pallor or absence of hairs, all being evidence of impaired circulation. The legs should be inspected when elevated to 45° above the horizontal; a poor arterial supply is shown by rapid pallor, and then with legs dependent at 90° over the edge of the examination couch; impaired arterial supply is shown by a change to a dusky blue cyanosis (*Buerger's sign*).

Patients with Raynaud's phenomenon may have hands and feet of normal appearance if the atmosphere is warm; however, a typical attack may be precipitated by immersion of the hands in cold water, when the digits will go first pale and deathly white, then blue and finally a dusky red. Raynaud's disease affects the hands more commonly and more severely than the feet.

Careful recording of the peripheral pulses will often clearly delineate a blockage in the arterial system; for instance the presence of a good femoral pulse and absence of pulses distal to the femoral suggests a superficial femoral arterial block. Presence of all pulses including the radial and ulnar pulses, yet obvious ischaemia of the digits is a typical finding in Raynaud's disease.

In addition to the pulses, skin temperature can be readily assessed by palpation, which is especially sensitive when the dorsum of the hand is used; a difference between the temperatures of one part of the leg and another or between the two legs can be ascertained when it is as small as 1 °C. A clearly marked change of temperature may reveal the site of blockage of a main artery.

The return of capillary circulation after blanching produced by pressure is a very useful gauge of the peripheral circulation, and this can be shown by pressing on the pulp of the toe or depression of the toe nail. On release of the pressure in a normal person there is an almost immediate return of normal red colour to the flesh; however, in a patient with impaired circulation this return may be very slow.

The veins of the foot and leg in a patient with diminished arterial supply are often very inconspicuous compared with normal veins. Indeed, the veins may be so empty that they appear as shallow grooves or gutters.

If it is difficult to obtain a clear history of the exact severity of intermittent claudication, the patient should be taken for a walk with the doctor, observing the time and nature of the onset of symptoms. A walk upstairs will provoke symptoms of claudication much more quickly than on the flat, and the speed of the walking is also important; some patients have no symptoms of claudication if they walk slowly, but as soon as they hurry or run they have to stop due to the pain.

Gangrene

The presence of gangrene indicates a severe degree of vascular impairment. Typically, it occurs in the toes or at pressure areas on the foot — the heel, over the malleoli or on the plantar aspect of the ball of the hallux. Gangrene results from infection of ischaemic tissues. Minimal trauma, such as a nick of the skin while cutting the toe nails, or an abrasion from a tight shoe enables ingress of bacteria into the infarcted tissues; the combination of these two factors results in clinical gangrene.

Special investigations

1   *Urine* for sugar to exclude diabetes, a common accompaniment, of peripheral artery disease; if necessary, a fasting blood sugar estimation.

2   *Haemoglobin estimation* to exclude anaemia or polycythaemia.

3   *Serum cholesterol*, often raised in atherosclerosis.

4   *Electrocardiogram* to exclude associated coronary disease.

5   *Chest X-ray.*

6   *The Doppler ultrasonic probe* is a very useful 'non-invasive' investigation used in conjunction with a standard sphygmomanometer to measure blood pressure at sites where the arterial pulse cannot be palpated. In normal subjects, the blood pressure in the arm and at the ankle are roughly the same so that this finding virtually excludes arterial occlusive disease. However, a considerable lowering of

the ankle pulse compared with the brachial pulse gives a numerical estimate of the degree of arterial impairment.

7 *Arteriography* to determine the site and extent of blockage is only performed if reconstructive surgery is contemplated.

If peripheral pulses are palpable as far as the pedal pulses then arteriography is unlikely to be of help. However, in other cases arteriography will provide accurate anatomical localization of the disease.

Arteriography is of especial value in atherosclerotic disease. It will give evidence of the severity of the distribution of atheromatous plaques, the location of stenoses and complete blocks and also the appearance of the main arterial vessels distal to the occlusion. This last factor is particularly important in the lower leg. Thus reconstruction is possible if the popliteal artery is patent and the chances of success are most likely if the three main tributaries of the popliteal, namely the anterior tibial, posterior tibial and peroneal arteries, are also open and constitute a good outflow (or 'run off') for arterial reconstruction (Fig. 10.2).

At the time of arteriography, the radiologist may be able to dilate a stenosed segment of artery under X-ray control by means of a specially designed balloon catheter. This transluminal angioplasty is now commonly undertaken for coronary as well as peripheral arteries.

Principles of treatment

The treatment of ischaemic vascular disease of the leg is obviously an individual matter which will vary with each patient. It will depend on his general condition, his cerebral and cardiac state, the severity of his symptoms and his attitude to them. Nevertheless, a few general principles can be laid down. In general there are two possibilities of treatment, conservative management or surgery. Conservative management can be of great value but is limited in potential. Reconstructive surgery can produce most dramatic results but obviously has a risk, and sometimes reconstruction is not possible for anatomical reasons.

ATHEROSCLEROTIC DISEASE

Although the metabolic factors concerned in the genesis of atherosclerosis are unknown, certain associated phenomena may be of aetiological significance. Thus a familial tendency to the disease is common and atherosclerosis tends to affect people who are over-weight and indulge in heavy cigarette smoking; it is especially common in diabetics.

Smoking

The malign effects of smoking in atherosclerotic disease result from three components:

1 Nicotine, which induces vascular spasm.

2 Carbon monoxide, which is present in the inhaled smoke and is taken up by haemoglobin to form carboxyhaemoglobin, which dissociates slowly and therefore considerably lowers the oxygen-carrying capacity of the blood.

3 Increased platelet stickiness, which increases the risk of thrombosis.

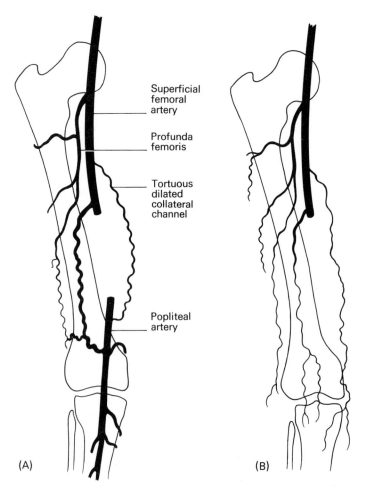

Superficial
femoral
artery

Profunda
femoris

Tortuous
dilated
collateral
channel

Popliteal
artery

(A)

(B)

Fig. 10.2. Tracings of arteriograms which demonstrate (A) an example of a good 'run off' with a patent popliteal artery; this is suitable for reconstructive surgery. In (B), however, the main arterial tree is obliterated and reconstruction cannot be carried out.

Diabetes

If a patient suffering from atherosclerosis has diabetes it is extremely important that this is satisfactorily controlled. Diabetics are liable to other forms of gangrene, namely infective gangrene associated with high blood sugar, diabetic micro-angiopathy and trophic ulcers due to diabetic neuropathy.

Treatment of claudication

The treatment of a patient with intermittent claudication due to atherosclerosis should be separated from the treatment of the patient with rest pain or gangrene since, in the latter group, the viability of the leg is obviously in immediate danger.

Conservative treatment

The conservative management of claudication requires first of all that the nature of the conditions be explained to the patient. If the patient can live a reasonably happy life with the claudication not limiting his activities unduly, then this is probably the most satisfactory state of affairs; claudication does not always progress, in fact in some patients claudication improves with time, presumably as collateral blood vessels enlarge. Approximately 10 per cent of patients with claudication eventually develop gangrene. A far higher proportion, however, succumb to the other complications of arteriosclerosis — coronary thrombosis, cerebral thrombosis, etc.

Patients with symptoms of impaired circulation to the legs, if overweight, should be strictly dieted in an attempt to limit the amount of work that the legs have to perform. Smoking produces vasospasm, increases platelet stickiness and replaces the oxyhaemoglobin in the blood with carboxyhaemoglobin; it must be prohibited.

If the claudication is limited to the calf, raising the heels of the shoes an inch may relieve the calf muscles of some work and therefore allow the patient to walk a greater distance.

Careful chiropody is important; gangrene can commence from the trauma of faulty nail or corn cutting.

Surgical treatment

If the claudication is so severe that it prevents the patient from working or makes his life a misery then the possibility of reconstructive surgery should be considered. The first essential is to determine whether this type of surgery can be carried out. Arteriography as outlined above will demonstrate the anatomy of the atherosclerotic disease.

If the popliteal artery is patent then reconstructive surgery is likely to be possible. However, the results will depend considerably on the severity of the atherosclerosis in the main tibial vessels. If these are occluded then the chance of success is low.

If the popliteal artery and its branches are blocked then reconstruction requires a long (and technically difficult) bypass below the knee.

Lumbar sympathectomy or destruction of the lumbar sympathetic chain by means of an injection of phenol may increase the flow of the blood to the skin but has no beneficial effect on claudication and may, in fact, make claudication worse by shunting blood from the muscles to the skin.

Summary of the treatment of claudication

Conservative

1 Stop smoking.
2 Learn to live within the claudication distance; this may involve change in employment.
3 Lose weight — less effort for the muscles.
4 Raise the heel of the shoe.

5   Take care of the feet to prevent minor trauma which may lead to gangrene.
6   Treat diabetes if present.

Surgical

Reconstructive surgery is indicated only if:
1   symptoms are very severe.
2   X-ray shows that reconstructive surgery is possible.
3   no serious coexisting disease (especially cardiovascular).

The two main types of operation are:
1   Removal of the stenosis and block (thromboendarterectomy) in which the patient's own vessel is still used as a conduit for the blood. The lumen may be increased by adding a patch graft to its circumference.
2   The diseased part of the vessel may be left intact and bypassed by a graft of vein or inert plastic material (Dacron or PTFE) from above to below the lesion. The graft most commonly employed is the patient's own saphenous vein which must be reversed so that its valves do not impede the flow of blood.

The radiologist may be able to dilate a stenosed vessel by means of a balloon catheter under X-ray control (balloon angioplasty), thus avoiding the need for open operation.

Treatment of rest pain and nutritional changes (gangrene)

Reconstructive surgery

A patient with ischaemic rest pain or frank or incipient gangrene is urgently in need of surgical treatment. If there is any prospect of reconstructive surgery from the anatomical point of view and the patient is considered to be a fair risk for surgery, then this should be carried out, since the alternative is amputation. The principles of reconstructive surgery are exactly the same as those outlined above. However, it is reasonable to subject these patients with severe occlusive disease of the arteries to this type of surgery even if the anatomical features of the disease are somewhat unsatisfactory.

Lumbar sympathectomy

If it is impossible for anatomical reasons to perform any kind of reconstructive surgery, then lumbar sympathectomy (or phenol injection into the lumbar chain) may abolish rest pain and occasionally improves the condition of the skin so that incipient skin necrosis does not lead to frank gangrene. If, however, there is already necrosis of tissues, sympathectomy may still have value in that it may improve the circulation to the skin adjacent to the gangrenous area and allow a more limited amputation than would otherwise be indicated. The results of lumbar sympathectomy are frequently disappointing.

Major amputation

The indication for major amputation is pain which cannot be controlled by sympathectomy or reconstructive surgery and also spreading infection of a gangrenous limb which is likely to threaten the life of the patient. The latter is rare nowadays since infection in these circumstances can usually be controlled by antibiotics.

EMBOLISM

Aetiology

In attempting to establish the source of an embolus it is useful to consider the possible sites of origin from the heart and the major vessels thus:

1   Left atrium: atrial fibrillation and mitral stenosis, atrial myxoma.
2   Valves: subacute bacterial endocarditis.
3   Left ventricular wall: mural thrombus after coronary thrombosis.
4   Aorta: from aneurysm or atheroma.
5   Rare paradoxical embolus via a septal defect, originating in the systemic veins.

Emboli tend to lodge at the bifurcation of vessels; their danger will depend upon the anatomical situation. Blockage of arteries of the central nervous system, retina and small intestine will produce dramatic effects. Emboli in the renal arteries will produce pain in the loin and haematuria. Emboli in the splenic artery will produce pain under the left costal margin.

The late results of embolism in limb vessels are similar to those of atherosclerosis and may, in fact, be associated or caused by this condition. However, acute embolism is a surgical emergency and prompt adequate treatment may produce a complete recovery.

Clinical features

The history and physical signs may reveal a cause for an embolus. The commonest causes of arterial emboli are atrial fibrillation due to rheumatic heart disease or myocardial ischaemia and dislodgement of a mural clot from a myocardial infarct. The history in acute blockage of a limb is usally one of sudden pain in the limb which soon becomes white and cold. Sensation may disappear and the muscles may become rapidly paralysed ('pain, pallor, pulselessness, paraesthesiae, paralysis, perishing with cold').

On examination the site of the block will usually be considerably proximal to the site at which pain is experienced. It is fairly common for the block to travel distally in the course of the first few hours, due to the embolus being dislodged or fragmented.

Treatment

The likelihood of surgical removal of an embolus being successful is inversely proportional to the time interval from the onset of the block to the operation and after 24 hours have elapsed successful disobliteration of the artery becomes less likely.

As soon as the diagnosis is made the patient should be systemically heparinized, so as to prevent propagation of clot from the site of blockage. The limb is exposed to room temperature and observed for signs of impairment to the circulation. If the block seems to be resolving, with the appearance of pulses that had previously been absent, then the collateral circulation may produce adequate

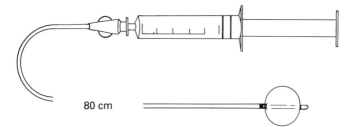

Fig. 10.3. A Fogarty catheter.

distal arterial blood supply and surgery may not be required. If the distal limb has apparently no blood supply and there are neurological changes, then urgent surgery is indicated.

Absent femoral, popliteal or aortic pulsations are indications that operation will probably prove necessary. The approach to the involved vessel will depend on physical findings; thus absence of both femoral pulses and a weak or absent aortic pulse will require mobilization of both femoral arteries so that these can be clamped and dislodgement of embolus fragments can be prevented.

The operative treatment is relatively simple; the vessel is exposed, opened and the clot removed. A special inflatable balloon catheter (designed by Thomas Fogarty when he was a medical student) is passed up into the aorta with the balloon collapsed — it is then distended and pulled back down the iliac and femoral vessels, the clot being expelled by the balloon via the femoral arteriotomy. Poor results will be due to propagation of clot beyond the embolus but removal of such propagated clot may be possible by passing the Fogarty catheter distally along the vessel through the arteriotomy. As the balloon is then withdrawn, the artery is cleared of clot (Fig. 10.3).

Emboli in the upper limb vessels usually produce less disability than those in the lower limb as a collateral circulation in the upper limb is better; surgery is less often indicated.

In some cases there is no obvious cause for an embolus and a spontaneous thrombosis *in situ* must be considered as the diagnosis.

It is most important that after the successful outcome of an embolectomy the cause of the embolism should be treated if this is possible. Especially pertinent in this regard is mitral stenosis, since mitral valvotomy will remove this source of emboli.

RAYNAUD'S PHENOMENON

This may be primary Raynaud's disease, almost invariably in females, or Raynaud's phenomenon secondary to some other lesion, e.g. scleroderma, poly-arteritis nodosa or other collagen diseases; it may occur in patients with cryoglo-bulinaemia, or it can result from work with vibrating tools. It is important to exclude other causes of cold, cyanosed hands, for instance pressure on the subclavian artery from a cervical rib (usually complicated by multiple emboli arising from the damaged artery wall at the site of rib pressure), or blockage of a main artery in the upper limb due to atherosclerosis or Buerger's disease.

Treatment

The management should be initially conservative. Patients should be exhorted to keep their hands and feet warm, to wear gloves and fur-lined boots in the winter, and make sure that the house, and especially the bed, are warm at night. They should also avoid immersion of the limbs in cold water. Treatment with vasodilator drugs is usually tried but the results are often disappointing.

Sympathectomy almost invariably produces a dramatic improvement in the symptoms, but unfortunately may not be long-lasting in the upper limbs.

Rarely Raynaud's phenomenon or disease leads to actual necrosis of tissues and gangrene of the digits. If this occurs local amputation may be necessary, but since the circulation of the proximal part of the hand is usually satisfactory, major amputations are seldom required.

Chapter 11
The Veins of the Legs

A comparatively small price that man has to pay for his upright posture is his liability to develop varicose veins. The normal flow of blood in the lower limbs is from the skin and the subcutaneous tissue to the superficial veins which drain via perforators to the deep veins, which in turn drain into the iliac veins and inferior vena cava. The passage of blood in the vein depends on the presence of competent valves, which prevent reflux, together with the contraction of the muscles in the limb which pump the blood towards the heart. Provided that the venous valves are competent, the return of blood to the heart is assured. However, the pressure to which these valves may be subjected can be very high; the maximum pressure is equal to a column of blood extending from the ground to the level of the heart, roughly equivalent to about a metre of water in an average adult man. One incompetent valve will put extra pressure on the next and will tend to make this incompetent and so once defects have arisen there is a tendency for the condition to get worse as further valves are involved.

VARICOSE VEINS

Varicose veins may be classified aetiologically into:

1 *Primary or idiopathic*: the great majority. This probably represents a primary valve defect and may be familial. Females are affected more than males. Symptoms are often accentuated by pregnancy, partly as result of pressure of the fetus on the iliac veins and partly due to hormonal relaxation of smooth muscle.

2 *Secondary*

(a) to a previous deep vein thrombosis; the veins subsequently recanalize but their valves are rendered incompetent

(b) to raised venous pressure due to a pelvic tumour (which includes the pregnant uterus)

Clinical features

Varicose veins are prominent and unsightly and patients may seek treatment on account of the unpleasant appearance. As the varicose veins become progressively worse there may be interference with venous return and oedema of the ankles occurs, especially at the end of a long period of standing. Eventually, the valves guarding the communications between the deep and superficial veins become incompetent (Fig. 11.1). When this happens there is an uninterrupted pressure column of blood directed to the foot; this results in the appearance of subcutaneous venules which tend to form a fan-like arrangement spreading over the malleoli (especially the medial). This flare of venules is a danger sign that gravitational ulcers may develop. Extravasation of red cells produces the typical varicose pigmentation (due to haemosiderin).

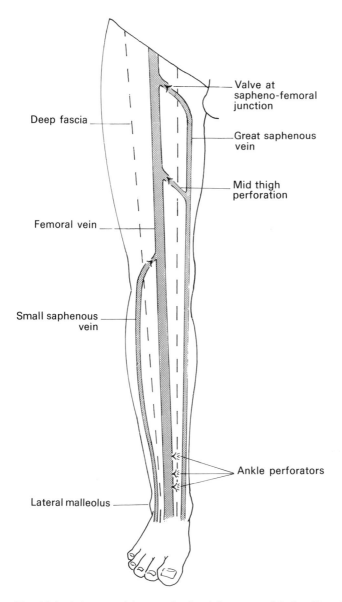

Fig. 11.1. A diagram of the superficial and deep veins of the leg. Note the two superficial systems — the great saphenous and small saphenous — each of which communicates with the deep veins by piercing the deep fascia.

At the points where there are incompetent valves between the superficial and deep veins, the varicosities tend to be extreme and are sometimes termed 'blow-outs'. Such a dilatation at the saphenous opening is called a *saphena varix* which may be confused with a femoral hernia. However, the varix has a fluid thrill, which can be elicited by tapping gently on the varicose veins lower down the thigh while an observing finger rests lightly on the varix. It disappears when the patient lies down.

Treatment

1 Injection of sclerosing agents with compression.
2 Ligation and stripping of the vein.
3 An elastic stocking — for the elderly, the pregnant, the unfit.

Injection treatment

Careful palpation determines the controlling points where the varicosities drain into the deep veins through the deep fascia. Sclerosant solution is injected at these points with the vein emptied and firm pressure maintained by bandaging for a period of 2 weeks to enable fibrosis to take place. This out-patient treatment is used for small or moderate sized varices below the knee. Recurrences can be treated by further injections.

Surgical treatment

Indicated for grossly dilated varices which extend into the thigh.

The most commonly practised operation for varicose veins is the Trendelen-burg operation which may be combined with stripping of the veins, and ligation or avulsion of incompetent deep perforators. In the Trendelenburg operation the saphenous vein is disconnected from the femoral vein and the terminal branches of the saphenous vein individually ligated and divided. The operation is very success-ful in treating the incompetent great saphenous vein but if in addition there are other incompetent communications, they need to be individually ligated or avulsed. Because of the frequency of coronary artery disease and the possible future need of vein grafts, the saphenous vein below the knee is preserved unless it is extensively dilated. Small varicose venules can be avulsed by twisting around a haemostatic clamp via a minute skin incision.

Diagnosis of further incompetence can be worked out by placing a venous tourniquet (a plain extensible rubber tube) around the thigh and leg at different levels. If compression of superficial veins in the region of the saphenofemoral junction completely prevents rapid filling of the varicosities when the patient stands up, the tourniquet having been applied when the patient was lying down, then the Trendelenburg operation can be expected to produce good results. If, however, there is fairly rapid filling of the varicosities, then there are probably other perforating veins and the exact level of these perforators can be sought by moving the tourniquet to different levels and finding at which level the varicosities are controlled. The perforators and severely dilated clumps of veins must be marked out before operation with the patient standing and then individually ligated and divided at the time of the operation.

Stripping of the varicose veins removes the unsightly veins and also discon-nects tributaries of the main saphenous system. This may be employed where there are gross varicosities extending from the knee to the groin.

Recurrence of varicose veins after operation is often due to incomplete operation, especially in failure to divide and excise all the groin tributaries of the saphenous vein. If this error is made these branches will dilate and form new varices. However, recurrence may be due to the development of further varices *de novo*, despite an adequate operation.

COMPLICATIONS OF VARICOSE VEINS

Haemorrhage

Usually due to minor trauma to the dilated vein. The bleeding is profuse due to the high pressure within the incompetent vein.

Treatment

The treatment is very simple; the patient is laid recumbent with the leg elevated and a pressure bandage is applied. Subsequent to the emergency, the varicose veins should be treated by operation.

Phlebitis

May occur spontaneously or may be secondary to trauma to the leg. A mild phlebitis is, of course, produced by the sclerosing fluid used in the injection treatment of varicose veins. Occasionally the reaction to this is quite violent and alarming; the varicose vein becomes extremely tender and hard and the overlying skin may be inflamed. The patient may have a constitutional disturbance with pyrexia and malaise. Secondary bacterial infection may occasionally complicate the thrombosis.

Treatment

Bed rest with the foot of the bed elevated and a pressure bandage on the leg, which compresses the superficial veins and increases the speed of flow of blood in the deep veins. If infection is present then antibiotics may be necessary, but this is unusual. In severe cases systemic anticoagulation may alleviate pain and prevent spread of the condition. Non steroidal anti-inflammatory drugs may give relief of symptoms but they can cause peptic ulceration.

Ulceration

Ulceration may be due to varicose veins, or to incompetent valves in the deep venous system. The latter is especially likely to occur after there has been a deep venous thrombosis. The deep veins recanalize, but the valves are irreparably damaged. A patient with a gravitational ulcer should always be asked if there has been any previous history of venous thrombosis, suggested by painful swelling of the leg after an operation, childbirth or immobilization in bed for any reason. If the valves of the deep veins are incompetent, then the pressure is transmitted as a column of blood from the heart to the lower leg and the valves that guard the superficial entrance to the deep veins (Fig. 11.1) become incompetent. The same sequence can follow primary varicose veins.

Why a gravitational ulcer is likely to occur around the malleoli and not in the foot itself is not fully explained. It is probably that in this area the subcutaneous tissue is less well supported than in the foot. The pressure of the column of blood and the consequent oedema and pericapillary fibrin cuffs result in ischaemia and very poor nutrition to this area so that the skin may break down either spontaneously or more commonly after minor trauma.

Gravitational ulcers have an edge which is either ragged or, if the ulcer is healing, the margins will be shelving with a faint blue rim of advancing epithelium. Rarely, a carcinoma can develop in the edge of a long-standing gravitational ulcer (*Marjolin's ulcer*).

Treatment

If the patient is confined to bed with the foot of the bed elevated, so that the high venous pressure is abolished, gravitational ulcers will heal fairly quickly, provided they are kept clean by careful toilet. Antibiotics should be administrated only in the unusual circumstances when the ulcer is grossly infected with a surrounding cellulitis. The antibiotics used will depend on the sensitivity of the bacteria cultured from the ulcer. Local chemotherapy should not be used; the incidence of sensitivity reaction is high.

This simple treatment is not often a practical one. The patients are mostly elderly and prolonged recumbency is obviously of some danger in these cases. Younger patients, from the economic point of view, do not wish to spend several weeks in hospital in bed.

In such cases healing can be obtained by either tight elastic bandaging of the leg or by using proprietary paste bandages over which elastoplast is applied. This firm pressure empties the dilated superficial veins and enables the leg muscle pump to act efficiently. Oxygenated blood is therefore able to reach the previously ischaemic tissues. A split skin graft may be useful in indolent cases, but grafting must only supplement the other treatment modalities.

Once the ulcer has healed the patient is fitted with a firm elastic stocking or advised to continue with the elastic bandage. Alternatively, especially in the younger and fitter patients, the incompetent perforating veins are ligated (Cockett's operation). Unless the incompetent veins are treated thus, either by support, or operation, recurrence is inevitable.

Gravitational ulcers account for approximately 90 per cent of all ulcers of the legs, but other, rarer, causes should always be considered.

Differential diagnosis of leg ulcers (rarer causes):

1   Ischaemic ulcer: due to impaired arterial blood supply; the peripheral pulses must always be examined.

2   Gummatous ulcer of syphilis: usually affects the upper one-third of the leg.

3   Malignant ulcer: a squamous carcinoma, often arising in a pre-existing chronic ulcer, or an ulcerated melanoma.

4   Ulcers complicating acholuric jaundice, ulcerative colitis and rheumatoid arthritis.

5   Infective ulcers in diabetics.

6   Ulcers complicating arterio-venous fistulae.

7   Ulcers caused by self-inflicted repetitive injury.

Chapter 12
The Lymph Nodes and Lymphatics

Enlarged lymph nodes are a common diagnostic problem. It is as well therefore to have a simple classification and clinical approach to this topic.

THE LYMPHADENOPATHIES

The lymphadenopathies are conveniently divided into those due to local, and those due to generalized disease:

Localized

1. *Infective*
   (a) *acute*, e.g. a cervical lymphadenopathy secondary to tonsillitis
   (b) *chronic*, e.g. tuberculous nodes of neck

2. *Neoplastic*
   Due to secondary spread of tumour.

Generalized

1. *Infective*
   (a) *acute*, e.g. glandular fever (mononucleosis), septicaemia
   (b) *chronic*, e.g. secondary syphilis, AIDS syndrome

2. *The reticuloses*
   Hodgkin's disease, non-Hodgkin's lymphoma, lymphatic leukemia.

3. *Sarcoidosis.*

Clinical examination

The clinical examination of any patient with a lymph node enlargement is incomplete unless the following three requirements have been fulfilled:

1 That the area drained by the involved lymph nodes has been searched for possible primary source of infection or malignant disease. Thus, if a patient has an enlarged lymph node in the groin, then the skin of the leg, buttock and lower abdominal wall below the level of the umbilicus must be scrutinized, together with the external genitalia and the anal canal.

2 That the other lymph node areas have been examined; if enlarged lymph nodes are found elsewhere, then obviously the condition must be part of some generalized lymphadenopathy.

3 That the liver and spleen have been carefully palpated; their enlargement will suggest a reticulosis, sarcoid or glandular fever.

Special investigations

In many instances the diagnosis of the cause of the lymphadenopathy will by now have become obvious. The following investigations may be required, however, in order to elucidate the diagnosis:

1 Examination of a blood film may clinch the diagnosis of glandular fever or leukaemia.

2 A chest X-ray may show evidence of enlarged mediastinal nodes or may reveal a primary occult tumour of the lung, which is the source of disseminated deposits.

3 The Wassermann reaction will be positive in secondary syphilis; the HIV antibody test is performed if AIDS is suspected.

4 Enlarged painless cervical lymph nodes should be X-rayed; tuberculous nodes often show typical spotty calcification.

5 Removal of one of the enlarged lymph nodes may be necessary for definite histological proof of the diagnosis. This is particularly so in Hodgkin's disease and non-Hodgkin's lymphoma.

LYMPHOEDEMA

Lymphoedema results from the obstruction of lymphatic flow, either because of congenital abnormalities of the lymphatics, their obliteration by disease or their operative removal. The causes of lymphoedema are:

1 *Congenital abnormalities of lymphatic channels of the lower limb:* lymphoedema in these cases may be present at birth (lymphoedema congenita) but usually develops at puberty (lymphoedema praecox). If delayed until adult life, it is termed lymphoedema tarda. Females are more affected than males and the condition may be familial (Milroy's disease). Lymphangiography reveals that three conditions may exist, aplasia, hypolasia or varicose dilatation of the lymphatics.

2 *Post-inflammatory:* the result of fibrosis obliterating the lymphatics following repeated attacks of streptococcal cellulitis.

3 *Filariasis:* the *Filaria bancrofti* infects lymphatics; a chronic inflammatory reaction is set up with consequent lymphatic obstruction. There is gross lymphoedema, especially of the lower limbs and genitalia.

4 *Following radical surgery,* e.g. after block dissection of the groin or neck in which extensive removal of lymphatics is performed.

5 *Post-irradiation fibrosis.*

6 *Malignant disease:* late oedema of the arm after radical mastectomy is often indicative of massive recurrence of tumour in the axilla occluding the residual lymphatic pathways.

Differential diagnosis

The diagnosis of lymphoedema depends first of all on the exclusion of other causes of oedema, for instance venous obstruction, cardiac failure or renal disease, and second, the demonstration of one of the causes mentioned above. It was previously taught that lymphoedema could readily be differentiated from other forms of oedema on the simple physical sign of absence of pitting in the lymphoedematous limb. However, lymphoedema of acute onset will initially pit on pressure although it is true that when it becomes chronic the subcutaneous tissues become indurated from fibrous tissue replacement and pitting will not then occur. But, indeed, oedema of any nature, if chronic, will have this characteristic.

Treatment

If the oedema is mild it may be controlled by well fitting elastic stockings. In more serious cases prolonged elevation of the limb, together with firm elastic bandaging may be of help, but if this fails the patient can be offered an operation which will restore the contour of the leg but leave it with considerable scarring. This consists of excision of the whole of the oedematous subcutaneous tissue down to the deep fascia, removal of the overlying skin as a split skin graft and its re-application directly to the deep fascia.

Occasionally the massive brawny arm which may occur after radical mastectomy and heavy post-operative radiation may be so burdensome to the patient that amputation has to be performed.

Chapter 13
The Brain and Meninges

SPACE-OCCUPYING INTRACRANIAL LESIONS

Space-occupying lesions within the skull may be:
1 Chronic subdural haematoma (see page 98).
2 Abscess.
3 Tumour (today by far the commonest).
Other causes are rare and include hydatid cyst, tuberculoma and gumma.

Clinical features

A space-occupying lesion manifests itself by the general features of raised intracranial pressure and by localizing signs.

Raised intracranial pressure

A space-occupying lesion within the skull produces a raised intracranial pressure partly by its actual pressure within the closed box of the cranium, by surrounding oedema excited by its presence, and sometimes by impeding the circulation or absorption of CSF with the production of hydrocephalus (see page 87); thus a tumour obstructing the posterior fossa may rapidly present with severe symptoms of raised intracranial pressure.

If the rise in intracranial pressure is slowly progressive, the following features may be found:
1 *Headache:* this is severe, often present when the patient wakes and is aggravated by straining or coughing.
2 *Vomiting:* often without preceding nausea.
3 *Papilloedema:* which may be accompanied by blurring of vision and may progress to permanent blindness.
4 *Mental deterioration.*
5 *Enlargement of the head:* in children before the suture lines have closed.

If raised intracranial pressure develops rapidly the clinical picture is one of intense headache with rapid progression into coma.

Localizing signs

Having diagnosed the presence of raised intracranial pressure, an attempt must be made on clinical findings to localize the lesion, although in some cases this is not possible. There may be upper motor neurone paralysis indicating a lesion of the pyramidal pathway; there may be cranial nerve signs, e.g. a bitemporal hemianopia indicating pressure on the optic chiasma. A lesion of the post-central cortex may produce loss of fine discrimination and stereognosis. Cerebellar lesions may produce coarse ataxia, muscular hypotonia, incoordination, and often nystagmus. A local fit may provide valuable localizing data. Motor aphasia (the patient knows what he wishes to say but cannot do so) suggests a lesion in Broca's area on the dominant side of the lower frontal cortex of the cerebrum.

Special investigations

Computerized axial tomography (CT scanning), MR scanning and radiological investigations are considered under cerebral tumours (page 84).

CEREBRAL ABSCESS

AETIOLOGY

There are three common causes of brain abscess:

1 *Penetrating wound* of the skull.

2 *Direct spread* from an infected middle ear or mastoid, either to the temporal lobe or the cerebellum, or from an infected frontal or ethmoid sinus to the frontal lobe.

3 *Blood-borne*, especially from a lung focus of infection such as bronchiectasis or lung abscess.

An abscess localized to the extradural or subdural space may result from the same aetiological factors, particularly direct spread of infection.

Clinical features

The clinical features are those of the underlying cause (for example chronic mastoiditis) together with evidence of the development of an intracerebral space-occupying lesion. There may also be localizing features, e.g. epilepsy or a focal neurological defect. Often the abscess is walled off by a relatively thick capsule so that the general manifestations of infection (fever, leucocytosis and toxaemia) are not evident. If, however, there is rapidly spreading cerebral infection then there is marked toxaemia, fever and meningism.

The accurate localization of the abscess can usually be made by CT scanning or magnetic resonance (MR).

Treatment

In the first instance the abscess is aspirated through a burr-hole by means of a brain needle. The pus is replaced with antibiotic together with a radio-opaque solution, which enables subsequent serial X-ray studies to be made of the abscess capsule. The aspirations may require to be repeated and systemic antibiotics are given, depending on the bacteriology report on the pus. Occasionally the abscess fails to respond to aspiration and its capsule must be excised.

A minority of patients may subsequently develop epilepsy and will therefore require anticonvulsant therapy.

INTRACRANIAL TUMOURS

Intracranial tumours can be divided into intrinsic tumours of the brain, arising from the supporting (glial) cells, and extra-cerebral tumours which originate from the numerous structures surrounding the brain — the meninges, cranial nerves, pituitary, pineal, blood vessels and skull.

It is important to remember that secondary deposits in the brain are common. In neurosurgical units they account for about 15 per cent of the cases seen, but many patients dying of widespread metastases have cerebral deposits and do not come under specialist care.

The incidence of the various intracranial tumours encountered at a neurosurgical unit is approximately:

Glioma — 45 per cent.
Meningioma — 15 per cent.
Metastases — 15 per cent.
Acoustic tumour — 5 per cent.
Pituitary tumours — 5 per cent.
All the others — 15 per cent.

Gliomas

The gliomas, arising from the glial supporting cells, account for some 45 per cent of intracerebral tumours. They are classified according to the principal cell component. The four important subgroups are:

1. Astrocytomas (80 per cent)

These vary considerably in their histological differentiation and invasiveness and about half are the highly anaplastic *Glioblastoma multiforme,* the name referring to the primitive cell structure of this tumour. The more benign forms are often cystic and are slow growing, although they may change over the years into less differentiated and more invasive tumours. Often a glioma may have cells of different grades of differentiation in different areas of the tumour. It is interesting that the glioblastoma tends to occur in the adult and in the cerebrum, whereas the well differentiated cystic glioma occurs frequently in children and usually arises in the cerebellum.

2. Medulloblastomas (10 per cent)

These are rapidly growing tumours of the cerebellum in children, usually boys. They may block the IV ventricle producing an obstructive hydrocephalus and may spread via the CSF to seed over the surface of the spinal cord. The cells appear to be embryonal in origin and form characteristic rosettes under the microscope.

3. Ependymomas (5 per cent)

These arise from the lining cells of the ventricles, the central canal of the spinal cord or the choroid plexus. They usually occur in children and young adults.

4. Oligodendrogliomas (5 per cent)

These are relatively slow growing and are usually found in the cerebrum and in adults.

Meningioma

These account for 15 per cent of intracranial tumours. They arise from arachnoid cells in the dura mater to which they are almost invariably attached and typically are found in middle-aged patients. Special sites are the lesser wing of the sphenoid, the olfactory groove, the suprasellar region, one or other side of the superior sagittal sinus and within the spinal canal. The majority are slow growing and do not invade the brain tissue but involve it only by expansion and pressure so they may become actually buried in the brain. The tumour may, however, invade the skull, producing a hyperostosis which may occasionally be enormous.

Acoustic tumours

Cranial nerve tumours arise from the Schwann cells of the nerve sheath. The great majority arise from the VIII nerve at the internal auditory meatus (acoustic tumour) which accounts for 5 per cent of all the intracranial tumours. It is usually found in adult patients between the ages of 30 and 60 and may project into the internal auditory meatus which may be demonstrated to be enlarged on imaging. It is occasionally associated with generalized neurofibromatosis (Von Recklinghausen's disease).

As the acoustic tumour enlarges it stretches the adjacent cranial nerves, VII and V anteriorly, and IX, X and XII over its lower surface. It also presses on the cerebellum and the brain stem, producing the 'cerebellopontine angle syndrome' with the following features:

1   Initially unilateral nerve deafness with tinnitus and giddiness (VIII).
2   Facial weakness with unilateral taste loss (VII).
3   Facial numbness and weakness of the masticatory muscles (V).
4   Dysphagia, hoarseness and dysarthia (IX, X and XII).
5   Cerebellar hemisphere signs and, later, pyramidal tract involvement.
6   Eventually features of raised intracranial pressure.

Pituitary tumours

These account for about 5 per cent of all intracranial tumours.

They have two special features: their endocrine disturbances and their relationship to the optic chiasma.

Chromophobe adenoma

This is the commonest pituitary tumour which, as it enlarges, compresses the optic chiasma, producing a bitemporal hemianopia. It is a non-secretory tumour which gradually destroys the normally functioning pituitary; there are therefore the added effects of hypopituitarism with loss of sex characteristics, hypothyroidism and hypoadrenalism. In childhood there is arrest of growth together with infantilism. As the tumour extends there may be involvement of the hypothalamus with diabetes insipidus and obesity.

Eosinophil adenoma

Secretes the pituitary hormones. If it occurs before puberty, which is unusual, it induces gigantism. After puberty acromegaly results.

Basophil adenoma

Small, produces no pressure effects and may be associated with Cushing's syndrome (see page 337).

Craniopharyngioma

(Suprasellar cyst, or cyst of Rathke's pouch) is a benign tumour, usually cystic, which arises in the remnant of the craniopharyngeal duct (the precursor of the anterior pituitary). It may present in childhood or adult life and lies above and/or within the sella turcica.

The tumour produces the signs of pituitary disfunction, raised intracranial pressure and optic chiasmal involvement.

Secondary tumours

These account for about 15 per cent of intracranial tumours seen on a neurosurgical unit but are more common on the general wards. Particular primary sites of origin are lung, breast and kidney.

Special investigations of cerebral tumours

The following investigations are required in the study of a suspected space occupying lesion:

1. X-rays of skull

10 per cent of tumours show calcification, most commonly in craniopharyngiomas and then in oligodendrogliomas. It is occasionally found in astrocytomas, meningiomas and vascular malformations.

In 70 per cent of adults the pineal gland is calcified. Inspection of the films of the skull may show shift of the pineal to one side, indicating a space occupying lesion.

The sella turcica should be examined; decalcification is evidence of raised intracranial pressure and expansion of the sella with erosion of the clinoid processes suggests the presence of a pituitary tumour.

In children, widening of the coronal sutures and increased convolutional markings may be seen (the 'beaten brass' appearance).

2. X-ray of chest

This must always be performed to exclude a symptomless primary bronchogenic carcinoma which is now reaching epidemic proportions in the cigarette-smoking population of this country.

3. CT scanning

A non-invasive and extremely accurate investigation for all cerebral tumours.

4. Magnetic resonance (MR)

This gives superb 'anatomical' localization of intracerebral space occupying lesions.

These investigations have all but superseded older established techniques, which include:

5. Gamma scan of the brain
A positive localizing diagnosis can be made in about 85 per cent of cases without any danger to the patient.

6. Air studies
Air may be introduced into the ventricles either through a burr-hole (ventriculography) or via a lumbar or cisternal puncture (air encephalography). Deformity or displacement of the ventricles may outline a space-occupying tumour.

7. Cerebral arteriography
An intracranial tumour may be localized directly by a vascular 'blush', or by inference, from displacement of the cerebral vessels from their normal positions.

8. The electroencephalogram
May give useful localizing information in brain tumours involving the cerebrum.

9. Aspiration biopsy
May be performed via a burr-hole. This enables tissue diagnosis to be established once tumour localization has been made.

Treatment

Treatment depends on both the localization and the degree of malignancy of the particular tumour. Of the extrinsic intracranial tumours, most meningiomas are removable. Acoustic neuromas can be removed completely, with some risk to facial nerve; alternatively, an intracapsular removal can be carried out with the knowledge that recurrence will occur eventually but with sparing of the facial nerve. Pituitary tumours which are producing pressure symptoms on the optic chiasma are submitted to intracapsular removal through either a trans-cranial or trans-sphenoidal route. Craniopharyngiomas are very difficult to remove completely because of their close relationship to the hypothalamus.

Of the gliomas, only the well-differentiated lesions are amenable to surgical removal. The more anaplastic growths have an extremely poor prognosis and are treated by palliative radiotherapy which may be combined with decompression by means of a small flap.

VASCULAR INTRACRANIAL LESIONS

Aneurysms

Pathology

Intracranial aneurysms are congenital in 95 per cent of cases. Only rarely are they due to arteriosclerosis, trauma or infection (mycotic aneurysms). The congenital aneurysms are saccular, generally arise near the bifurcation of a cerebral artery, and are probably due to aplasia or hypoplasia of the tunica media. About 30 per cent are situated on the middle cerebral artery, 30 per cent on the internal carotid proximal to its bifurcation, 20 per cent on the anterior cerebral or communicating arteries, and 20 per cent on the basilic or vertebral arteries. About 20 per cent are multiple. Males and females are equally affected.

Clinical features

These can be divided into two groups:

1 *Leakage of blood into the CSF*: intracranial aneurysms are the commonest cause of spontaneous subarachnoid haemorrhage with sudden onset of headache, neck stiffness and sometimes loss of consciousness, but they may also cause intra-cerebral or subdural bleeding with neurological signs depending on the site of the haematoma. Most cases occur after the age of 40, where increasing atheromatous degenerative changes in the arteries and hypertension are probably precipitating factors.

2 *Pressure symptoms due to the aneurysms*: especially III nerve palsy, but may also affect II, IV, V or VI.

Haemorrhage from a ruptured aneurysm is serious and a quarter of the patients die without recovering consciousness. Cerebral ischaemia is aggravated by intense spasm of the adjacent arteries. More than 50 per cent will bleed again within 6 weeks of the initial haemorrhage and the mortality of such bleeds is high. After 6 weeks the likelihood of haemorrhage becomes less but is still present and the rate never drops below 3 per cent per year.

Treatment

While the patient is in coma or has a dense hemiplegia, nursing care only is indicated. If the patient recovers from the initial bleed, cerebral angiography and CT scan are performed to locate the site of the aneurysm before the peak incidence of recurrent haemorrhage, which is after about 14 days.

When an aneurysm has been demonstrated, treatment comprises either ligation of the common carotid artery in those instances where the aneurysm is supplied by the internal carotid artery, or a direct attack on the aneurysm either by applying a silver clip to its base or its supplying vessels, excising the aneurysm or wrapping it in quick-setting plastic material.

About one-third of the angiograms are negative and probably indicate that thrombosis has taken place in a small aneurysm. Such cases are treated conservatively and the prognosis is good.

Angiomas

Developmental angiomatous malformations may occur in any part of the CNS, particularly over the surface of the cerebral hemispheres in the distribution of the middle cerebral artery. They comprise a tangle of abnormal vessels, often with arterio-venous fistulae.

They may produce focal epilepsy, headaches, slowly progressive paralysis or subarachnoid or intracerebral bleeding. The subarachnoid haemorrhage is less catastrophic than in rupture of an aneurysm, but accounts for about 10 per cent of all examples of spontaneous subarachnoid bleeding. About 50 per cent have a bruit which may be heard over the eye, the skull vault or over the carotid arteries in the neck.

Exact diagnosis and localization is made by cerebral angiography.

If producing marked symptoms or if there has been any preceding subarachnoid haemorrhage, an attempt should be made to excise the angioma; if technically impossible, then the feeding vessels are tied or clipped but this is much less satisfactory.

The Sturge—Weber syndrome is an association between an extensive venous angioma with a port-wine stain localized to one or more segments of the cutaneous distribution of the trigeminal nerve.

HYDROCEPHALUS

The circulation of the cerebro-spinal fluid (CSF)

CSF is produced by the choroid plexuses of the lateral, third and fourth ventricles. It escapes from the fourth ventricle through the median foramen of Magendie and the lateral foramina of Luschka into the cerebral subarachnoid space. About four-fifths of the fluid is reabsorbed via the arachnoid villi, which are minute projections of arachnoid which pierce the dural covering of the venous sinuses to lie immediately beneath their endothelium. Along the superior sagittal sinus these villi clump together in adults to form the Pacchionian bodies. The remaining one-fifth of the CSF is absorbed by the spinal arachnoid villi or escapes along the nerve sheaths into the lymphatics.

Obstruction along the CSF pathway produces rise in pressure and dilatation within the system proximal to the block.

Hydrocephalus can be divided into:

1 *Non-communicating or obstructive:* where fluid cannot escape from within the brain due to blockage within the duct system by tumour, chronic abscess, congenital stenosis or the Arnold—Chiari malformation, which is a congenital downward protrusion of the cerebellum into the foramen magnum (with consequent occlusion of the foramina of the fourth ventricle) frequently associated with spina bifida.

2 *Communicating:* CSF can escape from within the brain but absorption via the villi is prevented as a result of the obliteration of subarachnoid channels following meningitis, birth trauma or possible congenital failure of development of the arachnoid villi.

Clinical features

Clinically, hydrocephalus may be divided into two important groups. The first is the acquired variety, which presents with features of raised intracranial pressure described on page 80. The second comprises the congenital hydrocephalics who show the characteristic picture of enlargement of the skull, (comparison should be made with the size of an infant's skull of the same age obtained from standard charts), over which the scalp is stretched with dilated cutaneous veins. The fontanelles are enlarged, tense and fail to close at the normal times. Typical of this condition is the downward displacement of the eye balls and there may be an associated squint and nystagmus. Papilloedema is not present in these cases. There may be late epilepsy, and mental impairment may be considerable where there is extensive thinning of the cerebral cortex. There may be associated congenital deformities, especially spina bifida.

In some infants with congenital hydrocephalus, natural arrest occurs, presumably as a result of recanalization of the subarachnoid spaces. In the remainder there is steady progression with inevitable mental deterioration and high mortality unless adequate treatment is instituted.

Treatment

In cases of obstructive hydrocephalus obviously direct removal of the occluding tumour or abscess is desirable. Where this is impossible the block at the foramen of Munro, third ventricle or aqueduct of Sylvius can be short-circuited by the Torkildsen operation of ventriculocisternostomy in which a plastic tube is inserted into the lateral ventricle through a burr-hole, then carried subcutaneously to be placed into the cisterna magna through a cerebellar exposure.

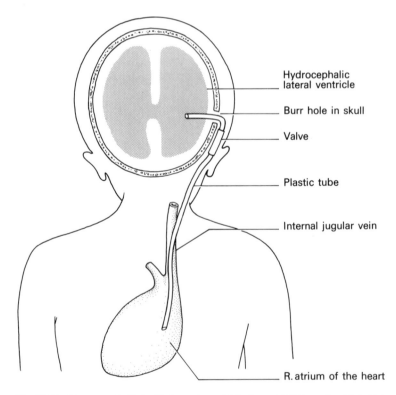

Fig. 13.1. Diagram of a Spitz-Holter valve, which shunts CSF from the dilated lateral ventricle into the right atrium. The valve prevents reflux of blood along the tube. (The child is viewed from behind.)

In congenital hydrocephalus of the progressive variety of Spitz-Holter plastic valve is inserted; this is an ingenious plastic tube passed from the lateral ventricle via the internal jugular vein into the right atrium. The valve mechanism allows CSF above a set pressure to pass into the vein without allowing reflux of blood into the subarachnoid space (Fig. 13.1).

Chapter 14
Head Injuries

Causes of coma

The casualty officer is often called upon to make a diagnosis of a patient in coma. The following are the common causes to be considered:

1 CNS
   (a) trauma
   (b) disease (e.g. cerebrovascular accident — the commonest — epilepsy, sub-arachnoid haemorrhage, cerebral tumour, abscess, meningitis, etc.)
2 Drugs, etc.
   (a) alcohol
   (b) carbon monoxide
   (c) barbiturates, aspirin, opiates, etc.
3 Diabetes
   (a) hyperglycaemia
   (b) hypoglycaemia
4 Uraemia.
5 Hepatic failure.
6 Hypertensive encephalopathy.
7 Profound toxaemia.
8 Hysteria.

It is usually easy enough to determine that unconsciousness is due to trauma, but it is important to remember that a drunk or an epileptic, for example, may have struck his head in falling so that his condition is complicated by a head injury.

MANAGEMENT OF THE UNCONSCIOUS HEAD INJURY

This should be considered under three headings:

1 Observation.
2 Nursing the unconscious patient.
3 Indications for surgery.

The first two apply to every case. Operative intervention is indicated in only some 10 per cent of head injuries. Although considered under separate headings, all three lines of management may be required at one and the same time.

Observation

Observation includes, of course, an immediate full general examination of the unconscious patient, who obviously cannot indicate if he has other injuries. Indeed, these often occur following an accident serious enough to produce a significant head injury. It is important to document and treat these associated injuries, especially if life-threatening. Priorities include: examination of the spine for fracture, of the chest for pneumothorax or haemothorax, of the abdomen for evidence of intra-abdominal bleeding and of the limbs for fractures.

Three things can happen to patients while under observation:

1   The great majority become progressively lighter and recover.

2   A small proportion remain in relatively deep coma as a result of severe cerebral trauma, often with brain-stem damage.

3   A small proportion pass into progressively deeper coma due either to intra-cranial bleeding, cerebral oedema, or, at a later stage, intracranial infection. The last is now fortunately rare except in some penetrating injuries.

Since it is extremely difficult to differentiate between the progressive coma of intracranial haemorrhage (which requires most urgent surgical intervention) and cerebral oedema, urgent CT scanning is essential. This may involve immediate transfer to a neurosurgical unit.

The purpose of careful observation in a head injury is centred on the need to detect that minority of patients who are developing features of cerebral compression.

In order of importance these features are:

1   The conscious level.

2   The reaction of the pupils.

3   The pulse, respiration and blood pressure.

4   CNS signs.

Conscious level

Vague terms such as comatose, semi-comatose, unconscious, stuporose, etc., should be avoided; they may be of value to a psychiatrist but not to a surgeon. Instead the conscious level is charted according to the patient's response to stimuli; these are very much the reactions of a patient recovering from deep anaesthesia:

1   No response to pain.

2   Incoordinated response to painful stimuli (e.g. the patient moves all four limbs).

3   Coordinated response to pain (e.g. the patient pushes away the examiner's hand).

4   Response to simple commands.

5   Talking but disorientated.

Any shift from a higher to a lower level in this scheme is highly significant of deepening coma.

Pupils

If a cerebral hemisphere is pressed upon by an enlarging blood clot, the third cranial nerve on that side becomes stretched by descent of the hippocampal gyrus over the edge of the tentorium cerebelli. Paralysis of III results in dilation of the corresponding pupil (due to the intact sympathetic supply) and failure of the pupil to respond to light. An important sign of cerebral compression is therefore dilation and loss of light reaction of the pupil on the affected side. Since the optic nerve pathway is intact, a light shone into this unreacting pupil produces constriction in the opposite pupil (consensual reaction to light). As compression continues, the contralateral third nerve becomes compressed, and the opposite pupil in turn dilates and becomes fixed to light. Bilateral fixed dilated pupils in a patient with head injury indicates very great cerebral compression from which the patient rarely recovers.

Pulse, respiration and blood pressure

With increasing cerebral compression the pulse slows, the respirations become stertorous and eventually Cheyne Stokes in nature and the blood pressure rises.

CNS Examination

Often the CNS signs in an unconscious patient following head injury are variable and difficult to interpret. Progressive unilateral weakness or Jacksonian epilepsy are, however, useful localizing signs.

Note that the clinical picture of decerebrate rigidity with small pupils and hyperpyrexia suggests severe brain stem damage, although it may be secondary to cerebral compression.

Special investigations

Comprehensive high quality skull and cervical spine X-rays should be obtained in all cases, supplemented by a CT scan. Haemorrhage and deepening coma are indications for urgent cerebral decompression, evacuation of the haematoma and arrest of haemorrhage. Intravenous urea or mannitol are given to reduce oedema; for severe cases hypothermia by ice packs and controlled respiration are employed.

Lumbar puncture should never be performed in an attempt to confirm the raised intracranial pressure; if the spinal CSF pressure is reduced by removing fluid from the spinal theca, the high intracranial pressure may force the brain stem downwards through the foramen magnum ('coning') with fatal consequences.

The nursing care of the unconscious patient

The airway

The most important single factor in the care of the deeply unconscious patient, whatever the cause, who has lost hish cough reflex is the maintenance of his airway. He is transported and nursed in the tonsil position, i.e. on one side with the body tilted head downwards, which allows the tongue to fall forward and bronchial secretions or vomit to drain the mouth rather than be inhaled (Fig. 14.1). Suction may be required to remove excessive secretions or vomit from the pharynx.

An endotracheal tube may be necessary if the airway is not satisfactory and if after some days it is still difficult to maintain an adequate airway tracheostomy may be required.

Restlessness

Morphia is contraindicated since this will depress respiration, disguise the unconscious level and will also produce constricted pupils which may mask a valuable

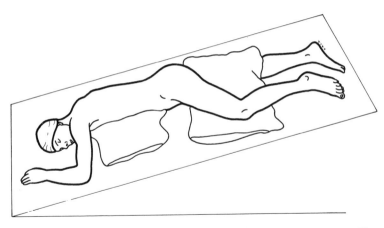

Fig. 14.1. The 'tonsil position' for transportation of an unconscious patient. Note the 'head down, feet up' inclination.

physical sign. Paracetamol, barbiturates or dihydrocodeine preparations may be necessary but often all that is required is to protect the patient from injuring himself by judicious restraint and padding.

A cause of restlessness may be a distended bladder; often if the retention is relieved the patient will then calm down.

Feeding

Many cases of head injury died in the past due to dehydration and starvation. Naso-gastric feeding is instituted if the patient remains unable to swallow after 12 hours.

Skin care

A deeply unconscious patient is liable to bed scores; careful nursing care and the use of an intermittently inflatable mattress is required for their prevention.

Sphincters

The unconscious patient may be incontinent; the resultant excoriation of the skin makes him still more liable to pressure sores. The use of Paul's tubing on the penis or of an indwelling catheter in the female patient will help in the nursing care. Retention of urine may require catheter relief.

Indications for surgery in head injuries

Early

1 The excision and suture of scalp lacerations.
2 Surgical toilet of a compound fracture.
3 Cerebral decompression and evacuation of the haematoma for intracranial bleeding.

Delayed
1 Repair of a dural tear with CSF rhinorrhoea.
2 Late repair of skull defects.
3 Late plastic surgery for deforming facial injuries.

FRACTURES OF THE SKULL

These are classified into:
1 *Closed*
2 *Compound*
   (a) external
   (b) via the nasal or aural cavities
The fracture itself may be:
   (a) fissured
   (b) comminuted
   (c) depressed

Depressed fractures in adults are nearly always compound; if the blow is severe enough to drive a fragment of the skull below its surrounds it is severe enough to tear the overlying scalp. In children, with their softer bones, 'pond' fractures may occur, over which the skin remains intact. In adults a common diagnostic trap is a large haematoma of the scalp which feels surprisingly like a closed-depressed fracture. The palpating fingers feel first the indurated edge of the haematoma and then drop into its soft centre, giving the sensation of a depression. No student really believes this; but he does later when he makes this mistake as a Casualty Officer.

A compound fracture to the exterior is treated like any other compound fracture, the wound edges are narrowly excised, dead tissue, bone deprived of periosteum and pulped brain removed, the dura repaired if possible and the skin then sutured. The patient is placed on sulphadimidine, since the sulphonamides readily pass across the blood–brain barrier.

External CSF leakage

A special variety of compound fracture is where continuity to the exterior is demonstrated by CSF rhinorrhoea or, less commonly, otorrhea. Occasionally air may enter the skull to produce an intracranial *aerocele*. In these instances a dural tear associated with a fracture of the base of the skull allows a ready pathway of infection to the meninges and brain. In such cases the patient is barrier nursed and placed on prophylactic antibiotic therapy. Since the pneumococcus is the most common infecting organism, penicillin is the drug of choice. After recovery from the immediate effects of head injury the leak is sealed in cases of persistent CSF rhinorrhoea by repairing the torn dura mater, using a fascia lata graft when required.

CSF dripping from the nose is to be differentiated from nasal secretion, although this in practice is very difficult; the CSF discharge is increased by jugular compression, as in a Queckenstedt's test, and CSF contains sugar and no mucin, unlike nasal discharge which contains little sugar and is rich in mucin.

The accompanying physical signs of fractures of the cranial fossae

Anterior fossa
1   Nasal bleeding.
2   Orbital haematoma (see below).
3   CSF rhinorrhoea.
4   Cranial nerve injuries I to VI.

Middle fossa
1   Orbital haematoma.
2   Bleeding from the ear.
3   CSF otorrhoea (rare).
4   Cranial nerve injuries VII to VIII.

Posterior fossa
1   Bruising over the suboccipital region which develops after a day or two.
2   Cranial nerve injuries IX, X, and XI (rare).

Differential diagnosis between an orbital haematoma and a black eye

Fractures of the anterior and middle cranial fossae are very frequently associated with orbital haematoma; blood tracks forward into the orbital tissues, into the eyelids and behind the conjunctiva. It may be difficult to differentiate this from a 'black eye', which is a superficial haematoma of the eyelid and surrounding soft tissues produced by direct injury.

An orbital haematoma is suggested by the following features:
1   Absence of grazing of the surrounding skin.
2   The haematoma is confined to the margin of the orbit (due to its fascial attachments) whereas a black eye frequently extends onto the surrounding cheek.
3   There is an associated subconjunctival haemorrhage.
4   There is usually an associated mild exophthalmos and a degree of ophthalmoplegia.
5   The orbital haematoma is usually bilateral.

There may also be some confusion in making a diagnosis between a subconjunctival and conjunctival haemorrhage. The subconjunctival haemorrhage extends from the orbit forwards deep to the conjunctiva; there is therefore no posterior limit to the haemorrhage. A conjunctival haemorrhage results from a direct blow on the eye and produces a small haematoma clearly delimited on the conjunctiva itself (Fig. 14.2).

INTRACRANIAL BLEEDING

Classification

Haemorrhage within the skull following injury may be classified as follows:
1   Extradural.
2   Subdural.

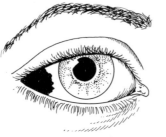 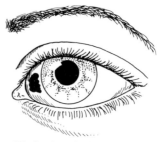

(A) Subconjunctival haemorrhage
    No posterior limit

(B) Conjunctival
    haemorrhage'
    Posterior limit seen

Fig. 14.2. The differential diagnosis between (A) subconjunctival and (B) conjunctival haemorrhage.

    (a) acute
    (b) chronic
3 Subarachnoid.
4 Intracerebral.
5 Intraventricular.

Extradural haemorrhage

This is sometimes badly named 'middle meningeal haemorrhage'. It may indeed arise from a tear of the middle meningeal artery or vein, but an extradural collection of blood may also develop from a laceration of one of the other meningeal vessels, from the torn sagittal sinus or oozing from the diploe, bone and stripped dura mater on each side of any associated fracture (Fig. 14.3A).

Clinical features

The classic story is of a relatively minor head injury producing temporary concussion, recovery ('the lucid period') then, some hours later, the development of headache and progressively deeper coma due to cerebral compression by the extradural clot. This picture may give rise to the tragedies of the drunk who is put into the cells for the night and is found dead in the morning, or the cricketer who goes home to bed after being mildly concussed by a cricket ball and perishes during the evening. It is important to note, however, that this classic picture only accounts for about half the cases. Often there is no lucid period; the patient progressively passes into deeper coma from the time of the initial injury.

    The physical signs are those of rapidly increasing intracerebral pressure which have already been discussed (page 80).

    In addition there are certain localizing signs which may help the surgeon decide on which side to explore the skull. These are:

1 The pupils: a good neurosurgical aphorism is 'explore the side of the dilated pupil' (see page 91).

2 Hemiparesis or hemiplegia (common) or Jacksonian fits (uncommon) indicate contralateral compression.

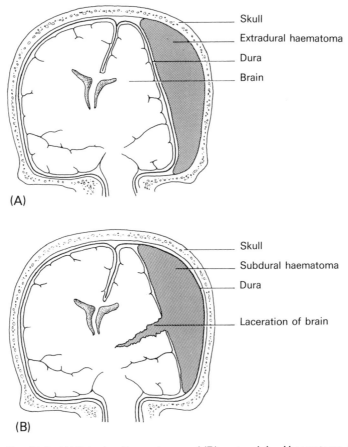

Skull
Extradural haematoma
Dura
Brain

(A)

Skull
Subdural haematoma
Dura

Laceration of brain

(B)

Fig. 14.3. (A) Extradural haematoma and (B) acute subdural haematoma. The latter is associated with a severe brain laceration.

3 A boggy haematoma of the scalp usually overlies the extradural clot; this is because some of the extradural blood escapes through the fracture line into the subcutaneous tissues.

Special Investigations

X-rays of the skull may be entirely normal. However, the clot tends to be on the side of the fracture if one is visible. A calcified pineal gland may be seen to be pushed over from the midline in a good anteroposterior film. A CT scan is invaluable and allows accurate localization of the position and of the size of the clot.

Treatment

An extradural haemorrhage is one of the few surgical emergencies where minutes really do matter. A burr-hole is made over the suspected site of the clot, the opening enlarged with nibbling forceps and the clot evacuated. The major bleeding point on the dura is controlled either with silver clips, diathermy or by undersewing. Bleeding from the bone edges is plugged by means of Horsley's wax. Only rarely, if ever, is the operation which every student seems to know, that of plugging the foramen spinosum with a sharpened and boiled matchstick, actually required.

Subdural haematoma

Acute

This results from bleeding into the subdural space from lacerated and pulped brain; it is usually part of an overwhelming head injury (Fig. 14.3B). The patient is frequently in deep coma from the moment of injury but his condition deteriorates still further.

Treatment

Release of the subdural clot through burr-holes or a bone flap may give some improvement in the neurological state, but the condition is often fatal because of the severity of the underlying brain trauma.

Chronic subdural haematoma or hygroma

This follows a trivial (often forgotten) injury sustained weeks or months before. There is a small tear in a cerebral vein as it traverses the subdural space. Whenever the patient coughs, strains or bends over a little blood extravasates. The resulting haematoma becomes encapsulated; as the clot breaks down, smaller molecules are formed with a rise in the osmotic pressure within the haematoma. Consequent absorption of tissue fluid produces gradual enlargement of the local collection which may comprise liquid blood, clot or clear yellow fluid (hygroma).

Clinical features

Those of a rapidly developing intracerebral 'tumour'. There is mental deterioration, headaches, vomiting and drowsiness which progresses to coma. Moderate papilloedema is seen in about half the cases. The condition is indeed often confused with an intracerebral tumour but cerebral angiography and, particularly, CT scanning demonstrate the outline of the clot.

Treatment

Comprises the evacuation of the clot through burr-holes. Since 50 per cent are bilateral, both sides of the skull are explored unless the CT scan positively excludes a contralateral collection.

Subarachnoid haemorrhage

Clinical features

Blood in the CSF after head injury is incidental, not surprisingly, to most severe head injuries and gives the clinical picture of meningeal irritability with headache, neck stiffness and a positive Kernig's sign. There may be a mild pyrexia.

If there is any doubt about the diagnosis it can be confirmed by lumbar puncture which will reveal bloodstained or later yellow (xanthochromic) fluid.

Treatment

Analgesics and bed rest until the severe headache has subsided, followed by rapid rehabilitation.

Intracerebral haemorrhage

Scattered small haemorrhages throughout the brain substance are a common post-mortem finding in severe head injuries and may be demonstrated at CT scanning in extensive cerebral injury. Occasionally a local clot may develop within the brain substance; sometimes it is possible to evacuate this successfully through a burr-hole by means of a brain needle, but usually it is best to leave the damaged brain undisturbed.

Intraventricular haemorrhage

Haemorrhage into a ventricle may occur from tearing of the choroid plexus at the time of injury or rupture of an intracerebral clot into the ventricle. It occurs particularly in childhood and is usually part of an overwhelming head injury.

OTHER COMPLICATIONS

Meningitis

Infection of the meninges may complicate a fracture of the skull which is compound either directly to the exterior or via a dural tear into the nasal or aural cavities (see page 94).

Confirmation of the diagnosis of meningitis is the only positive indication for performing a lumbar puncture on a patient with a head injury.

Treatment

The treatment of established meningitis is antibiotic therapy. Infection via the nasal route is probably due to the pneumococcus; here penicillin should be the first drug of choice, given both systemically and intrathecally. For infection complicating a compound fracture, sulphadimidine should be used in the first instance, since this readily passes the blood-brain barrier. The antibiotic may have to be changed when the sensitivity of the organism obtained on lumbar puncture becomes known.

Hyperpyrexia

The temperature of a patient with severe brain stem injury may soar to 40°C (105°F) or more as a result of injury to the heat-regulating centre. This is a serious complication and must be treated vigorously by means of ice-packs applied to the limbs and trunk.

Late complications

Neurosis following a head injury is not uncommon. Unless reassured and rapidly rehabilitated, the patient who has had concussion is easily led to believe that his brain has been damaged and that he will never be fit to lead a normal life again.

Some idea of the severity of the injury is given by the period of amnesia, both the retrograde amnesia up to the time of the accident and the post-traumatic amnesia following injury. If this period amounts to only minutes or a few hours the ultimate prognosis is good. Amnesia of several days or even weeks is of grave import with regard to ultimate return of full mental function.

Persistent epilepsy may especially complicate penetrating compound wounds with resultant cortical scarring. It is good practice to give all such cases anticonvulsive therapy, e.g. phenytoin or phenobarbitone, for at least 6 months following injury. Established post-traumatic epilepsy is treated medically by means of anti-convulsants. Occasionally success may follow excision of a cortical scar.

Brain death: the medical and nursing care of patients with severe brain damage due to trauma, haemorrhage or intracranial tumour is now so good that the doctors and nurses are often faced with the sad case of a patient whose brain is completely and irreversibly destroyed, but whose heart and circulation are intact provided the lungs are mechanically ventilated. This state of affairs may persist for many weeks with severe distress to the patient's relatives and to the ward staff.

The diagnosis of brain death depends on the demonstration of permanent and irreversible destruction of brain stem function. *All brain stem reflexes should be absent:*

1 The pupils are fixed in diameter and do not respond to sharp changes in the intensity of incident light.

2 There is no corneal reflex.

3 The vestibulo-ocular reflexes are absent. There are lost when no eye movement occurs during or after the slow injection of 20 ml of ice-cold water into each external auditory meatus in turn, clear access to the tympanic membrane having been established by direct inspection. This test may be contraindicated on one or other side by local trauma.

4 No motor responses within the cranial nerve distribution can be elicited by adequate stimulation of any somatic area.

5 There is no gag reflex response to bronchial stimulation by a suction catheter passed down the trachea.

6 No respiratory movements occur when the patient is disconnected from the mechanical ventilator for long enough to ensure that the arterial carbon dioxide tension rises above the threshold for stimulating respiration — that is the $P_a\text{co}_2$ must normally reach 6.7 kPa (50 mmHg).

If this situation persists over an observational period of 24 hours, death can be certified.

The decision to stop mechanical ventilation rests on the above factors. However, once this decision has been made, the possibility of the patient becoming an organ donor for transplantation should be considered. This should be discussed fully and sympathetically with available relatives so that their informed consent is obtained for the removal of organs.

Chapter 15
The Spinal Cord

SPINA BIFIDA

The neural tube develops by an infolding of the neural ectoderm to become the spinal cord. The surrounding meninges and vertebral column derive from mesodermal tissue. Failure of embryonic fusion may result in the following anomalies (Fig. 15.1):

1 *Spina bifida occulta:* failure of the vertebral arch fusion only; meninges and nervous tissue normal.

2 *Meningocele:* protrusion of the meninges through a posterior vertebral defect without nervous tissue involvement.

3 *Myelomeningocele:* neural tissue (the cord or spinal roots) protrudes into, and may be adherent to, the meningeal sac.

4 *Myelocele (rachischisis):* failure of fusion of the neural tube; an open spinal plate occupies the defect as a red, granular area weeping CSF from its centre.

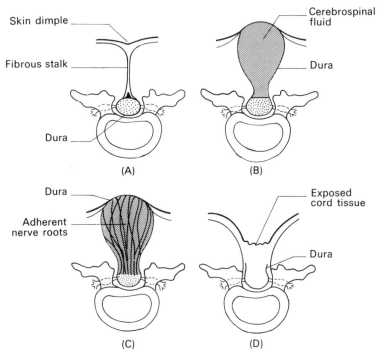

Fig. 15.1. The varieties of spina bifida: (A) spina bifida occulta; (B) meningocele; (C) myelomeningocele; (D) myelocele or rachischisis.

Ante-natal screening (alpha-feto protein in the amniotic fluid and ultrasound) enables a high degree of accuracy in intra-uterine diagnosis of neural tube defects, and gives the opportunity for termination of the pregnancy. The number of infants born with severe spinal abnormalities has, in consequence, greatly declined.

Clinical features

Since the neural tube closes progressively from above downwards, these defects are particularly common in the lumbo-sacral area, although any part of the spine may be involved. There may be an associated overlying lipoma, tuft of hair or skin dimple which may be an important clue to the astute clinician of the underlying defect. Where nervous tissue is involved there may be paraparesis, paraplegia, sensory disturbances in the limbs and loss of sphincter control.

Hydrocephalus nearly always coexists with the myelomeningocele due to the *Arnold–Chiari malformation*, in which the medulla, fourth ventricle and cerebellum are dragged caudally into the foramen magnum with consequent obstruction of the CSF pathway.

As with any other congenital deformity there may be multiple developmental anomalies, e.g. congenital dislocation of the hip, talipes equinovarus, cleft lip or palate, cardiac lesions or supernumary digits.

Treatment

Minor degrees of spina bifida are left alone. Skin covered lesions require only cosmetic surgery. All cases with an exposed neural plate should be repaired within a few hours of birth to prevent progressive neurological damage. Associated hydrocephalus should be drained within the next 1 or 2 weeks provided there is no ascending meningitis (see page 87). The most grossly malformed are better left untreated.

SPINAL INJURIES

Injuries to the spinal cord and its nerve roots are intimately connected with, and cannot be divorced from, damage to the vertebral column.

Fractures of the dorso-lumbar region

The great majority of fractures of the spine involve either the cervical vertebrae, or the lower thoracic and upper lumbar vertebrae, especially T 12, L 1 and 2. In civilian practice these dorsolumbar fractures are usually flexion injuries; a fall from a height landing on the feet or the buttocks, forward flexion of the spine in a decelerating car crash, or a heavy weight falling on the shoulders. Compound fractures due to gunshot wounds are unusual except in times of war; however in these days of increasing civilian violence, their incidence is rising.

Classification

1 Wedge compression.
2 Comminution, often associated with crushing of the intervertebral disc.
3 Fracture dislocation with forward or lateral displacement and with rupture of

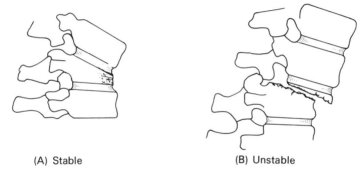

(A) Stable   (B) Unstable

Fig. 15.2. Fractures of the spine fall into two main categories: (A) the stable wedge fracture and (B) the unstable fracture-dislocation; it is in the latter that the spinal cord and nerve roots are usually injured.

the interspinous ligaments, accompanied by fracture or dislocation of the inter-articular facets.

From the practical point of view fractures are divided into *stable* and *unstable* (Fig. 15.2); if the interspinous and the posterior longitudinal ligaments are intact, as in most wedge and some comminuted fractures, the spinal column is stable. The cord may be contused but usually recovers and is not in danger of further injury from increasing displacement at the fracture line. Most of the comminuted fractures and all the fracture dislocations are unstable; the spinal cord and nerve roots are frequently damaged and may be further injured by increasing displacement unless careful treatment is instituted.

Injuries of the cervical spine

The cervical spine is usually injured by flexion, such as a fall upon the head in diving, or acute flexion of the neck is a deceleration injury. Hyperextension ('whiplash') injuries are also common.

A wedge fracture or comminuted fracture may occur as in the thoraco-lumbar injuries, but more often dislocation or fracture dislocation occurs. If the facets do not lock, occasionally there is spontaneous reduction and nothing is seen on radiological examination, although complete transection of the cord has taken place. More often the articular processes slip forward over the ones below into the locked position. Because of the much closer fit of the cervical cord within the vertebral canal compared with the wider lumbar region, the incidence of cord damage in these injuries is extremely high with resultant tetraplegia.

Clinical features

There is the typical history of injury followed by localized pain, bruising, tenderness and often a kyphus.

Careful neurological examination is of course imperative (see below). The exact type of fracture is shown by radiological examination, of which the lateral films are the most important. In suspected cervical injuries, the lateral films are taken in flexion and extension (if the patient is conscious), the surgeon applying traction meanwhile, in order to demonstrate any instability of the cervical spine.

It is obligatory to examine every head injury for suspected spinal fracture since this is easily overlooked in the unconscious patient. Unskilful handling of such a case may produce an irreparable spinal injury.

Nervous system lesions

Paraplegia following vertebral column injury may be due to:

1. Spinal concussion

Nervous continuity is not lost, paraplegia is only partial and recovery commences with a few hours. Full return of function can be anticipated.

2. Cord transection

This occurs in the cervical and thoracic zones. Loss of function due to anatomical division of the cord is irrecoverable since the axons within the cord have no power of regeneration. There is an initial period of spinal shock with complete flaccid paralysis below the line of cord section, loss of tendon reflexes, atonicity of the bladder (which becomes distended), faecal retention and priapism. This phase lasts for days or weeks. The cord below the line of transection then recovers reflex function so that the paralysis becomes spastic with muscle spasms, the plantar responses become extensor and bladder and bowel commence to empty reflexly.

3. Cauda equina injury.

This may complicate fractures below the level of termination of the spinal cord at the lower border of the first lumbar vertebra. The cauda equina nerve roots are the roots of peripheral nerves and therefore possess the power of regeneration providing that continuity of the nerve trunk is not lost.

4. Combined cord and cauda equina injury

Since many spinal injuries take place at the thoraco-lumbar junction, there is usually a combination of spinal cord and nerve root injury. For example, a fracture dislocation at the T 12/L 1 junction will divide the cord at the first sacral segment but clinical examination may reveal paralysis being due to damage to the spinal roots as they pass the site of the fracture dislocation (Fig. 15.3). In this instance, the roots may recover with return of knee and hip movement although the sacral paralysis will be permanent.

Treatment in the absence of neurological damage

Stable fractures of the spine are treated by 2 to 3 weeks' bed rest, to allow the associated soft tissue injury to subside, followed by early exercise and active mobilization. There is no need to reduce the fracture by hyperextension and prolonged fixation; often this results in permanent residual pain.

If the fracture is unstable, immobilization is indicated in order to secure bony stability and thus to protect the cord from later damage.

Unstable cervical fractures are immobilized by traction using Crutchfield's

Vertebrae   Nerve roots

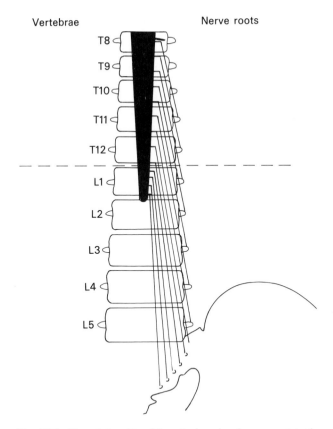

Fig. 15.3. The relationship of the spinal cord and nerve roots to the vertebrae. Because of the disparity between the two, a fracture dislocation at the dorso-lumbar junction, shown here by the dotted line, will miss the lumbar cord but may transect the *sacral* segments of the cord together with injury to the *lumbar* nerve roots (after Holdsworth).

tongs applied to the skull for 6 weeks. This is followed by a cervical collar for a further month.

Unstable thoraco-lumbar fractures are treated by operative reduction and internal fixation.

Treatment with paraplegia or tetraplegia

The patient is transported in a neutral position (so that flexion and extension are not possible), to a spinal or neurosurgical centre, the spine being supported by suitable arranged pillows and the patient being moved frequently from side to side to prevent bed-sore formation. The distended bladder is best left alone until catheterization can be carried out under full aseptic precautions.

The following are the main headlines of treatment in special centres:

1. The management of the fracture

Plaster casts or beds are avoided since pressure sores are almost inevitable.

Two techniques of management may be employed. The conservative approach, favoured in most centres in the United Kingdom, comprises nursing the patient on a circo-electric bed or a Stryker frame. This allows regular turning of the paraplegic (thus avoiding pressure sores), while maintaining the fracture immobilized. This is continued for six weeks. Once the fracture has become stable, the patient can progress to the rehabilitation stage of his treatment. The surgical approach, more often used on the Continent and in the USA, consists of open reduction and Harrington rod fixation of the unstable fracture.

2. Care of the skin

Pressure sores may develop with extraordinary rapidity in the first weeks because of the combination of anaesthesia and immobilization. Two-hourly turning, aided by use of the circo-electric bed, and meticulous skin care are required.

3. The bladder

In the initial phase of complete bladder paralysis, continuous catheter drainage by means of a fine polythene urethral or suprapubic catheter is instituted. With recovery from spinal shock the patient may develop an automatic bladder wherein stroking the side of the thigh or abdominal compression may evoke reflex bladder emptying.

4. The rectum

This is best managed by regular enemata; faecal impaction must be watched for and treated by digital evacuation.

5. Rehabilitation

Active development of muscles with an intact or partial innervation by expert physiotherapy can restore 80 per cent of paraplegic patients to walk again. However, they require calipers and crutches so that they can swing their paralysed legs by the use of abdominal, flank and shoulder muscles. At the same time vocational training can be commenced and a large percentage of these unfortunate patients can be restored to useful activity.

PROLAPSED INTERVERTEBRAL DISC

Disc herniation comprises a protrusion of the nucleus pulposus posteriorly, or more commonly posterolaterally, through a defect in the annulus fibrosus. It is probable that these ruptures are nearly always initiated by trauma, which may be severe but which is more often mild or repetitive. It is probably for this reason that the great majority of prolapsing discs occur in the active adult male.

By far the commonest sites are between the fourth and fifth lumbar vertebrae and between the fifth lumbar vertebra and the sacrum. Cervical disc protrusion may occur between C 5 and 6 or between C 6 and 7. The cervical lesion is often associated with degenerative changes in the spine and is therefore usually found in older patients than the lumbar disc prolapse. Disc herniation elsewhere may occur but is unusual.

Lumbar disc herniation

Clinical features

There is often lumbar pain early in the history, with exacerbations as a result of straining or heavy lifting. The majority of patients complain of sciatic pain, usually unilateral and radiating from the buttock along the back of the thigh and knee and then down the lateral side of the leg to the foot. This pain is aggravated by coughing, sneezing or straining (which raise the intrathecal pressure) or by straight leg raising (which stretches the sciatic nerve). Sometimes there is the complaint of weakness of ankle dorsiflexion (L 5) or plantar flexion (S 1). There may be paraesthesiae or numbness in the foot. The unusual central prolapse of the lumbar disc may produce bilateral sciatic pain, sphincter disturbance and complete or incomplete paraplegia.

Examination reveals flattening of the normal lumbar lordosis, scoliosis with a tilt away from the side of the pain, and limited spinal flexion. The erector spinae muscles are in spasm and straight leg raising is limited and painful. There may be weakness of plantar or dorsiflexion of the ankle and there may be disuse muscle wasting of the leg on the affected side. Sensory loss on the medial side of the dorsum of the foot and the great toe (L 5 innervation) suggest an L 4/5 disc lesion. Sensory loss on the lateral side of the foot (S 1 innervation) may occur in L 5/S 1 disc lesions. The ankle jerk may be diminished in the latter cases.

Special investigations

1 *X-rays of the spine* may be or may not reveal narrowing of the affected disc space on the lateral view.

2 *CT scanning* or *magnetic resonance* more sensitive and may demonstrate a laterally placed disc protrusion not otherwise visualized.

3 *A radiculogram* may occasionally be required to confirm the diagnosis. This is performed by injecting a water soluble contrast material (omnipaque or niopam) at lumbar puncture. This passes down the dural sheaths of the nerve roots and can demonstrate displacement due to quite a minor degree of disc prolapse.

4 *ESR* is normal — and is helpful in the differential diagnosis.

Differential diagnosis

This includes the other common spinal lesions; sacro-iliac strain, osteoarthritis, spondylolisthesis, spinal tumours and tuberculosis. Particularly in the elderly patient one should consider an intrapelvic tumour, e.g. of the prostate or rectum, involving the sacral plexus; never omit a rectal examination in any patient with sciatica. Intermittent claudication is readily differentiated by careful history and examination.

Treatment

The majority of cases respond to conservative treatment. In the acute episode of pain three weeks bed rest on a hard bed is prescribed. In less severe cases a lumbosacral corset is fitted. Operative removal of the prolapsed disc is indicated if conservative measures fail, if repeated attacks occur, if there are severe neurological disturbances and particularly if a large central protrusion is diagnosed. If bladder sphincter disturbance occurs, surgical decompression must be performed urgently.

Cervical disc herniation

Clinical features

There is cervical pain which is usually overshadowed by a more severe pain radiating into the arm and accompained by numbness and tingling in the fingers.

Differential diagnosis

There is an extensive differential diagnosis of the many causes of pain in the arm, including cervical spondylosis, spinal tumour, cervical rib, the carpal tunnel syndrome and angina pectoris.

Treatment

In the majority of cases this is conservative. A severe episode may require a period of neck traction, otherwise the neck is supported in a plastic collar. Operative removal of the prolapsed cervical disc has the same indications as lumbar disc protrusions.

EXTRADURAL SPINAL ABSCESS

An abscess in the extradural spinal compartment usually represents a metastatic infection as part of a *Staphylococcus aureus* septicaemia. Occasionally it is secondary to an osteomyelitis of the spine.

Clinical features

Clinical features are local pain and tenderness, fever, malaise and anorexia, and a rapidly progressive paraplegia. The white blood count is raised and the ESR is elevated.

Treatment

Urgent: the abscess is drained via a laminectomy and antibiotic therapy is commenced. Provided that surgery is performed in the initial stages the paraplegia recovers but delay carries with it the risk of permanent cord damage.

SPINAL TUMOURS

Spinal tumours are conveniently classified, both from the pathological and clinical points of view, into those which occur outside the spinal theca (extradural), those within the theca but outside the cord itself (intradural extramedullary) and those occurring within the cord (intramedullary).

The tumours which are most commonly encountered are:

1 *Extradural:*
   (a) Secondary deposits in the spine — by far the commonest
   (b) primary vertebral bony tumours (e.g. osteoclastoma, myeloma)

(c) lymphomas (Hodgkin's disease, non-Hodgkin's lymphoma)
2 *Intradural extramedullary:*
  (a) meningioma
  (b) neurofibroma
3 *Intramedullary* (rare):
  (a) glioma
  (b) angioma
  (c) ependymoma

Clinical features

The three groups of spinal tumours listed above tend each to have a fairly distinctive clinical picture.

The *extradural tumours* are usually fast growing and malignant; they therefore give a picture of rapidly progressive cord compression leading to paraplegia, although symptoms of root irritation (see below) may also be present.

The *intradural extramedullary tumours* are usually slow growing and benign. Initially there is irritation of the involved nerve roots; pain occurs in the localized area of nerve distribution which is often aggravated by recumbency and by factors such as coughing, sneezing or straining which raise the CSF pressure. There may be hyperalgesia in the affected cutaneous segment. Motor symptoms due to anterior root pressure are not a feature if only one nerve segment is involved since most major muscle groups are innervated from several segments; however, if more than one segment is affected there may be localized flaccid paralysis.

As the tumour increases in size, cord compression takes place. There may be features of the *Brown–Séquard syndrome* with spastic paralysis on the compressed side (involvement of the pyramidial tract), loss of position and vibration sense also on the affected side (posterior column involvement) and loss of pain and temperature sensation on the opposite side to the lesion (involvement of the spinothalamic tract). Further compression results in complete paraplegia of the spastic type with increased tendon jerks and extensor plantar response, together with overflow retention of urine and severe constipation.

Cauda equina tumours produce a lower motor neurone lesion: flaccid paralysis with diminished reflexes and paralysis of the anal and bladder sphincters with incontinence.

The *intramedullary tumours* may be accompanied by pain, but much more frequently give a picture very similar to that of syringomyelia. Progressive destruction of the cord produces bilateral motor weakness below the lesion and, since the crossed spinothalamic tracts are the first to be involved, there may be dissociation of sensory loss below the lesion, with abolition of pain and temperature but with persistence of vibration and position sense until late on in the progress of the disease.

Differential diagnosis

Spinal tumours are relatively uncommon and are great impersonators of other diseases; indeed a correct diagnosis made *ab initio* is something of a rarity. The root pain, if it occurs in the thoracic or abdominal segments, is often mistaken for intra-thoracic or intra-abdominal disease; if the pains radiate to the leg they may be at first diagnosed as a prolapsed disc or intermittent claudication. The intrameduallary lesions closely simulate syringomyelia and it may be difficult at first to differentiate them from disseminated sclerosis or other intraspinal lesions.

Special investigations

1 *Lumbar puncture* is most informative. Queckenstendt's test may show either no rise or else a very slow rise and fall of the CSF pressure on jugular compression, indicating a complete or partial block within the spinal canal. The protein in the CSF is nearly always raised above the normal 40 g/l (40 mg per cent) and may indeed be grossly elevated with yellow (xanthochromic) fluid which may actually clot in the container.

2 *X-rays of the spine* may show obvious bony deposits within the vertebral bodies. In other cases pressure erosion from the enlarging tumour may scallop the posterior aspect of the vertebral body, erode one or more vertebral pedicles or enlarge the intervertebral foramen. Occasionally calcification is seen within a meningioma.

3 *A radiculogram,* in which radio-opaque omnipaque or niapam is injected into the theca, will confirm the presence of a space-occupying lesion and localize its position accurately.

4 *Magnetic resonance* (MR) scanning has now become the definitive investigation and gives almost anatomically perfect imaging of spinal tumours.

Treatment

A laminectomy is required to confirm the pathological nature of the tumour and also to decompress the cord. Wherever possible the tumour is completely excised; this is usually confined to the benign meningiomas and neurofibromas, in which case complete recovery can be anticipated. In the malignant tumours radiotherapy is usually the only practical treatment and the prognosis is poor.

Chapter 16
Peripheral Nerve Injuries

Although there is no regeneration of divided tracts in the central nervous system, injured peripheral nerve fibres may recover to a varying extent, depending on the severity of the trauma.

Pathological classification

It is convenient to consider three types of injury:

1 *Neurapraxia* is damage to the nerve fibres without loss of continuity of the axis cylinder and is analogous to concussion in the central nervous system. The conduction along the fibre is interrupted for only a short period of time. Recovery usually commences within a few days and is complete in 6 to 8 weeks.

2 *Axonotmesis* is injury to the axon without disruption of the continuity of its sheath. The axon distal to the lesion degenerates and regrowth of the axon occurs from the node of Ranvier proximal to the injury. Since the sheath is intact, the correct axon will grow into its original nerve ending. The rate of regeneration is approximately one millimetre a day, therefore the more proximal the injury the longer it will be before functional recovery occurs.

3 *Neurotmesis* refers to actual physical disruption of the peripheral nerve. Regeneration will take place provided that the two nerve ends are not too far apart, but functional recovery will never be complete.

The distal part of the severed nerve undergoes degeneration. The medullary sheath is depleted of myelin and the axis cylinders vanish; the empty sheaths remain as tubules composed of proliferating neurilemmal cells. The muscles atrophy and their response to electrical stimulation changes so that, after a few weeks, although they continue to respond to galvanic shocks, they lose their response to faradic stimulation (the reaction of degeneration). The proximal end of the nerve degenerates up to the first uninjured node of Ranvier. New axis cylinders proliferate from this point and grow into the empty neurilemmal tubules. However, there is no selection of tubules for the appropriate axon; the distal growth is governed solely by the position of the nerve fibres. Thus, with most mixed nerves, there is likely to be considerable wastage due to regenerating fibres growing into endings which will be functionless, i.e. motor nerve fibres growing into sensory nerve endings, and vice versa. Even when a motor nerve grows into a motor nerve ending it may not supply the original muscle and the patient will have to relearn the affected movement.

Since a peripheral nerve contains a large number of individual fibres it is quite possible in a nerve injury for some fibres to suffer from neuropraxia, others axonotmesis and others neurotmesis. However, a distinction between the first two and the last may be quite clear in that if the nerve is found to be severed at surgical exploration then neurotmesis must have occurred.

Partial nerve injury may occur as the result of pressure or friction, for instance from a crutch, a tightly applied plaster cast or a tourniquet, as well as from closed injuries or open wounds.

Special investigations

Electromyography plays an important part in the diagnosis and assessment of nerve injuries. Serial studies are useful in demonstrating the amount and rate of regeneration. The EMG is also useful in the diagnosis of nerve compression syndromes.

Treatment

The treatment of neuropraxia and axonotmesis is to splint those joints whose muscles have been paralysed in the position of function and to put them through passive movements several times a day so that, when recovery of the nerve lesion occurs, the joints will be fully mobile.

With neurotmesis, operative treatment is usually required and here, the operating microscope is useful. If the injury is a fresh, clean, incised wound, a razor slash for example, then primary suture of the divided nerve is performed. If the wound is at all contused or contaminated, no attempt is made to deal wtih the nerve at this stage; the aim is to excise the wound and to achieve rapid skin cover without infection. Then 3 to 4 weeks after the original injury the wound is re-explored and the nerve is gently dissected. The two ends are cut square with a sharp scalpel blade and are then approximated with a few fine nylon stitches passed through the epineurium. If there has been loss of a section of the nerve, which precludes approximation, then the nerve must be freed proximally or even moved from its original position to a new anatomical plane where more length will be available; thus the ulnar nerve can be transposed from the posterior to the anterior aspect of the elbow joint to allow compensation for a distal loss of nerve substance.

When important nerves are divided, sometimes useful function can be obtained by grafting sections of non-essential nerves to act as conduits for the axons or, alternatively, by grafting a less essential motor nerve into the distal end of an important severed motor nerve; thus the hypoglossal nerve can be sutured to the distal stump of the divided facial nerve.

After nerve suture, recovery cannot be expected to take place until the time for regeneration has been allowed for, at the rate already mentioned of 1 mm per day. Eventual recovery will seldom be full.

If restoration of nerve functions cannot be achieved after injury, then tendon transfers may allow the patient to perform movements that were otherwise impossible. Thus, wrist drop after a radial nerve lesion may be treated by transposing some of the flexor tendons into the extensor group.

It is outside the scope of this book to discuss lesions of all the individual nerves, but a few important peripheral nerve injuries will be mentioned.

Brachial plexus injuries

1. Upper lesions (Erb's paralysis)
Due to the head being forced away from the shoulder, a common injury in motor

cyclists; it may also occur as an obstetric injury. C5 and 6 are damaged and there is paralysis of the biceps, brachialis, brachioradialis, supinator, supraspinatus, infraspinatus and deltoid. The limb will assume the 'waiter's tip' position, being internally rotated with the forearm pronated. There will be an area of impaired sensation over the outer side of the upper arm.

2. T1 Injury (Klumpke's paralysis)

May occur with a cervical rib lesion or dislocation of the shoulder. The small muscles of the hand are wasted and there is loss of sensation on the inner side of the forearm and medial 3½ fingers. In addition there may be a Horner's syndrome due to associated damage of sympathetic fibres passing to the inferior cervical ganglion (see page 116).

Radial nerve injuries (Fig. 16.1A)

Usually the radial nerve is injured by a fracture of the humerus involving the spiral groove where the nerve is closely applied to the bone. The nerve supply to the triceps comes off the radial nerve before it enters the spiral groove, and the lesions distal to that point will not affect extension of the elbow. However, there will be wrist drop due to paralysis of the wrist extensors and also loss of sensation over a small area on the dorsum of the hand at the base of the thumb and index finger. This surprisingly small sensory loss is due to considerable overlap from the medial and ulnar nerves.

Median nerve injuries (Fig. 16.1B)

This nerve may be damaged in fractures around the elbow joint or laceration of the

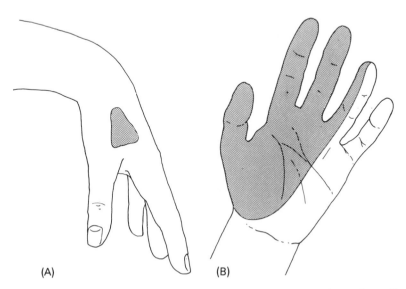

(A)   (B)

Fig. 16.1. (A) Radial nerve injury — wrist drop, together with anaesthesia of a small area of the dorsal aspect of the hand at the base of the thumb and index finger. (B) Median nerve injury — thenar eminence paralysis with anaesthesia of the palmar aspect of the radial 3½ digits and corresponding palm.

forearm or wrist. In high lesions the pronators of the forearm and flexors of the wrist and fingers will be involved, with the exception of the flexor carpi ulnaris and the medial half of the flexor digitorum profundus, which are supplied by the ulnar nerve and which produce ulnar deviation of the wrist. When the patient clasps his two hands together the index finger on the affected side remains extended — the 'pointing sign' of a high median nerve injury. Whether the injury is in the forearm or wrist, there will be paralysis of the small muscles of the thumb so that the thenar eminence is wasted. The patient is unable to abduct the thumb, i.e. to lift it at right angles to the plane of the hand. The sensory loss with a median nerve lesion is serious. There is anaesthesia over the palmar aspects of the thumb and the lateral 2½ fingers, and the loss extends onto the dorsum of the distal phalanges of these digits. This sensory defect makes it difficult to perform fine and delicate tasks.

Median nerve compression at the wrist (carpal tunnel syndrome) commonly occurs in middle-aged women. It is associated with wasting of the thenar eminence, diminished sensation and most often unpleasant pain, (characteristically at night), and paraesthesia in the thumb and lateral two fingers, and sometimes paraesthesia extends up into the arm. The reason for this latter symptom is not clear.

Treatment consists of dividing the flexor retinaculum at the wrist deep to which the median nerve is compressed.

Ulnar nerve injuries (Fig. 16.2)

Like the median, this nerve is also injured by fractures around the elbow joint and by lacerations of the forearm and wrist.

The ulnar nerve supplies all the intrinsic muscles of the hand apart from the three muscles of the thenar eminence (abductor pollicis brevis, opponens, and

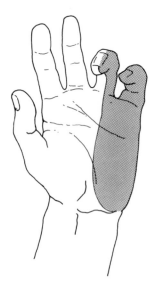

Fig. 16.2. Ulnar nerve injury — 'main en griffe' with anaesthesia of the ulnar 1½ digits and ulnar border of the hand on both palmar and dorsal aspects.

flexor pollicis brevis) and the two lateral lumbricals, all of which are supplied by the median nerve. The affected intrinsic muscles are the adductor pollicis, the muscles of the hypothenar eminence, the medial two lumbricals and the interossei, which are the abductors and adductors of the fingers and which also extend the i.p. joints. In the forearm the ulnar nerve supplies flexor carpi ulnaris and the medial half of flexor digitorum profundus.

Damage to the ulnar nerve produces the typical deformity of clawed hand or 'main en griffe'. The clawed appearance results from the unopposed action of the long flexors and extensors of the fingers. The flexor profundus and sublimis, inserted into the bases of the distal and middle phalanges respectively, flex the i.p. joints, while the long extensors, inserted into the bases of the proximal phalanges, extend the m.p. joints.

If the nerve is injured at the elbow, flexor digitorum profundus to the fourth and fifth finger is paralysed so that the clawing of these fingers, rather anomalously, is less intense than in injuries at the wrist. Paralysis of flexor carpi ulnaris produces a tendency to radial deviation at the wrist. In late cases, wasting of the intrinsic muscles is readily evident on inspecting the dorsum of the hand. Sensory loss occurs over the dorsal and palmar aspects of the ulnar 1½ digits and the ulnar border of the hand on both palmar and dorsal aspects. If the ulnar nerve is divided at the level of the wrist, the sensory loss is confined to the palmar surface, since the dorsal branch of the ulnar nerve, supplying the dorsal aspects of the ulnar one-and-a-half fingers, is given off 5cm above the wrist and thus escapes injury.

Division of the ulnar nerve leaves a surprisingly efficient hand. The long flexors enable a good grip to be taken; the thumb, apart from the loss of adductor pollicis, is intact, and the important sensation over the palm of the hand is largely maintained. Indeed, it may be difficult to be certain clinically that the nerve is injured. A reliable test is loss of the ability to abduct and adduct the fingers wtih the hand laid flat, palm downwards, on the table. This eliminates the trick movements of adduction and abduction of the fingers brought as part of their flexion and extension respectively.

Differential diagnosis of flexion deformities of the fingers

Ulnar nerve lesion
This has been described above: there is hyperextension of the metacarpophalangeal joints and clawing of the hand, with sensory loss along the ulnar border of the hand and ulnar one-and-a-half fingers.

Dupuytren's contracture
This is a common condition in the elderly, usually male, subject in which there is fibrosis of the palmar aponeurosis which produces a flexion deformity of the finger at the metacarpo-phalangeal and proximal interphalangeal joints, usually starting at the fourth digit and spreading to the fifth and sometimes the third finger. Since the aponeurosis only extends distally to the base of the middle phalanx, the distal interphalangeal joint escapes. The contracture is often bilateral and may occasionally affect the plantar fascia also.

Volkmann's contracture due to ischaemic fibrosis of flexors of the fingers

The fingers will be curled up in the hand with m.p. extension and wrist flexion. This deformity can to some extent be relieved by flexion of the wrist when the shortened tendons are no longer so taut and the fingers can be partially extended (see page 59).

Congenital contracture

Usually affects the little finger and produces very little, if any, disability. The proximal interphalangeal joint is typically affected, the condition is usually bilateral and, of course, dates from birth.

Mallet finger

Follows trauma (common in cricketers) with flexion deformity of the distal interphalangeal joint due to avulsion of the extensor tendor insertion.

Trauma

Scar formation following burns, injury or surgery to the fingers or the palm may produce gross flexion deformities.

Sciatic nerve injuries

This nerve may be wounded in penetrating injuries or torn in posterior dislocation of the hip associated with fracture of the posterior lip of the acetabulum, to which the nerve is closely related. Injury is followed by paralysis of the hamstrings and all the muscles of the leg and foot; there is loss of all movement below the knee joint with foot drop deformity. Sensory loss is complete below the knee, except for an area extending along the medial side of the leg over the medial malleolus, which is innervated by the saphenous branch of the femoral nerve.

Common peroneal nerve injuries

The common peroneal nerve is in a particularly vulnerable position as it winds around the neck of the fibula. It may be injured at this site by the pressure of a tight plaster cast, by skin traction applied without padding over the fibular head, or may be torn in severe adduction injuries to the knee. Damage is followed by the foot drop (due to paralysis of the ankle and foot extensors) and inversion of the foot (due to paralysis of the peroneal muscles with unopposed action of the foot flexors and invertors). There is anaesthesia over the anterior surface of the leg and foot. The medial side of the foot, innervated by the saphenous branch of the femoral nerve, and the lateral side of the foot, supplied by the sural branch of the tibial nerve, both escape.

Cervical sympathetic nerve injuries

If the T1 contribution to the cervical sympathetic chain is damaged the result is known as *Horner's syndrome*, in which there is:

1 Paralysis of the dilator pupillae, resulting in constriction of the pupil.
2 Ptosis due to paralysis of the sympathetic muscle fibres transmitted via the oculomotor nerve to the upper eyelid.

3 Loss of sweating on the affected side of the face and neck.

Horner's syndrome may follow operations on, or injuries to, the neck in which the cervical sympathetic trunk is damaged, malignant invasion from lymph nodes or adjacent tumour, or spinal cord lesions at the T1 segment.

Chapter 17
The Mouth and Tongue

It is a useful exercise (and a favourite examination topic) to consider what can be learned by examining a specific anatomical site in making a clinical diagnosis: for example, the finger, the nails, or the eye. The mouth and tongue can conveniently be used to illustrate how best to deal with this subject, which can be considered under three headings:

1. *Information about local disease*

   Tumours of the mouth and tongue, congenital anomalies, etc., are obviously diagnosed by local examination.

2. *Local manifestations of diseases elsewhere*

   The smooth tongue of pernicious anaemia, the ulcerated fauces of agranulocytosis or of severe glandular fever, the hemiatrophy of the tongue in XIIth nerve palsy, the pigmentation of Addison's disease, the pigmented spots of the Peutz–Jeghers syndrome and the gingivitis, the swollen bleeding gums and loosened teeth of vitamin C deficiency, are examples of intra-buccal signs of more widespread diseases.

3. *Information given about the general condition and habits of the patient*

   For example, the dry tongue of dehydration, the brown dry tongue of uraemia, the coated tongue with foetor oris of acute appendicitis and the typical response of the hypochondriac to the command 'show me your tongue', upon which he opens his mouth to an extraordinary degree and enables the nethermost recesses of his buccal cavity to become exposed.

CYSTS WITHIN THE MOUTH

Mucous retention cysts

These result from leakage of mucus due to minor trauma of the mucous glands and are better termed extravasation cysts. They are commonly found on the inside of the lips and inner aspects of the cheek. They are blue in appearance and contain glairy mucoid fluid. Their nuisance value is that they tend to be chewed upon by the patient.

Ranula

A large mucous extravasation cyst on one or other side of the floor of the mouth arising from the sublingual salivary gland. Often the submandibular duct can be seen passing over the cyst. The word ranula means a small frog and the lesion is so-called because it resembles a frog's belly.

Mid-line dermoid

This occupies the floor of the mouth and may project below the chin. It represents a congenital implantation of ectoderm during the process of fusion of the two mandibular processes.

Treatment

All these cysts are dealt with by excision.

Leukoplakia

This condition may occur anywhere within the mouth, particularly on the tongue. Other sites are the larynx, the anus and the vulva. The affected area of mucous membrane is thickened, white, cannot be rubbed off and may show cracks or fissures.

Under the microscope there is hyperplasia of the squamous epithelium with hyperkeratosis. It is usually found in middle-aged or elderly subjects and may result from chronic irritation. One invokes the well-known list of S's — syphilis, smoking, sepsis, sore tooth, spirits and spices — but it must be confessed than often no cause at all can be found.

The importance of the condition is that it is often pre-malignant; carcinomatous change especially occurs within the fissures and should be suspected if there is local thickening, pain or bleeding or areas of erythema.

Treatment

Remove any underlying cause. Any area suspicious of malignancy should be subjected to biopsy. Superficial areas of leukoplakia are usually satisfactorily treated by excision, with skin grafting if the area is large.

ULCERS OF THE TONGUE

Traumatic

Due to a sharp edge of a tooth or a denture; healing rapidly takes place when the cause is removed. Rarely seen nowadays is the ulcer produced on the under-aspect of the tongue as this is rubbed against the lower incisor teeth in whooping-cough.

Aphthous

A small round white painful ulcer which may occur singly or in crops anywhere in the mouth but particularly on the edge of the tongue. Its cause is unknown, but it may possibly have an auto-immune aetiology. For some unknown reason this is also called a dyspeptic ulcer, but in fact it occurs rather more in adolescents and young adults than in the chronic dyspeptic. The ulcer will usually heal rapidly if a hydrocortisone tablet is held against it.

Tuberculous

Usually multiple and situated along the dorsum or edges of the tongue. The ulcers are undermined and are extremely painful. Since this condition is associated with advanced pulmonary tuberculosis, it is rarely seen today in the United Kingdom.

Herpes simplex

Multiple small painful ulcers of the mouth and lips associated with severe constitutional symptoms. Commonly found in children. Can be extensive in the oropharynx, nose, oesophagus and larynx in patients on immunosuppressive drugs or infected with HIV.

Syphilitic ulcers

May occur in the first, second and third stages of syphilis; a chancre in the first, a 'snail track' ulcer in the second and a midline punched out gumma in the third. In addition, tertiary syphilis may produce leukoplakia or diffuse fibrosis of the tongue. All these conditions are extremely rare now that early syphilis is efficiently treated.

Carcinoma

See page 123.

CLEFT LIP AND PALATE

These developmental abnormalities are very common. Cleft lip occurs in one in every 750 live births, cleft palate in one in every 2000; in half the cases the cleft of lip and palate coexist, in a quarter the cleft of the lip is the only anomaly and in a quarter the cleft of the palate occurs alone. It is important here, as in all congenital anomalies, to make a careful search for other developmental defects; 10 per cent of patients with clefts have some other malformation.

Embryology

These deformities can only be understood if the embryological development of the face and palate is revised (Fig. 17.1).

Around the primitive mouth or stomodaeum there develop:

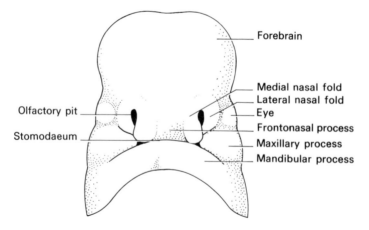

Fig. 17.1. The ventral aspect of a fetal head showing the three processes — frontonasal, maxillary and mandibular — from which the face, nose and jaw are derived.

1 *The fronto-nasal process,* which projects downwards from the cranium. Two olfactory pits develop in this process, then rupture into the pharynx to form the nostrils. The fronto-nasal process forms the nose, the nasal septum, the nostril, the philtrum of the upper lip and the premaxilla; this is the V-shaped anterior portion of the upper jaw which usually bears the four incisor teeth.

2 *The maxillary processes* on either side, which fuse with the frontonasal process to become the cheeks, the upper lip (exclusive of the philtrum), the upper jaw and the palate apart from the premaxilla.

3 *The mandibular processes,* which meet in the midline to form the lower jaw.

Cleft lip (Fig. 17.2)

Once termed hare-lip, but only rarely is the cleft a median one, like the upper lip of a hare, although this may occur as a failure of development of the philtrum from the fronto-nasal process. Much more commonly the cleft is on one side of the philtrum as a result of failure of fusion of the maxillary and fronto-nasal process. In 15 per cent of cases the cleft is bilateral. The cleft may be a small defect in the lip or may extend into the nostril, split the alveolus or even extend along the side of the nose as far as the orbit as a very rare anomaly. Associated with the deformity is invariably a flattening and widening of the nostril on the same side.

Cleft of the lower lip occurs very rarely but may be associated with a cleft of the tongue and of the mandible.

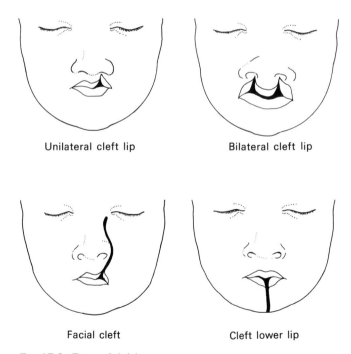

Unilateral cleft lip   Bilateral cleft lip

Facial cleft   Cleft lower lip

Fig. 17.2. Types of cleft lip.

Cleft palate

A failure of fusion of the segments of the palate. The following stages may occur (Fig. 17.3):

1   A bifid uvula, which is of no clinical importance.

2   A partial cleft which may involve the soft palate alone or the posterior part of the hard palate also.

3   A complete cleft. This may be unilateral, running the full length of the maxilla and then alongside one face of the premaxilla, or bilateral in which the palate is cleft with an anterior V which separates the premaxilla completely; this floats forward to produce a hideous deformity.

Principles of management

The details of surgical repair belong to the realms of the specialist plastic surgeon, but the principles underlying management are of importance to the pediatrician and the general practitioner.

Cleft lip alone presents no feeding or nursing problems. Repair is required at an early stage so that normal moulding of the bones of the face may occur during growth. Providing the baby is otherwise healthy the lip is repaired between the third and sixth month.

Cleft palate interferes with the normal suckling mechanism. The infant is fed either by using a spoon or by dripping milk into the mouth from a bottle provided

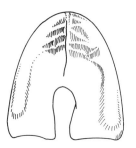
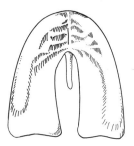

Partial clefts of palate

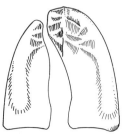

Unilateral complete
cleft palate

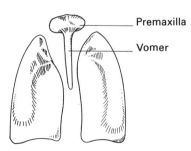

Premaxilla

Vomer

Bilateral complete
cleft palate

Fig. 17.3. Types of cleft palate.

with a large hole in the teat. The defect is repaired at between 6 months and one year in order to allow normal speech to develop. If delayed beyond this time the child will develop bad speech which will require considerable rehabilitation to restore to normal.

Where both defects coexist, the lip is repaired at about 10 weeks and the palate then operated upon at a second stage at the age of about 6 months.

MALIGNANT DISEASE OF THE MOUTH AND PHARYNX

In broad principles the pathology, diagnosis and treatment of malignant disease of lips, tongue, floor of mouth, gums, inner aspects of the cheek, the hard and soft palate, tonsils, fauces and the pharynx can be considered as one.

Pathology

Sex distribution

For the most part these tumours are more common in males than in females, but in tumours of the hard palate and posterior one-third of the tongue the sex distribution is equal and in the post-cricoid region females are more often affected than males.

Predisposing factors

These can be divided into three groups:

1   *Chronic irritation:* there is the well-known list commencing with 's': smoking, syphilis, sepsis, spices, sore tooth and spirits. A positive WR was once an extremely common accompaniment of carcinomas of the mouth, but it is now comparatively rare. Certainly mouth cancer is particularly seen among old men of poor social class with gross dental caries and heavy smoking. habits. Especially at risk is the heavy smoker who is also a heavy drinker. In Southern India betel nut chewing is associated with a high incidence of mouth cancer.

2   *Leukoplakia:* a definite pre-cancerous condition (see page 119).

3   *Iron deficiency:* the Plummer-Vinson syndrome with smooth tongue, cracks at the angles of the mouth (cheilosis), koilonychia, dysphagia and an iron deficiency is often present in oral and pharyngeal cancer in the female.

Macroscopically malignant tumours of the mouth present as one of three types:

1   A nodule.

2   An ulcer or fissure, usually feels hard to the palpating finger.

3   A warty or papilliferous growth.

Microscopically by far the commonest tumours are keratinizing squamous-cell carcinomas. In addition two other types may be seen, particularly in the posterior third of the tongue, the tonsil and the nasopharynx. These are:

1   *Transitional cell carcinoma*, made up of undifferentiated epithelial cells which simulate the transitional carcinomas of the urinary tract.

2   *Lymphoepithelioma*, comprising sheets of rather anaplastic epithelial cells pervaded with a diffuse lymphocytic infiltration. Probably both these variations are merely examples of undifferentiated squamous cell tumours.

Malignant tumours may also arise in the minor salivary glands which are abundantly distributed over the mucous membrane of the mouth.

Spread

Occurs by local infiltration which often transgresses nearby anatomical boundaries; thus a carcinoma of the tongue may invade the floor of the mouth, the gum and the fauces. Cervical lymph node involvement is common and indeed is frequently presenting symptom. Distant bloodborne spread, e.g. to the lung and liver, is late and relatively uncommon.

Causes of death

Tumours of the mouth and pharynx are particularly horrible in their late stages. The patient becomes cachectic from a combination of difficulty in swallowing and anorexia resulting from the infected, foul-smelling, fungating ulcer within the mouth. As a result of this sepsis, inhalation bronchopneumonia is a common termination. Fatal haemorrhage may occur, either from the primary ulcerating growth or from the breaking down of cervical lymph nodes which may erode the jugular vein or carotid artery.

Principles of treatment

The diagnosis must first be confirmed by biopsy. The search for predisposing factors will include a Wasserman reaction and haemoglobin estimation. A chest X-ray is taken to exclude the rare pulmonary secondary spread. Where relevant, X-rays of the skull and mandible and a CT scan may be required to estimate bony invasion. In every case treatment must be considered with respect: (a) to the primary tumour itself, and (b) to the regional lymph nodes.

Management of the primary tumour

The treatment of choice is radiotherapy. Where the tumour is readily accessible, e.g. the lip, the anterior part of the tongue and the buccal mucosa, this is conveniently carried out by implantation of radium needles. More posteriorly placed tumours are treated by supervoltage therapy.

With conventional X-ray therapy invasion of the mandible or maxilla by the tumour was a contra-indication to treatment because bone necrosis almost invariably took place; in such circumstances only radical surgery could be offered. Fortunately supervoltage therapy applied carefully does not damage the bone so that jaw involvement is no longer a bar to treatment.

Irradiation is abandoned under two circumstances; first if the tumour proves to be radio-resistant and second if recurrence takes place subsequent to satisfactory regression. In these circumstances it may be necessary to consider radical surgical excision, e.g. a hemiglossectomy or mandibulectomy and in continuity block disection of the cervical nodes.

Management of the regional lymph nodes

If the lymph nodes are not enlarged, the patient is kept under close regular observation. Experience has shown that little is to be gained by prophylactic block dissection. These patients are usually elderly and a major operation should obviously be avoided whenever possible. Moreover, since lymphatic drainage tends to be bilateral, prophylactic block dissection should logically be performed bilaterally — a still more formidable undertaking. In those cases where this technique has been employed, a surprisingly small percentage of lymph nodes have, in fact, been found to contain tumour deposits on histological examination.

If the lymph nodes are enlarged but mobile and obviously operable, block dissection is performed providing the primary tumour is controllable; clearly there is little point in carrying out a radical block dissection of the neck in the presence of a hopelessly inoperable carcinomatous mass within the mouth.

If the lymph nodes are enlarged but are fixed and clinically irremovable, then palliative deep X-ray therapy is given and may be combined with cytotoxic treatment.

Prognosis

Prognosis becomes increasingly worse as we pass backwards into the mouth; the outlook is best in tumours of the lip, then of the anterior two-thirds of the tongue, but it is usually grave in tumours of the pharynx, tonsil, etc. As with tumours elsewhere, the prognosis also depends on the degree of differentiation of the tumour on histological examination and on the extent of spread, particularly whether or not the lymph nodes are involved.

The local pathological and clinical features at specific sites can now be considered. In every case the management of the tumour and the regional lymph nodes are as described in the above scheme.

The lips

Clinical features

This disease commonly affects men (90 per cent); nearly always elderly, and those exposed to a weather-beaten outdoor life associated with sunlight exposure. The lower lip is by far the commonest site, accounting for 93 per cent of the tumours. 5 per cent occur on the upper lip and 2 per cent at the angle of the mouth — these last have a peculiarly bad prognosis. The lesion appears either as a fissure, a typical malignant ulcer or a warty papilliferous tumour. The majority are slow growing and spread to the regional lymph nodes is comparatively late; first to the submental, then the submandibular and finally the internal jugular chain of nodes. Distant metastasis is rare.

Differential diagnosis

The differential diagnosis of carcinoma of the lip conveninetly sums up the other swellings that may be found in this situation. They are:

1 *Simple papilliferous wart*, which may itself be premalignant.

2 *Molluscum sebaceum (keratoacanthoma):* see page 357.

3 *Chancre:* the lip is the commonest extragenital site for a chancre. Usually the upper lip is affected; it is accompanied by considerable local oedema and exuberant enlargement of the regional lymph nodes.

4 *Haemangioma.*

5 *Lymphangioma.*

6 *Herpes simplex.*

7 *Mucous cyst:* this results from blockage of a labial mucous gland and presents as a dome-shaped bluish swelling. Excision reveals a thin-walled cyst containing mucous, sticky clear fluid. This is probably the commonest swelling to be found upon the lip (see page 118).

Tongue

Carcinoma of the tongue once had a very strong predilection for the male; this is now less so because of the decline in the incidence of the tumour in the elderly syphilitic. The incidence among females remains relatively constant. The tumours are conveniently divided into those of the anterior two-thirds and those of the posterior one-third of the tongue.

Clinical features

The anterior tumours commence as a nodule, fissure or ulcer, although occasionally a widely-infiltrating type of tumour is seen. At first the lesion is painless but becomes painful as it invades and becomes grossly septic. The pain often radiates to the ear, being referred from the lingual branch of the trigeminal nerve, supplying the tongue, along its auriculotemporal branch. Ulceration is accompanied by bleeding; thus the typical picture of late disease is an old man sitting in the outpatient department spitting blood into his handkerchief and with a plug of cotton wool in his ear. As the tumour extends onto the floor of the mouth and the alveolus, speech and swallowing become difficult because of fixation of the tongue (*ankyloglossia*). Palpation is especially valuable. Malignant ulcers in the mouth, as in the rectum, feel hard with surrounding induration.

Lymphatic spread occurs to the submental, submandibular and deep cervical nodes. Unless the primary tumour is situated far laterally on the margin of the tongue this lymphatic spread may be bilateral.

Tumours of the posterior third of the tongue are rapidly growing and of the lymphoepitheliomatous type with early spread bilaterally to the cervical nodes.

Any nodule or chronic ulcer of the tongue must be regarded with great suspicion of malignant disease particularly if there is any predisposing factor such as leukoplakia.

Differential diagnosis

This is to be made from the other ulcers of the tongue discussed on page 119, from the comparatively rare benign tumours of the tongue (papilloma, haemangioma, lymphangioma and fibroma) and from the still rarer lingual thyroid which occurs as a midline nodule. More commonly the nervous patient may suddenly discover a circumvallate papilla which he sees on his tongue in the mirror, and presents to the surgeon having decided that he has a cancer of the tongue.

Soft palate and fauces

These tumours usually resemble in their behaviour those of the posterior third of the tongue.

Hard palate

Tumours in this region are usually warty, spread over the palate and later invade the bone. Differential diagnosis must be made from secondary involvement of the palate from an antral tumour and from mixed salivary tumours which arise from the small accessory salivary glands scattered over the hard palate.

Floor of mouth, alveolus and cheek

Here the tumour is commonly an ulcerating carcinoma which often involves more than one of these structures; thus an ulcer is often found wedged in the floor of the mouth extending upwards onto the gum and backwards to involve the root of the tongue. There is early spread to the regional nodes.

In addition, adenomas or adenocarcinomas occasionally arise in the mucous and salivary accessory glands of this region.

Tonsil

About 85 per cent of the tumours of the tonsil are squamous carcinomas, about 10 per cent are due to involvement of the lymphoid tissue of the tonsil in one of the lymphomas and 5 per cent are lymphoepitheliomas which show rapid lymph node spread.

Nasopharynx

As elsewhere the predominant tumour is a squamous carcinoma. In addition a rapidly growing lymphoepithelioma occurs in younger subjects and for some unexplained reason is particularly common among the Chinese with a high incidence of raised antibody titres to the EB virus; indeed in this race it is second in frequency only to uterine cancer. Rarely a fibrosarcoma of the nasopharynx arises from the periosteum of the basi-occiput.

These tumours may present with nasal obstruction and bleeding, Eustachian tube blockage with deafness, involvement of one or more of the cranial nerves and severe deeply-situated headache. Tumours at this site are notoriously difficult to locate even on careful inspection and palpation under anaesthesia. One-third present first as a cervical node mass.

Oro- and laryngopharynx

Carcinomas at these sites present first with discomfort in the throat, excessive salivation and expectoration of blood-stained mucus, which then becomes foetid. Later there may be alteration of the voice progressing to hoarseness and then dysphagia. Often, however these tumours present with enlarged cervical lymph nodes. The hypopharyngeal tumours (postcricoid carcinoma) are almost always confined to women, many of whom present features of the Plummer–Vinson syndrome (see page 123). Diagnosis is confirmed by oesophagoscopic examination and biopsy.

Chapter 18
The Gums and Jaws

There are a number of general conditions which produce gum changes:
1   Vitamin C deficiency, which results in the spongy bleeding gums of scurvy.
2   Phenytoin therapy, which causes gum swelling in epileptics.
3   Immunosuppressive drugs (e.g. cyclosporin), which often cause gum swelling and bleeding associated with chronic infection.
4   Acute leukaemia, haemophilia, aplastic anaemia and thrombocytopenia may all be associated with bleeding from the gums.

EPULIS

Epulis is a non-specific term applied to a localized swelling of the gum. This may be:
1   Fibrous: a nodule of dense fibrous tissue covered by epithelium and which arises from the sub-mucosa of the gum.
2   Giant cell: with the histological appearance of an osteoclastoma.
3   Granulomatous: peculiarly likely to occur in pregnancy and probably arises as a result of minor trauma followed by chronic infection.
4   Denture granuloma: originates from the persistent irritation of an ill-fitting denture.
5   Dental abscess: while not a true epulis, it initially presents as an acute inflammatory swelling of the mucosa adjacent to the diseased tooth.

CYSTS OF JAWS

Developmental cyst

Congenital cysts may arise at the lines of fusion in the developing maxilla or mandible. The commonest is the globulomaxillary cyst between the pre-maxilla and maxilla; this lies between the upper lateral incisor and the canine.

Cyst of eruption

A bluish cystic swelling which occurs most commonly over an erupting deciduous molar.

Dental cyst

A cyst related to the root of an erupted non-vital tooth. The cyst may be residual after the tooth itself has been extracted and may become infected.

Dentigerous cyst

A squamous-lined cyst containing the unerupted crown of a tooth and characterised by a swelling in the jaw of a young adult in which a count reveals that one tooth is missing.

Odontogenic keratocyst

A multi-locular cyst which arises from a developing tooth germ prior to its calcification. It is lined by a stratified squamous epithelium and is characterised by much keratin production. The cyst has considerable tendency to recur after local removal due to daughter cyst formation and therefore treatment comprises wide excision, which may necessitate jaw resection with bone grafting for the advanced case.

ODONTOMES

This term was once applied to any cystic or solid abnormality derived from a tooth or its embryonic precursor. It is now given to the mass of dental tissue of composite character arising from a developing tooth made up of a densely hard, irregular mass lying within the jaw and associated with an erupted tooth.

LEONTIASIS OSSEA

A descriptive term for the gross thickening that takes place in the maxillary and frontal bones with consequent gross deformity. In the past it has been considered to be due to syphilis or chronic pyogenic infection but the condition probably represents either a variant of Paget's disease or monostotic fibrous dysplasia.

TUMOURS OF THE JAW

Tumours of the jaw are of extremely wide pathological variety because they may arise from the bone of the jaw itself, from the tissues over the surface of the jaw or, in the case of the maxilla, from the mucosa lining the maxillary antrum.

Tumours of the bone itself

These may originate from any of the histological structures forming the bone, e.g. osteogenic sarcoma or osteoma from the bone itself, chondroma and chondrosarcoma from the cartilage, osteoclastoma from the osteoclasts, myeloma from the marrow cells, haemangioma from the blood vessels and fibrosarcoma from the periosteum. In addition to this, the jaw is the occasional site for secondary deposits, the common sources of which are lung, breast, prostate, thyroid and kidney.

Ameloblastoma (adamantinoma)

This is an interesting benign tumour which is derived from the epithelial cells of the enamel organ; its histological appearance resembles these cells arranged in clumps within a fibrous stroma. Gradual destruction of the jaw takes place but the tumour metastasizes only rarely. It is multilocular, and usually involves the lower jaw towards its angle. Any age may be affected, but the majority present in the second and third decades with equal sex distribution.

Surface tumours

Carcinoma, mixed salivary tumour, or rarely melanoma of the palate, gum, cheek or floor of the mouth may invade the underlying bone.

Central tumours

Probably the commonest tumour of the upper jaw is the squamous carcinoma arising from the mucous membrane of the maxillary antrum.

The antral carcinoma occurs in middle-aged and elderly subjects; the sex distribution is equal.

Clinical features of antral carcinoma

Symptoms and signs are late in manifesting themselves, indeed the tumour must burst through the bony walls of the antrum before it becomes obvious. Presentation then depends on the direction of growth of the tumour and can be deducted by the application of some knowledge of the anatomy of the region:

1 Medially there may be blockage of the ostium of the maxillary antrum with consequent infection of the sinus, or there may be nasal obstruction and epistaxis.

2 Lateral extension may present as a swelling of the face which often has an inflammatory appearance and may well be mistaken for an acute infection.

3 Upward extension invades the orbit with proptosis, diplopia and lacrimation due to blockage of the tear duct. Anaesthesia of the cheek may result from invasion of the maxillary branch of the trigeminal nerve.

4 Inferior extension produces bulging and ulceration into the palate. Metastases to the upper jugular lymph nodes occur at a relatively late stage.

X-ray usually reveal decalcification and erosion of the maxilla. There may be opacification of the normally translucent maxillary antrum. CT scan and MRI are valuable in indicating the exact spread of the tumours.

Treatment

Benign tumours are treated by local excision, in the case of the lower jaw this may require bone graft to the resected portion of the mandible.

Malignant tumours of the mandible and of the maxillary antrum are treated initially by radiotherapy, followed by hemimandibulectomy or maxillectomy.

Chapter 19
The Salivary Glands

The salivary glands comprise the parotid, submandibular and sublingual glands, together with tiny accessory salivary glands scattered over the walls of the buccal cavity.

The two principal surgical conditions of the salivary glands are inflammation, with or without calculus, and neoplasm.

CALCULI

Stone formation is common in the submandibular gland and its duct, rare in the parotid and unknown in the sublingual. The submandibular gland secretes a highly mucous saliva, the parotid much less so; moreover the submandibular duct has a long and upward course in the floor of the mouth. The sublingual gland produces a watery secretion and, unlike the other main salivary glands, drains by a series of very short ducts into the floor of the mouth. These factors probably account for this distribution of calculi.

It is surprising that calculi are nearly always associated with a clean and well-kept mouth, the teeth being either in nearly perfect condition or the patient being edentulous; stones are rare in patients with gross caries. A possible explanation may be that the calculi develop around minute fragments of toothpaste which find their way into the duct.

The stones consist of calcium phosphate and carbonate, and are therefore radio-opaque.

Clinical features

There is painful swelling of the affected gland, aggravated by food (classically by sucking a lemon) and there may be an unpleasant taste in the mouth due to the purulent discharge. On examination the obstructed gland is enlarged and tender, its duct is seen to be red and swollen and gentle pressure on the gland may produce a purulent exudate from the orifice of the duct. The stone is usually palpable on bimanual examination.

X-rays invariably confirm the presence of the stone.

Treatment

If the stone lies within the submandibular duct it can be removed from within the mouth. If one or more stones are impacted in the gland substance, excision of the gland is required.

INFLAMMATION OF THE SALIVARY GLANDS

Aetiology

1 *Associated with calculus:* usually submandibular gland (see above).

131

2   *Mumps:* usually parotid; rarely submandibular.
3   *Post-operative:* usually parotid.
4   *Chronic recurrent:* usually parotid.
5   *Mikulicz's syndrome:* involving all the salivary and the lacrimal glands.

Mumps

An infectious viral disease (incubation period 17 to 21 days), which is usually bilateral, usually occurs in children, and usually affects the parotid glands. Rarely the submandibular or sublingual glands may be involved.

Mumps is of interest to the surgeon for the following reasons:

1   As an occasional puzzling cause of parotid swelling in an adult.

2   As an occasional cause of acute orchitis, especially when mumps occurs in adolescents or young adults. (Orchitis complicating this condition is rare before puberty). Pain and swelling in the testicle occur 7 to 10 days after the onset of the parotitis and may lead to testicular atrophy. If bilateral orchitis occurs there may be sterility or eunuchoidism. Very rarely the orchitis occurs without prodromal parotitis.

3   As a rare cause of pancreatitis, mastitis, thyroiditis or oöphoritis

Post-operative parotitis

Ascending infection of the parotid gland via its duct may occur after major surgical procedures. Aetiological factors include dental sepsis, dehydration, the presence of a naso-gastric tube for a prolonged period and poor oral hygiene. This complication may also occur in any severe debilitating illness and in uraemia.

Clinical features

Clinically there is swelling and intense pain in one or both parotid glands which are hard, enlarged and tender. There may be a purulent discharge from the duct. Suppuration occasionally occurs.

Treatment

Prophylaxis is important; elimination of the above aetiological factors has rendered this complication rare nowadays. In the established case the patient must be kept fully hydrated and the flow of saliva encouraged by sucking sweets or chewing gum. Antibiotic therapy is commenced. Occasionally surgical drainage is required.

Chronic recurrent parotid sialadenitis

Repeated episodes of pain and swelling in one or both parotids is not uncommon and is caused by a combination of obstruction and infection of the gland. There may be an associated dilation of the duct system and alveoli of the gland, termed *sialectasia* (which resembles bronchiectasis), associated with a stricture of the duct or a stone. These changes are best demonstrated by performing a sialogram.

Treatment

An associated stricture is treated by dilation or plastic enlargement, and if stones are present these must be removed. Massage of the gland, several times a day, and the use of sialogogues (such as acid drops) encourage drainage. Occasionally, in severe and refractory cases, excision of the gland with preservation of the facial nerve is required.

Mikulicz's syndrome

Enlargement of all of the salivary glands, together with the lacrimal glands, is unusual. It may occur in the following conditions:

1 Sarcoid (commonest).
2 The lymphomas
3 Tuberculosis.
4 Sjögren's syndrome (middle-aged females with associated conjunctivo-keratitis, due to diminished lachrymal secretion, and rheumatoid arthritis).

SALIVARY TUMOURS

Classification

Benign

(a) 'mixed salivary tumour': pleomorphic adenoma.
(b) adenolymphoma.

Malignant

1 *Primary carcinoma.*
2 *Secondary:* direct invasion from skin or from secondarily involved lymph nodes.

PLEOMORPHIC ADENOMA

Ninety per cent occur in the parotid, although occasionally they are found in the submandibular, sublingual or accessory salivary glands. Ninety per cent present before the age of 50, although any age may be affected. Sex distribution is equal.

Pathology

Macroscopically
A lobulated tumour lying within a false capsule of compressed salivary tissue. The cut surface is glistening and translucent; the consistency is crumbly.

Microscopically
The tumours vary in a spectrum from a typical adenoma to a frank carcinoma. The majority show glandular acini within a blue-staining stroma which gives the appearance of a cartilage but which is, in fact, mucus. The appearance of epithelial cells and 'cartilage' gave rise to the older concept of a 'mixed tumour'.

Other considerations

If treated by enucleation, at least 25 per cent of the tumours recur, because:

1   The capsule surrounding the tumour is a false one, which itself is incomplete and may contain tumour cells.

2   Serial sections show that the tumour often has 'amoeboid' processes which may be left behind.

3   Implantation of tumour cells may occur into the wound.

Although slow growing, these tumours cannot be considered benign because of the lack of encapsulation, the occasional wide infiltration of surrounding tissues and the tendency to recur. Moreover, the less differentiated tumours, which are extremely difficult to distinguish from frank carcinoma, may metastasize to the regional lymph nodes and even by the blood stream.

Clinical features

The patient presents with a slowly growing swelling anywhere within the parotid gland, but usually in the lower pole and in the region of the angle of the jaw. The lump is well defined, usually firm or hard but sometimes cystic in consistency. It is usually placed in the superficial part of the gland but may occasionally be in its deep prolongation and indeed may project into the pharynx. The VIIth nerve is never involved, except by frankly malignant tumours.

Treatment

Wide excision of the tumour and the surrounding parotid tissue, with careful preservation of the fibres of the facial nerve (conservative partial parotidectomy). Some centres advise local excision followed by radiotherapy, especially in elderly patients.

Where the tumour involves one of the other salivary glands complete excision of the gland is performed.

Prognosis

Providing the tumour is completely excised the prognosis is excellent but inadequate surgery is followed by a recurrence in a high percentage of cases.

ADENOLYMPHOMA

Adenolymphomas (Warthin's tumour) account for about 10 per cent of parotid tumours, and are very rare elsewhere. The tumour is soft and cystic, usually occuring in men over the age of 50. Occasionally they are bilateral.

Microscopically the tumour consists of columnar cells forming papillary fringes which project into cystic spaces, and which are supported by a lymphoid stroma. These tumours probably arise from the salivary duct epithelium, the lymphoid tissue originating from the lymphoid aggregates which are present in the normal parotid gland. Prognosis is excellent after local removal.

CARCINOMA

Clinical features

Again this usually affects the parotid. Sex distribution is equal, and the patients are usually over the age of 50. The tumour is hard and infiltrating; clinically the diagnosis is based on rapid growth, pain, involvement of the facial nerve and of the regional lymph nodes. Eventually surrounding tissues are infiltrated and the overlying skin becomes ulcerated.

Treatment

When the tumour lies in the parotid, radical parotidectomy is performed with sacrifice of the facial nerve. This is combined if necessary with block dissection of the regional lymph nodes if these are involved, and is followed by radiotherapy. When the tumour arises in the other sites of salivary tissue, wide local excision is performed, again with block dissection if this is indicated by the presence of enlarged but mobile lymph nodes.

The prognosis is not good for this tumour, particularly when the submandibular gland is the site of origin.

DIFFERENTIAL DIAGNOSIS OF A PAROTID SWELLING

A swelling in the parotid region may be one of the following:

1 Swelling of the parotid gland itself:
   (a) parotitis
   (b) mixed salivary tumour or adenolymphoma
   (c) carcinoma
2 Swelling in other anatomical structures in the vicinity:
   (a) sebaceous cyst
   (b) lipoma
   (c) enlarged pre-auricular or parotid lymph nodes
   (d) neuroma of facial nerve
   (e) ameloblastoma (adamantinoma) and other tumours of the mandible.

Examination of a parotid swelling is incomplete unless the following have been performed:

1 Inspection of the parotid duct: redness, oedema of the duct or exudation of pus indicate parotitis.
2 Testing the integrity of the facial nerve: it is invariably intact in benign swelling, but may be paralysed in malignant disease.
3 Inspection and palpation of the fauces: a parotid tumour may plunge into the pharynx.
4 Palpation of the regional lymph nodes: they may be involved with secondary deposits from a parotid carcinoma.

Chapter 20
The Oesophagus

DYSPHAGIA

Dysphagia is difficulty is swallowing; the causes may be local or general. The local causes of obstruction of any tube in the body are subdivided into those in the lumen, those in the wall and those outside the wall.

Local causes

1 *In the lumen:* foreign body
2 *In the wall:*
    (a) congenital atresia
    (b) inflammatory stricture, secondary to reflux oesophagitis
    (c) caustic stricture
    (d) achalasia
    (e) Plummer–Vinson syndrome with oesophageal web
    (f) pharyngeal pouch
    (g) tumour of oesophagus or cardia
3 *Outside the wall:*
    (a) pressure of enlarged lymph nodes (malignant or one of the lymphomas)
    (b) thoracic aortic aneurysm
    (c) bronchial carcinoma
    (d) retrosternal goitre

General causes

1 Myasthenia gravis
2 Bulbar palsy
3 Bulbar poliomyelitis
4 Diphtheria
5 Hysteria

Investigation of dysphagia

History

The subjective site of obstruction is not always exact; the patient often merely points vaguely to behind the sternum. The diagnosis may be given by a history of swallowed caustic in the past. A previous story of reflux oesophagitis suggests peptic stricture. Patients with achalasia tend to be young and the history is often long, usually without loss of weight.

Malignant stricture has a short history, occurs usually in elderly people and is associated with severe weight loss.

Examination

Often this is negative, but search is made for clinical evidence of Plummer–Vinson syndrome (a smooth tongue, anaemia and koilonychia), secondary nodes from a carcinoma of the oesophagus may be felt in the neck and the upper abdomen is carefully palpated, since a carcinoma of the cardia is a common cause of dysphagia in elderly patients and indeed is commoner in this country than carcinoma of the oesophagus.

Special investigations

Barium swallow and oesophagoscopy, the latter now rendered much safer by the use of flexible fibre-optic instruments.

CONGENITAL ABNORMALITIES

The oesophagus develops as a derivative of the foregut, from the floor of which the larynx and trachea become separated by the laryngo-tracheal groove. This close developmental connection explains the commonest oesophageal anomaly; oesophageal atresia with an associated tracheo-oesophageal fistula (Fig. 20.1). Much more rarely an oesophageal atresia or a fistula occurs alone.

Clinical features

Atresia occurs in 1:2500 births and, as with nearly all developmental anomalies, is often associated with other congenital malformations. Half the cases are associated with maternal hydramnios.

Swallowed saliva and the first attempted feed distend the blind pouch of oesophagus which then regurgitates into the trachea, so that the child presents at the day of birth with attacks of cyanosis, excessive salivation and coughing. The

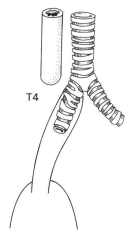

Fig. 20.1. The usual form of oesophageal atresia. The upper oesophagus ends blindly; the lower oesophagus communicates with the trachea at the level of the 4th thoracic vertebra.

upper abdomen may be distended by air passing via the tracheal fistula into the stomach.

Differential diagnosis

Must be made from cerebral birth injury and from intestinal obstruction — here vomiting rather than choking is the presenting feature (see page 173).

Diagnosis is confirmed by the inability to pass a soft catheter more than an inch or so into the oesophagus. A drop of radio-opaque contrast fluid is then injected and an X-ray clinches the diagnosis as the fluid remains in the blind oesophageal pouch. If the X-ray of the abdomen shows gas in the stomach this establishes also the presence of a tracheo-oesophageal fistula which has enabled air to pass into the alimentary tract.

Treatment

Unless this is rapidly instituted the child will die of an aspiration pneumonia. Transthoracic repair of the fistula and reconstruction of the oesophagus by end-to-end anastomosis is performed immediately on diagnosis; delays of much more than 24 hours from birth are usually fatal.

SWALLOWED FOREIGN BODIES

Foreign bodies are swallowed either accidentally, usually in children, or deliberately by lunatics, prison inmates and circus sideshow performers. Obstruction of the oropharynx and tracheal opening by a large portion of meat can rapidly become fatal. A sharp blow on the xiphoid, Heimlich's manoeuvre, may lead to dislodgement of the plug and save the patient's life.

Unless they are sharp or irregular, amazingly large foreign bodies will pass into the stomach. If a smooth object, such as a bolus of food, impacts in the oesophagus, one must suspect the presence of a stricture. Occasionally, for example, a carcinoma of the oesophagus presents as an acute dysphagia when a morsel of food lodges above it.

The presenting feature is painful dysphagia. The danger is perforation with mediastinitis; rarely perforation of the aorta occurs with fatal haematemesis. The diagnosis may be confirmed by a plain X-ray if the body is radio-opaque, otherwise it may be shown up on a barium swallow.

Treatment

Oesophagoscopic removal; occasionally oesophagotomy is required.

The great majority of foreign bodies, once they have passed into the stomach, proceed uneventfully along the alimentary canal and are passed per rectum. Occasionally, a sharp foreign body penetrates the wall of the bowel (there is an especial tendency for it to lodge in, and pierce, a Meckel's diverticulum).

The treatment of a foreign body which has passed the cardia is initially conservative. The patient is watched and serial X-rays taken to observe its progress if it is radio-opaque. Operation is performed if a sharp object fails to progress or if abdominal pain or tenderness develop.

PERFORATIONS OF THE OESOPHAGUS

Classification

1 *From within:*
   (a) swallowed foreign body (may occur anywhere)
   (b) rupture at oesophagoscopy (usually at the level of cricopharyngeus)
   (c) bouginage or biopsy, usually at the lower end of the oesophagus and especially likely in the present of oesophageal disease (carcinoma or stricture)
2 *From without:* perforating wounds (rare).
3 *Spontaneous:* lower thoracic oesophagus.

Clinical features

After instrumentation, perforation is suspected if the patient complains of pain in the neck, chest, or upper abdomen, together with dysphagia and pyrexia. Diagnosis is certain if surgical emphysema is felt in the supraclavicular area.

Spontaneous rupture of the oesophagus occurs rarely and is associated with violent vomiting after a large meal (Boerhaave's syndrome). There is severe pain in the chest, the dorsal region of the spine or the upper abdomen. The patient is collapsed and cyanosed; the abdomen may be rigid and often a false diagnosis of perforated peptic ulcer or myocardial infarction is made. However, there is usually surgical emphysema in the neck due to gas escaping into the mediastinum.

Special investigations

X-rays show gas in the neck and mediastinum and there may be fluid and gas in the pleural cavity. Swallowed water-soluble contrast fluid will confirm the perforation and define its position.

Treatment

Cervical perforation is managed conservatively: antibiotics, nil by mouth and intravenous drip. Abscess formation in the superior mediastinum requires drainage via a supraclavicular incision.

Thoracic rupture is treated by immediate suture (or resection if a carcinoma is instrumentally perforated).

CAUSTIC STRICTURE OF THE OESOPHAGUS

This follows accidental or suicidal ingestion of strong acids or alkalis (particularly caustic soda and ammonia). It often occurs in children.

In the acute phase there are associated burns of the mouth and pharynx. The mid and lower oesophagus are usually affected since these are the sites of temporary hold-up of the caustic material where the oesophagus is crossed by the aortic arch and at the cardiac sphincter.

Treatment

In the acute phase this is to neutralize the alkali with vinegar or acid with bicarbonate of soda. The damaged oesophagus is rested by instituting feeding via a gastrostomy, nil being given by mouth. Systemic steroids are given to reduce scar formation. If a stricture develops, gentle dilatation with bougies is commenced after 3 or 4 weeks. An established, impassable stricture is treated by a by-pass operation, a loop of colon or small bowel being brought up on its vascular pedicle between the stomach below and the upper oesophagus above, either in front of, or more usually behind, the sternum.

ACHALASIA OF THE CARDIA (CARDIOSPASM)

This is a neuromuscular failure of relaxation at the lower end of the oesophagus with progressive dilatation, tortuosity, incoordination of peristalsis and often hypertrophy of the oesophagus above.

Clinical features

Achalasia may occur at any age but particularly in the third decade. The ratio of female to male is 3:2.

There is progressive dysphagia. Regurgitation of fluids from the dilated oesophageal sac may be followed by an aspiration pneumonia. There may be an associated hiatus hernia and, occasionally, malignant change occurs in the dilated oesophagus.

Special investigations

1 *A plain X-ray of the chest* in an advanced case may reveal a mediastinal mass produced by the dilated oesophagus, and pneumonitis from aspiration of oeso-phageal contents.

Note that there are three other 'pseudo-tumours': scoliosis, tuberculous para-vertebral abscess and thoracic aortic aneurysm, all of which may simulate a mediastinal tumour on X-ray of the chest (see page 44).

2 *Barium swallow* shows gross dilatation and tortuosity of the oesophagus leading to an unrelaxing narrowed segment at the lower end.

3 *Oesophagoscopy* demonstrates an enormous sac of oesophagus containing a pond of stagnant food and fluid.

Treatment

Satisfactory results are obtained by Heller's operation, which is a cardiomyotomy dividing the muscle of the lower end of the oesophagus and the upper stomach down to the mucosa in a similar manner to Ramstedt's operation for congenital pyloric hypertrophy.

In some centres the same effect is achieved by forcible dilatation of the oesophago-gastric junction by means of a hydrostatic bag. Although this avoids open operation, it is accompanied by the risk of rupture of the oesophagus.

PLUMMER–VINSON SYNDROME

A syndrome actually described by Paterson and Kelly before Plummer and Vinson, which sometimes rejoices in all four names, comprising dysphagia and iron deficiency anaemia (with its associated smooth tongue and koilonychia) usually in middle-aged or elderly females.

The dysphagia is associated with hyperkeratinization of the oesophagus and often with the formation of a web in the upper part of the oesophagus. The condition is premalignant and is associated with the development of a carcinoma in the cricopharyngeal region.

Treatment

The dysphagia responds to treatment with iron, although the web may require dilatation through an oesophagoscope.

OESOPHAGEAL DIVERTICULA

The only common diverticulum of the gullet is the pharyngeal pouch.

Pharyngeal pouch

This is a mucosal protrusion between the two parts of the inferior pharyngeal constrictor — the thyropharyngeus and cricopharyngeus (Fig. 20.2). The weak area between these portions of the muscle is situated posteriorly (Killian's dehiscence). The pouch is believed to originate above the spasm of cricopharyngeus; it develops first posteriorly but cannot then expand in this direction and protrudes to one or other side, usually the left. As the pouch enlarges it displaces the oesophagus laterally.

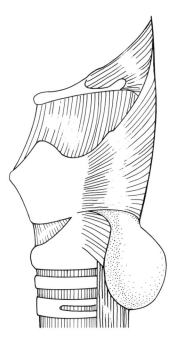

Fig. 20.2. A pharyngeal pouch emerging between the two components of the inferior constrictor muscle.

Clinical features

It occurs more often in men and usually in the elderly. There is dysphagia, regurgitation of food, which collects in the pouch, and often a palpable swelling in the neck which gurgles. Diagnosis is confirmed by a barium swallow.

Treatment

Excision of the pouch combined with myotomy of the cricopharyngeus.

Other diverticula

Other oesophageal diverticula are very rare.

Traction diverticula may occur in association with fixation to tuberculous nodes or to pleural adhesions.

Pulsion diverticula may be associated with cardiospasm and occur at the lower end of the oesophagus.

Occasionally congenital diverticula are found. These are usually X-ray findings only, although they may occasionally produce dysphagia.

Reflux oesophagitis. See page 148.

TUMOURS OF THE OESOPHAGUS

Classification

Benign

Leiomyoma

Malignant

1. *Primary*
   (a) carcinoma
   (b) leiomyosarcoma

2. *Secondary*
Direct invasion from lung or stomach.

CARCINOMA OF THE OESOPHAGUS

Post-cricoid carcinoma usually occurs in females and is associated with the Plummer–Vinson syndrome (see above). Ninety per cent of the remaining oesophageal growths occur in males, usually elderly. The commonest site is the mid-oesphagus, then the lower, then the upper oesophagus.

Predisposing factors include iron deficiency (Plummer–Vinson syndrome), achalasia of the cardia, caustic stricture and excessive intake of alcohol.

Pathology

The tumour commences as a nodule which then develops into either an ulcer, a papilliferous mass or an annular constriction.

Microscopically the majority are squamous carcinomas, but adenocarcinoma may occur at the lower end of the oesophagus, either arising in a gastric rest or as a result of an invasion of the oesophagus from a tumour developing at the cardiac end of the stomach.

Spread

1   *Local:* into the mediastinal structures: the trachea, aorta, mediastinal pleura and lung.

2   *Lymphatic:* to para-oesophageal, tracheo-bronchial, supraclavicular and sub-diaphragmatic nodes.

3   *Blood stream:* to liver and lungs (relatively late).

Clinical features

Carcinoma of the oesophagus may present:

1   *With local symptoms:* dysphagia.

2   *As a result of secondary deposits:* enlarged neck nodes, occasionally jaundice or hepatomegaly.

3   *With general manifestations of malignant disease:* loss of weight, anorexia, anaemia.

Dysphagia in an elderly male with a short history is almost invariably due to carcinoma of the oesophagus or the upper end of the stomach.

Special investigations

A barium swallow shows an irregular filling defect; oesophagoscopy enables the tumour to be inspected and a biopsy taken. Chest X-ray is carried out together with bronchoscopy to exclude a primary tumour of the lung invading the oesophagus or oesophageal invasion of the mediastinum. Ultrasound examination of the liver screens for hepatic deposits.

Differential diagnosis

Other causes of dysphagia (page 136).

Treatment

Resection – restoration depends on the defect. Most often the mobilized stomach is brought into the chest and anastomosed to residual oesophagus or to the pharynx in the neck.

If the tumour is inoperable, dysphagia may be relieved by intubation. This may be performed using the fibreoptic oesophagoscope after preliminary dilatation of the malignant stricture. If this is impossible, a Mousseau–Barbin plastic tube can be threaded through the stricture by means of a bougie threaded up through a gastrotomy incision. Intubation may be supplemented by deep X-ray therapy. The average expectation of life is in the region of three months with a maximum survival of about a year, but at least the patient is spared the misery of total dysphagia.

Chapter 21
The Diaphragm

This is of principal importance as the site of herniae.

Classification of diaphragmatic herniae
1 Congenital
2 Acquired
   (a) traumatic.
   (b) hiatal.

CONGENITAL DIAPHRAGMATIC HERNIAE

Embryology
These herniae can best be understood by reference to the embryology of the diaphragm (Fig. 21.1). The diaphragm is developed by fusion of:

1 *The septum transversum*, which forms the central tendon, and which develops from mesoderm lying in front of the head of the embryo. With the folding of the head, this mesodermal mass is carried ventrally and caudally to lie in its definite position at the anterior part of the diaphragm. During this migration, the cervical myotomes and cervical nerves contribute muscle and nerve supply respectively, thus accounting for the long course of the phrenic nerve (C3, 4, 5) from the neck to the diaphragm.

2 *The dorsal oesophageal mesentery.*

3 *The pleuro-peritoneal membranes*, which close the primitive communication between the pleural and peritoneal cavities.

4 *A peripheral rim* derived from the body wall.

In spite of this complex story congenital abnormalities of the diaphragm are unusual. They may be:

1 Hernia through the foramen of Morgagni; between the xiphoid and costal origins.

2 Hernia through the foramen of Bochdalek; a defect in the pleuroperitoneal canal.

3 Hernia through a deficiency of the whole central tendon.

4 Hernia through a congenitally large oesophageal hiatus.

Clinical features
Herniae through the foramen of Morgagni are usually small and unimportant. Those through the foramen of Bochdalek or through the central tendon are large and present as respiratory distress shortly after birth; urgent surgical repair is required.

The congenital hiatal herniae present with regurgitation, vomitting, dysphagia

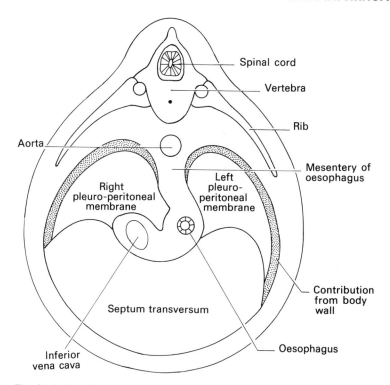

Fig. 21.1. The development of the diaphragm. The drawing shows the four contributory elements; septum transversum, dorsal mesentery of oesophagus, body wall and pleuroperitoneal membrane.

and progressive loss of weight in small children; they usually respond to conservative treatment, nursing the child in a sitting position. If this fails, surgical repair is necessary.

TRAUMATIC DIAPHRAGMATIC HERNIAE

These are comparatively rare and follow crush injuries to the chest or penetrating injuries, such as stab wounds, which implicate the diaphragm. The left diaphragm is far more often affected than the right (which is protected by the liver) and is accompanied by herniation of the stomach into the thoracic cavity.

Treatment comprises urgent surgical repair.

ACQUIRED HIATAL HERNIAE

Classification

These are divided into:
1 Sliding (90 per cent).
2 Rolling (10 per cent).

In the sliding variety the stomach slides through the hiatus and is covered in its anterior aspect with a peritoneal sac; the posterior part is extra-peritoneal. It thus

(A) Sliding hernia

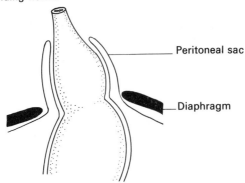

Peritoneal sac

Diaphragm

(B) Rolling hernia

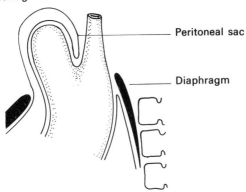

Peritoneal sac

Diaphragm

Fig. 21.2. (A) Sliding hiatus hernia; the stomach and lower oesophagus slide into the chest through a patulous oesophageal hiatus. (B) Rolling hiatus hernia; the stomach rolls up through the hiatus alongside the lower oesophagus (paraoesophageal hernia).

resembles an inguinal hernia en glissade (Fig. 21.2A). This type of hernia produces both the effects of a space-occupying lesion in the chest, and also disturbances of the cardio-oesophageal sphincter mechanism.

In the rolling (or para-oesophageal) hernia the cardia remains in position but the stomach rolls up anteriorly through the hiatus, producing a partial volvulus. Since the cardio-oesophageal mechanism is intact, there are no symptoms of regurgitation (Fig. 21.2B).

These herniae probably represent a progressive weakening of the muscles of the hiatus. They occur in the obese, middle-aged and elderly, and are four times commoner in women than men.

Clinical features

Most are symptomless, but when they occur, these fall into three groups:

1   *Mechanical:* produced by the presence of the hernia within the thoracic cavity; cough, dyspnoea, palpitations, hiccough.

2 *Reflux:* resulting from incompetence of the cardiac sphincter; burning retretrosternal or epigastric pain which is aggravated by lying down or stooping, and which may be referred to the jaw, or arms, thus simulating cardiac ischaemia. There is relief from alkalis. In severe cases, spill-over into the trachea may cause pneumonitis.

3 *The effects of oesophagitis:* stricture formation with dysphagia and bleeding, which may be acute or occult.

Reflux oesophagitis

Is produced by the reflux of peptic juice through the incompetent cardiac sphincter into the lower oesophagus, resulting in ulceration and inflammation and eventually to stricture formation. The exact mechanism of the cardio-oesophageal sphincter is not understood; it is sufficient to prevent regurgitation into the oesophagus when standing on one's head or in forced inspiration, when there is a pressure difference of some 80 mmHg between the intra-gastric and intra-oesophageal pressure, but yet it can relax readily to allow vomiting or belching to occur. The mechanism is probably a complex affair comprising:

1 Physiological muscle sphincter at the lower end of the oesophagus.

2 Plug-like action of the mucosal folds at the cardia.

3 Valve-like effect of the obliquity of the oesophago-gastric angle.

4 Pinch-cock effect on the lower oesophagus of the diaphragmatic sling when the diaphragm contracts in full inspiration.

5 Positive intra-abdominal pressure acting on the lower (intra-abdominal) oesophagus, maintaining a high pressure zone at the cardia.

The diaphragm is an important but not essential part of the cardiac sphincter mechanism, since sliding hiatus herniae are not necessarily accompanied by regurgitation. Similarly free regurgitation occurs in some subjects with a normal oesophageal hiatus, presumably because of some defect in the function of the physiological sphincter.

Reflux oesophagitis may also occur in association with:

1 Repeated vomiting, especially in the presence of a duodenal ulcer with high acid content of gastric juice.

2 Long continued naso-gastric intubation.

3 Resections of the cardia with gastro-oesophageal anastomosis.

4 The presence of ectopic acid-secreting gastric mucosa within the oesophagus ('gastric-lined oesophagus').

Investigations

Barium meal: the patient is examined in the head down position, which shows the hernia to pass up through the hiatus. Not only will this demonstrate the outline of the hernia, but will also indicate reflux and the presence of any associated stricture.

Oesophagoscopy (by fibre-optic endoscopy) demonstrates the presence of oesophagitis, which shows as a red oedematous mucosa with streaky haemorrhages. Any associated stricture can be inspected and a biopsy taken to exclude carcinoma.

Differential diagnosis

The pain of hiatus hernia may be confused with cholecystitis, peptic ulcer or angina pectoris; indeed, these conditions often coexist.

The obstructive symptoms of an associated stricture must be differentiated from carcinoma of the oesophagus or of the cardia.

Treatment

This may be medical or surgical.

Medical treatment comprises weight loss and the abandonment of corsets. Regurgitation is discouraged by avoiding stooping or lying and by sleeping propped up in bed. H_2 receptor antagonist drugs, (cimetidine or ranitidine), or the gastric acid secretion inhibitor omeprazole are prescribed to reduce gastric acidity. Many patients with mild symptoms obtain considerable relief from this regime.

Surgical repair of the hernia through a transthoracic or abdominal approach is undertaken when medical treatment fails. This may be supplemented by the Nissen plication operation; the fundus of the stomach is sutured around the lower oesophagus in an ink-well fashion in order to produce an anti-reflux valve.

In the presence of stricture surgical treatment is indicated. In a mild case, repair of the hernia will prevent reflux and enable a good deal of the associated oedema to subside with relief of symptoms. In the advanced case repeated dilatation may control the condition or, if this fails, resection of the stricture may be necessary.

Chapter 22
The Stomach and Duodenum

CONGENITAL HYPERTROPHIC PYLORIC STENOSIS

Aetiology

The aetiology of this condition of pyloric obstruction in infants due to a pyloric muscle 'tumour' is unknown. It may result from an abnormality of the ganglion cells of the myenteric plexus; failure of the pyloric sphincter to relax may then produce an intense work hypertrophy of the adjacent circular pyloric muscle.

Eighty per cent occur in male infants, 50 per cent are first-born and the condition often occurs in siblings.

Clinical features

The child usually presents at 3 to 4 weeks of age, although symptoms may be present rarely at or soon after birth. It is extremely uncommon for a previously healthy infant to develop this condition after 12 weeks of age.

The presenting symptom is projectile vomiting; the vomit does not contain bile and the child takes food avidly immediately after vomiting, i.e. it is always hungry. There is failure to gain weight and, as a result of dehydration, the baby is constipated (the stools resembling the faecal pellets of a rabbit).

The infant may be dehydrated and visible peristalsis of the dilated stomach may be seen in the epigastrium. Ninety-five per cent have a palpable pyloric tumour which is felt as a firm 'bobbin' in the right upper abdomen, especially after vomiting a feed.

Differential diagnosis

1 Enteritis: diarrhoea accompanies this.
2 Neonatal intestinal obstruction from duodenal atresia, volvulus neonatorum or intestinal atresia: symptoms commence within a day or two of birth and the vomit contains bile.
3 Cranial birth injury.
4 Overfeeding: here there are no other features to suggest pyloric stenosis apart from vomiting.

Investigations

If the clinical features are characteristic and a pyloric mass is palpable, no further investigations are necessary.

In doubtful cases, a plain X-ray of the abdomen reveals a dilated stomach with minimal gas in the bowel, in contrast to dilated coils of bowel in intestinal obstruction. Ultrasound can demonstrate the thickened pylorus. A barium meal reveals the pyloric obstruction with characteristic shouldering of the pyloric antrum due to the impression made on it by the hypertrophied pyloric muscle.

Treatment

This is anomalous in that the more seriously ill the child, the less urgent is the operation; in such cases a day or two must be spent in gastric lavage and fluid replacement, either by the subcutaneous or intravenous route. The otherwise healthy child can be submitted to operation soon after admission.

Surgical treatment

Ramstedt's operation

A longitudinal incision is made through the hypertrophied muscle of the pylorus down to mucosa and the cut edges are separated (Fig. 22.1). The operation is preceded by gastric aspiration and is conveniently performed under either local or general anaesthetic.

The infant is given glucose water 3 hours after the operation and this is followed by 3-hourly milk feeds which are steadily increased in amount.

Results are excellent and the mortality is extremely low.

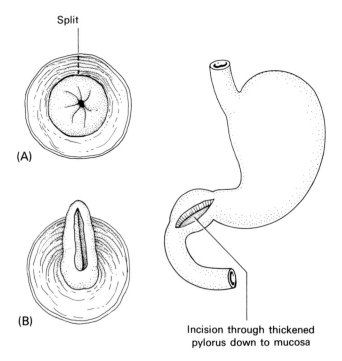

Fig. 22.1. Ramstedt's operation. The thickened muscle at the pylorus is split down to the mucosa. The inset diagrams show the pathology and the operative procedure in transverse section.

Post-operative complications

1   Gastro-enteritis, especially in debilitated children: rare with modern aseptic feeds and good nursing techniques.

2   Peritonitis from perforation through the mucosa: avoided by carefully testing the integrity of the mucosa at operation and repairing any puncture.

3   Bleeding from the pyloric incision: prevented by undersewing any bleeding point that may be encountered at operation.

4   Persistence of vomiting post-operatively: this occasionally requires re-operation and division of residual strands of muscle.

5   Wound infection.

6   Burst abdomen.

Medical treatment

Comprises gastric lavage together with 5 ml of 1/10 000 Eumydrin (atropine methyl nitrate) given as an antispasmodic 15 minutes before frequent feeds. Medical treatment is used only in babies with a long history and satisfactory weight gain or when the diagnosis is in doubt and should not be persisted with for more than 48 hours if symptoms continue.

ADULT PYLORIC HYPERTROPHY

This is occasionally seen. There is the typical hypertrophied pyloric tumour as in infants and there may be a long history of gastric symptoms leading to frank pyloric obstruction. It may be that in these cases the congenital pyloric hypertrophy has persisted and only become manifest in adult life. The condition is usually misdiagnosed as the far commoner carcinoma of the pylorus.

DUODENAL ATRESIA

Duodenal atresia may be:

1   A complete absence of the duodenum.

2   Fibrous band.

3   A diaphragm.

4   Partial diaphragm (stenosis).

Clinical features

The common bile duct usually enters above the obstruction and the vomit therefore usually contains bile.

Vomiting occurs from birth and the stomach may be visibly distended. There is a high incidence of Down's syndrome.

Differential diagnosis

1   Oesophageal atresia: there is choking rather than vomiting (page 137).

2   Pyloric stenosis: bile is absent from the vomit, there is a palpable pyloric tumour and onset is later.

3   Congenital intestinal obstruction: there is abdominal distension and X-rays show multiple distended loops of bowel with fluid levels (see page 173).

Plain X-ray of the abdomen is diagnostic and shows distension of the stomach and proximal duodenum with absence of gas throughout the rest of the bowel. (The 'double bubble' sign).

Treatment

Duodeno-jejunostomy or gastro-jejunostomy is performed after rehydration and gastric aspiration.

PEPTIC ULCER

Pathology

Peptic ulcers occur in situations where peptic acid digestion can take place, i.e. the oesophagus (peptic oesophagitis), stomach and duodenum, at the stoma of a gastro-jejunal anastomosis or in a Meckel's diverticulum when ectopic oxyntic cells are present. The ulcer may be acute or chronic.

The acute peptic ulcer

May be single or multiple (multiple erosions), may occur without apparent cause, or may be associated with ingestion of alcohol, aspirin, indomethacin or butazolidine, steroid therapy, acute stress, a major operation, or severe burns (Curling's ulcer). It may present with sudden pain, haemorrhage or perforation. A proportion of acute ulcers probably go on to become chronic.

The chronic peptic ulcer

At least 80 per cent occur in the duodenum. Duodenal ulcers may occur at any age but especially in the thirties to forties; about 80 per cent occur in males. Females are relatively immune to duodenal ulceration before the menopause and especially during pregnancy.

Gastric ulcers occur predominantly in males, but the sex preponderance is less marked, about 3:1 male to female. Any age may be affected but especially the forties to fifties (i.e. a decade later than the peak for duodenal ulceration).

Duodenal ulcers particularly occur among the executive and business classes in the United Kingdom, whereas there is a higher incidence of gastric ulcer among poorer patients.

Aetiology

The pathogenesis of peptic ulcer appears to involve a disturbance in the balance between the secretion of acid and pepsin on the one hand and mucosal defence mechanisms on the other.

Increased acid secretion appears to be of more importance in duodenal than in gastric ulceration. A proportion of patients with duodenal ulcer have high basal gastric acid secretion due to vagal overactivity, which can be abolished by vagotomy. Duodenal ulcers are almost always confined to the first part of the duodenum, beyond which the acid is neutralised by the pancreatic and biliary juices.

In a small group of patient duodenal ulcers are due to the Zollinger-Ellison syndrome in which a non-insulin secreting islet cell tumour of the pancreas produces a potent gastrin-like hormone (see page 264). In these patients ulceration can be more widespread within the small bowel.

A number of factors decrease the effectiveness of the mucosal defences against gastric juice. Non-steroidal anti-inflammatory drugs inhibit the production of protective prostaglandins in the mucosa. In a high proportion of patients with peptic ulcer it is possible to culture *Helicobacter pylori* from mucosal biopsies taken at endoscopy. This infection is associated with an inflammatory response which may impair mucosal defences. Both smoking and stress are thought to have an effect on both acid secretion and mucosal defences.

Clinical features

Physical signs in the uncomplicated case are absent or confined to epigastric tenderness; clinical diagnosis depends on the careful history.

The pain is typically epigastric, occurs in attacks which last for days or weeks and is interspersed with periods of relief. Pain which radiates into the back suggests a posterior penetrating ulcer. Peptic ulcer pain may come on immediately after a meal but more typically commences about 2 hours after food so that the patient says it precedes a meal ('hunger pain'). Quite characteristically, it wakes the patient at 2 a.m., so much so that he may adopt the habit of taking a glass of milk or an alkali preparation to bed with him. It is a myth to say that one can differentiate between a gastric and a duodenal ulcer merely on the time relationship of the pain. The pain is aggravated by spicy foods and relieved by milk and alkalis, although the relief is lost in deep and penetrating ulcers.

There may be associated heartburn, nausea and vomiting; the patient may lose weight because of the pain produced by food but equally often may gain weight because of his high intake of milk.

Special investigations

1 *Barium meal:* Gastric ulcers show the following features: a niche along the otherwise quite smooth line of the lesser curvature, usually in the typical position above the incisura, often associated with a notch of spasm immediately opposite on the greater curvature. A blob of barium may be left behind in the ulcer crater when the stomach empties. Normal peristaltic waves are seen, but there is distortion of adjacent mucosal folds around the ulcer.

Duodenal ulcers are often associated with a large hypermotile stomach with thick mucosal folds. The duodenal cap is deformed and tender to palpation; an ulcer crater may be visualized. If there is stenosis there is excess of resting juice, dilatation of the stomach, gross narrowing of the first part of the duodenum and delay in gastric emptying of 6 hours or more.

2 *Gastroscopy:* the modern fibre-optic instruments enable the oesophagus, stomach and duodenum to be examined with safety and with little discomfort in the sedated, conscious patient. The ulcer can not only be identified but, particularly in the case of a gastric lesion, biopsy material can be obtained to enable differentiation between a benign and malignant ulcer.

3 *Occult blood* examination of the stools is often positive.

Treatment

Treatment of a peptic ulcer is medical in the first instance; surgery is indicated when complications supervene. These are *chronicity, perforation, stenosis, haemorrhage* and, in the case of gastric ulcer, malignant change. They are considered in detail later in this chapter.

Principles of medical treatment

These are to neutralize acid secretion (using alkalis and milk), to reduce acid secretion or to improve mucosal defence in order to relieve pain and to aid the remissions which are a feature of the natural history of peptic ulcers.

Acid secretion can be reduced by the histamine H_2 receptor antagonists (cimetidine and ranitidine) or the newer H^+K^+-ATPase pump inhibitor (omeprazole) which blocks the enzyme which occurs almost exclusively in the gastric parietal cell and which mediates the final stage of gastric acid secretion. All these drugs result in rapid reduction in acid secretion and the majority of ulcers heal within one to two months. Ulceration, however, frequently recurs on cessation of treatment, so that long-term maintenance therapy may be required.

In ulcers that are refractory to the above treatment, and where *Helicobacter pylori* infection can be demonstrated, eradication of the organism with a six-week course of metronidazole and colloidal bismuth may promote healing.

Synthetic prostaglandins (e.g. misoprostol) have been shown to have ulcer-healing properties. The main use of this type of therapy is in the prevention of peptic ulceration in patients taking non-steroidal anti-inflammatory drugs, especially in those who give a past history of peptic ulcer or of bleeding while previously taking these preparations.

There is little evidence in controlled studies that conventional strict diets are of value. However, violent gastric stimulants should be avoided. Rest, sedation, avoidance of smoking and dealing with underlying anxiety states are helpful. Aspirin and non-steroidal anti-inflammatory drugs should be avoided wherever possible.

Results of medical treatment

The uncomplicated duodenal ulcer can be controlled in the majority of cases. Long-term results for gastric ulcer are not so good. In addition, there is a small, but definite risk of treating a gastric carcinoma under the mistaken diagnosis of benign gastric ulcer; this error is perhaps in the region of 1 per cent even with the help of the most skilled radiologist and fibre-optic endoscopic biopsy.

The clinician is thus more readily inclined to advise surgery in a gastric, as compared with a duodenal ulcer.

Principles of surgical treatment

Gastric ulcers are best treated by removing the ulcer together with the gastrin-secreting zone of the antrum; this is effected by the Billroth I gastrectomy (Fig. 22.2). The results are 90 per cent satisfactory with a mortality in the region of 1 per cent.

A duodenal ulcer will heal providing the high acid production of the stomach is abolished. This can be effected either by removing the bulk of the acid-secreting area of the stomach (the body and the lesser curve) or dividing the vagi. Since total vagotomy interferes with the mechanism of gastric emptying, this operation must be accompanied by a drainage procedure, either gastro-jejunostomy or pyloroplasty (Fig. 22.2). If the branches of the vagus that supply the pyloric sphincter (the nerves of Latarjet) are left intact, the remaining vagal fibres can be divided without the necessity of gastric drainage but nevertheless the goal of reduction in the vagal phase of acid secretion is achieved. This operation, variously termed

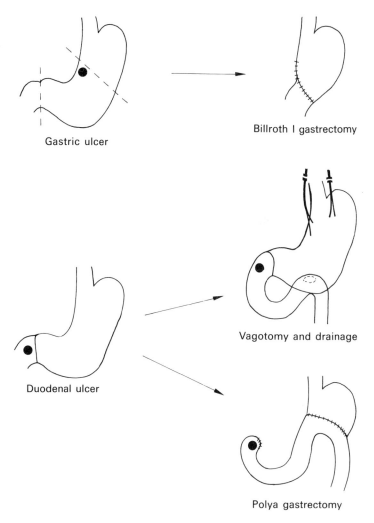

Gastric ulcer

Billroth I gastrectomy

Duodenal ulcer

Vagotomy and drainage

Polya gastrectomy

Fig. 22.2. The principcal operations for a peptic ulcer. For a gastric ulcer the Billroth 1 gastrectomy with gastro-duodenal anastomosis. For a duodenal ulcer, either vagotomy with some type of drainage procedure — a gastro-jejunostomy (as shown here) or pyloroplasty — or alternatively the Polya type of gastrectomy with gastro-jejunal anastomosis. If highly selective vagotomy is performed, a drainage procedure is not necessary.

highly selective, proximal or parietal cell vagotomy, has a low incidence of post-vagotomy symptoms (see page 157) but is associated with a higher ulcer recurrence rate than truncal vagotomy and drainage. It is also a time-consuming and technically difficult operation with a risk of incomplete denervation of the parietal cells. Indeed, the recurrence rate following this operation is directly proportional to the skill and experience of the surgeon.

The Billroth I type of gastrectomy for duodenal ulcer has a high incidence of recurrent stomal ulceration unless combined with vagotomy; probably this is because removal of the bulk of the acid-secreting part of the stomach is alone insufficient, and requires in addition the neutralizing effect of the bile to protect the stoma. This is produced by a gastro-jejunal anastomosis — the Polya gastrectomy (Fig. 22.2).

Gastro-jejunostomy alone will produce healing in a percentage of duodenal ulcers by the alkalinating effect of the bile and pancreatic juices shunted into the acid stomach. However, at least a quarter of cases will develop stomal ulcers and the operation is no longer used in this condition.

Pre-operatively patients with peptic ulcer should be checked for four things:

1   The haemoglobin level; these patients have often been on a diet low in iron and may also have had occult bleeding.

2   The teeth; these often require dental treatment — it is unlikely that the patient will be able to enjoy a normal diet if he cannot chew his food properly. Moreover gross dental caries predisposes to post-operative parotitis and there is always the risk of dislodgement and inhalation of a loose and septic tooth during induction of anaesthesia.

3   Vitamin C; peptic ulcer patients are often deficient in this vitamin because of their long use of a diet which lacks fruit and vegetables.

4   A chronic cough caused by heavy smoking. Smoking is forbidden and intensive chest physiotherapy given in the pre- and post-operative period, with reduction in the incidence and severity of post-operative pulmonary collapse.

Post-gastrectomy syndromes

Although about 85 per cent of patients are highly satisfied following Polya partial gastrectomy for peptic ulcer, a large number of unpleasant sequelae may occur.

These may be classified into:

1   *The 'small stomach' syndrome:* a high gastrectomy is associated with feeling of fullness after only a moderate sized meal. There may be accompanying loss of weight due to the impaired appetite.

2   *Bilious vomiting* due to emptying of the afferent loop of a Polya gastrectomy into the stomach remnant. If severe, this is corrected by conversion into a Billroth gastrectomy or by fashioning a Roux loop together with a vagotomy.

3   *Anaemia* due usually to iron deficiency (HCl is required for adequate iron absorption) or occasionally B_{12} deficiency due to loss of intrinsic factor with extensive gastric resection. The latter invariably occurs in total gastrectomy after a lag period of about 2 years in which the body's stores of B_{12} are depleted.

4   *The 'dumping syndrome':* comprises attacks of fainting, vertigo and sweating after food, rather like a hypoglycaemic attack. This is probably an osmotic effect due to gastric contents of high osmolarity passing rapidly into the jejunum, absorbing fluid into the gut lumen and producing a temporary reduction in circulating blood volume. The patient may have to lie down and rest for half an hour or so after a meal.

5 *Steatorrhoea* may occur, particularly in the presence of a long afferent loop; food passing into the jejunum traverses the bowel without mixing adequately with pancreatic and biliary secretions. Occasionally calcium deficiency and osteomalacia may occur.

6 *Stomal ulceration* complicates about 2 per cent of gastrectomies for duodenal ulcer; it is extremely rare after resection for gastric ulcer. It may be due to inadequate removal of the acid-secreting area of the stomach, or, rarely, because of the Zollinger—Ellison syndrome (page 264).

A stomal ulcer, like any other peptic ulcer, may perforate, stenose, invade surrounding structures or bleed. It is treated either by vagotomy or higher gastric resection.

Post-vagotomy syndromes

1 *Steatorrhoea and diarrhoea* may occur. Frequently these complications are transient or episodic but may be severe and persistent in about 2 per cent of patients; the reason for this is not understood but may be more the result of the gastric drainage procedure than of the vagotomy itself. Certainly the incidence is reduced in patients subjected to highly selective vagotomy without drainage.

2 *Stomal ulceration* may occur if vagotomy is incomplete. Failure to divide the whole vagal supply of the stomach may be tested post-operatively by the insulin test meal. A dose of insulin sufficient to produce hypoglycaemia produces a brisk vagal reflex secretion of HCl in the normally innervated stomach; this response is abolished if the vagotomy has been complete.

COMPLICATIONS OF PEPTIC ULCERATION

Peptic ulcer at any site may undergo the following complications:

1 *Chronicity* due to formation of fibrous tissue in the ulcer base.

2 *Perforation* either into the general peritoneal cavity or into adjacent structures, e.g. the pancreas, liver or colon.

3 *Stenosis.*

4 *Haemorrhage.*

5 *Malignant change* does not occur in duodenal ulcers but may rarely take place in a gastric ulcer; a long history does not necessarily mean that the ulcer was not malignant *de novo*. Both gastric ulcer and gastric carcinoma are common conditions and there may merely be a chance association between the two. It would seem that about 1 per cent of all gastric carcinomas arise in a gastric ulcer.

PERFORATED PEPTIC ULCER

Pathology

Perforation of a peptic ulcer is still a relative common and important emergency. The incidence of perforations fell steadily from the 1950s (i.e. before the introduction of the H$_2$ receptor antagonists), but has been relatively constant for the past 10 years. Male preponderance, once very high, is now about 2:1. Until recently, perforation occurred especially in young adults, but now the shift is towards the older are groups, especially in patients who are either on steroids or non-steroidal anti-inflammatory drugs (aspirin, indomethacin, phenylbutazone etc.).

Gastric carcinomas occasionally present with perforation.

Clinical features

A previous history of peptic ulceration is obtained in about half the cases, although this may be forgotten by the patient in his agony. Typically the pain is of sudden onset and of extreme severity, indeed the patient can often recall the exact moment of the onset of the pain. Subphrenic irritation may be indicated by referred pain to one or both shoulders, usually the right. The pain is aggravated by movement and the patient lies rigidly still. There is nausea, but only occasionally vomiting; sometimes there is accompanying haematemesis or melaena.

Examination reveals a patient is severe pain, cold and sweating with rapid, shallow respirations. Yet, in the early hours, there is no clinical evidence of true shock; the pulse is steady and the blood pressure normal. In the early stages also the temperature is either normal or a little depressed. The abdomen is rigid and silent, although in some instances an occasional bowel sound may be heard. Liver dullness is diminished in about half the cases due to escape of gas into the peritoneal cavity. Rectal examination may reveal pelvic tenderness.

In the delayed case, after 12 hours or more, the features of later peritonitis with paralytic ileus become manifest; the abdomen is distended, effortless vomiting occurs and the patient is extremely toxic and in oligaemic shock.

X-ray of the abdomen with the patient erect shows free gas below the diaphragm in 70 per cent of cases.

Differential diagnosis

The four conditions with which perforated ulcer is most commonly confused are: perforated appendicitis, acute cholecystitis, acute pancreatitis and coronary thrombosis.

Treatment

The stomach is emptied by means of a nasogastric tube; this diminishes further leakage and is essential as a pre-anaesthetic measure. Morphia is given to relieve pain and an intravenous drip in commenced. Antibiotics are given to contend with the peritoneal infection. Most surgeons are in favour of immediate operative repair of the perforation.

Prognosis

The mortality for perforated peptic ulcer lies between 5 and 10 per cent. Most deaths are in patients incorrectly diagnosed, with consequent delay in correct treatment, or too ill for operation; the subjects who die are typically either over the age of 70 or reach hospital 12 hours or more from the time of perforation.

The late prognosis following perforation depends on whether or not the ulcer is chronic. If there is a previous history of peptic ulcer, about 50 per cent have further serious symptoms and usually come to later elective surgery; if the ulcer is acute with no previous history this figure falls to 20 per cent. A second perforation or later haemorrhage are not rare.

PYLORIC STENOSIS

This is an inaccurate term when applied to duodenal ulceration, since the obstruction is in the first part of the duodenum.

Pathology

At first, fibrotic scarring is compensated by dilatation and hypertrophy of the stomach muscle. Eventually failure of compensation occurs, much like the failure of a hypertrophied ventricle of the heart with valvular stenosis.

Clinical features

During the phase of compensation there is nothing in the history to suggest stenosis. Once failure occurs, there is characteristic profuse vomiting, which is free from bile and the vomitus may contain food eaten one or two days previously. Because of copious vomiting there is associated loss of weight, constipation (because of dehydration) and weakness due to electrolyte disturbance.

On examination the patient may appear dehydrated and wasted. The progressive dilatation and hypertrophy of the stomach can be summed up as 'The stomach you can hear, the stomach you can hear and see and the stomach you can hear, see and feel'. At first a gastric splash can be elicited by shaking the patient's abdomen several hours after a meal; as the stomach enlarges, visible peristalsis can be seen also, passing from left to right across the upper abdomen. Finally the grossly dilated, hypertrophied stomach, full of stale food and fluid, can actually be palpated.

Gastric aspiration yields a morning resting juice of over 100 ml. In advanced cases it may amount to a litre or more of foul-smelling gastric contents. The barium meal shows dilatation of the stomach, a narrow outlet and considerable delay in emptying.

Biochemical disturbances

Patients with duodenal ulcer have a high gastric acidity. Pyloric obstruction with copious vomiting therefore results not only in dehydration from fluid loss, but also alkalosis due to loss of hydrogen ions; the alkalosis may be made worse if, at the same time, the patient is taking large doses of alkali in an attempt to relieve his ulcer pain. Initially the alkalotic tendency is compensated by the renal excretion of sodium bicarbonate, which may keep the blood pH within normal limits. At this phase, the dehydration results in diminished volume and increased concentration of the urine whose chloride content is first diminished and then disappears and whose reaction is alkaline. If vomiting continues, a large sodium deficit now becomes manifest. This loss of sodium is partly accounted for by loss in the vomitus but it is mainly due to urinary excretion consequent upon the bicarbonate lost in the urine as sodium bicarbonate. As the body's sodium reserves become depleted, hydrogen and potassium ions are substituted for sodium as the cations which are excreted with the bicarbonate. This results in the paradox that the patient with advanced alkalosis now excretes an acid urine. The blood urea arises, partly as a result of dehydration and partly because of renal impairment secondary to the electrolyte disturbances. Eventually, the patient may develop tetany as a result of a shift of the ionized, weakly alkaline calcium phosphate to its un-ionized state, in attempted compensation for the alkalosis. The concentration of calcium ions in the plasma therefore falls, although the total calcium concentration is not affected.

The metabolic disturbances may be summarized as follows:

1   The patient is dehydrated and the haematocrit level is raised.

2   The urine is scanty, concentrated, initially alkaline, but later acid; its chloride content is reduced or absent.

3   Serum chloride, sodium and potassium are lowered and the plasma bicarbonate and urea are raised.

Differential diagnosis

Carcinoma of the pylorus is by far the most important; other causes of pyloric obstruction are unusual in the adult and may be adult hypertrophy of the pylorus (see page 151), scarring associated with a benign gastric ulcer near the pylorus, invasion of the pylorus by malignant nodes, or infiltration from carcinoma of the pancreatic head.

The differential diagnosis from a pyloric carcinoma cannot always be established until laparotomy, but a reasonable attempt can be made on the following points:

1   Length of history: a history of several years of characteristic peptic ulcer pain is in favour of benign ulcer. A cancer usually has a history of only months and indeed may be painless.

2   Gross dilatation of the stomach favours a benign lesion since it may take several years for this to develop.

3   The presence of a mass at the pylorus indicates malignant disease, although rarely a palpable inflammatory mass in association with a large duodenal ulcer can be detected.

Treatment

The treatment of established pyloric obstruction is invariably surgical. Before operation dehydration and electrolyte depletion are corrected by intravenous replacement of saline together with potassium. Daily gastric lavage is performed to remove the debris from the stomach, in addition this often restores function to the stomach and allows fluid absorption to take place by mouth. Vitamin C is given, since the patient with a chronic duodenal ulcer is often deficient in ascorbic acid.

Surgical correction is carried out after a few days of pre-operative preparation. The choice of treatment lies between a partial gastrectomy of the Polya type and a vagotomy with drainage; the latter is to be preferred.

GASTROINTESTINAL HAEMORRHAGE

Management

The management of patients presenting with haematemesis and/or melaena is threefold:

1 The assessment and replacement of the blood loss.
2 The diagnosis of the source of the bleeding.
3 The treatment and control of the source of bleeding.

Blood loss

The indications for blood transfusion are the general condition of the patient (i.e. whether he demonstrates features of shock with pallor, sweating, etc.), a pulse rate above 100 and a blood pressure which has a systolic below 100. The last two are general rules which may be varied with the general condition of the patient, i.e. if he is a known hypertensive then obviously a systolic pressure well above 100 may still be a strong indication for transfusion. Every case is grouped on admission and blood made available by cross-matching.

It may be possible to assess blood loss by direct inspection of the amount of blood vomited. The haemoglobin estimation on admission is of only limited value since it may be more than 24 hours before haemodilution will reduce the haemoglobin level from its normal value.

Diagnosis

Bleeding may be from some local source or result from a general bleeding diathesis (haemophilia, leukaemia, anticoagulant therapy, or thrombocytopenia).

It is useful to consider the possible local causes anatomically:

1 *Oesophagus:* peptic oesophagitis (associated with hiatus hernia), oesophageal varices (associated with portal hypertension).
2 *Stomach:* gastric ulcer, acute erosions (including those associated with aspirin, indomethacin, butazolidine and cortisone), Mallory-Weiss syndrome, gastric tumours, benign and malignant.
3 *Duodenum:* duodenal ulcer, erosion of the duodenum by a pancreatic tumour.
4 *Small intestine*
   (a) tumours.
   (b) Meckel's diverticulum.
5 *Large bowel*
   (a) carcinoma.
   (b) diverticulitis.
   (c) angiodysplasia

About 85 per cent of patients with gastrointestinal bleeding of an acute form in this country have a peptic ulcer or erosion of the stomach or duodenum, chronic duodenal ulcer heads the list. About 5 per cent of patients have oesophageal varices and the remainder are accounted for by the other causes listed above.

Diagnosis is made on history, examination and special investigations.

History

There may be a typical story of peptic ulceration and perhaps the patient has had a positive barium meal in the past. It is important to take a history of drug habits since many obscure bleeds are found to be due to recent ingestion of aspirin, anticoagulants, butazolidine, etc. A story of alcoholism or previous virus hepatitis may suggest cirrhosis and an alcoholic debauch may also have precipitated an acute gastric erosion. Repeated violent vomits after a large meal or alcohol followed by a bright red haematemesis is typical of the Mallory—Weiss syndrome, in which a stress mucosal tear in the upper part of the stomach may result in a sharp haemorrhage.

Clinical examination

This is usually negative apart from the clinical features which enable assessment of blood loss. However, a bleeding tendency may be suggested by purpura, or oesophageal varices due to cirrhosis by enlargement of the liver and spleen, the presence of spider naevi and liver palms.

Investigations

1 *The haemoglobin* percentage is estimated as a baseline but, as mentioned above, the first estimate is not an accurate guide as to the extent of blood loss.

2 *Fibre-optic endoscopy* of the oesophagus, stomach and duodenum is a most valuable investigation, and can be carried out as an emergency. It will usually identify the exact site of the bleeding in upper gastro-intestinal haemorrhage. Some actively bleeding peptic ulcers may be treated endoscopically by injection of adrenaline or alcohol into the ulcer bed or by laser coagulation.

3 *A barium meal* can be performed as soon as active bleeding has ceased.

4 *Selective visceral angiography* using a Seldinger catheter inserted through the femoral artery may localize the source of haemorrhage in an obscure case.

Treatment

In the first instance this is on medical lines.

1 The patient is reassured, and reasurance is supplemented with morphia if he is restless.

2 Shock is treated, if present, by blood transfusion.

3 A careful watch is kept on the general condition, pulse and blood pressure.

4 Intravenous cimetidine is commenced to reduce acid secretion to a minimum.

5 As soon as active bleeding ceases, milk is allowed by mouth in the form of regular hourly or 2-hourly milk drinks. As soon as possible the patient is transferred to a semi-solid gastric diet.

On this regime three out of four patients with gastro-intestinal haemorrhage settle down.

Indications for surgery

The mortality of gastro-intestinal haemorrhage is in the region of 10 per cent. This is almost confined to patients over the age of 45, especially the elderly, who continue to bleed, or in whom bleeding recurs, while in hospital on the above regimen. It is common sense therefore that surgery is advised in patients over the age of 45 under medical treatment in hospital in whom haemorrhage obviously continues (i.e. continued melaena or haematemesis, rising pulse or falling blood pressure) or recurs.

In these cases blood transfusion is continued and urgent preparation made for laparotomy. At operation the source of bleeding is found and controlled. This usually takes the form of a gastrectomy for chronic gastric ulcer and vagotomy, pyloroplasty and undersewing of the ulcer for duodenal ulceration. In other cases it may be possible to undersew an acute erosion or bleeding ulcer, particularly in the desperately ill patient who is unfit for gastrectomy.

In most cases, the surgeon will know the cause of the haemorrhage pre-operatively, thanks to the high diagnostic accuracy of fibre-optic endoscopy. If the source of haemorrhage is not immediately obvious, the stomach is opened by a gastrotomy, the blood clot evacuated and the bleeding point sought by direct inspection of the gastric and duodenal mucosa.

In the patients who are treated medically and who settle down, careful assessment is made in the convalescent period. If the presence of a chronic duodenal or gastric ulcer is established, then surgery is usually advised as an elective procedure; once a chronic ulcer has bled, subsequent haemorrhages are likely to occur.

The management of haemorrhage from oesophageal varices This is considered on *page 245.*

STOMACH TUMOURS

Classification

Benign
> 1 Epithelial:
>> (a) adenoma:
>>> (i) single
>>> (ii) multiple (gastric polyposis)
>> (b) leiomyoma
> 2 *Connective tissue:*
>> (a) fibroma
>> (b) neurofibroma
> 3 *Vascular:* haemangioma.

Malignant
> 1 *Primary:*
>> (a) adenocarcinoma
>> (b) leiomyosarcoma
>> (c) lymphoma
>> (d) Hodgkin's disease
> 2 *Secondary:* invasion from adjacent tumours (pancreas or colon)

Benign tumours

These are rare, but the leiomyomas are an occasional cause of brisk haematemesis. Leiomyomas arise from the muscle of the gastric wall, project into the stomach lumen and ulcerate at their apex, producing a characteristic crater on a domelike projection. On cut section, they have a fibroid-like whorled appearance.

CARCINOMA OF STOMACH

Pathology

This is an extremely common and important tumour. In this country it is headed in incidence only by carcinoma of lung and large bowel in the male and by carcinoma of breast, uterus and large bowel in the female. For reasons quite unknown, its incidence is falling, both in Europe and the USA. Distribution is world-wide although it is particularly frequent in some races, especially the Japanese. Any age may be involved but it especially affects the 50 to 70 age group.

No absolute association has been shown with diet, alcohol or tobacco, although these have been implicated; the incidence is raised in patients with pernicious anaemia. There is a definite link with subjects having blood group A, which suggests a genetic factor. Occasionally a gastric carcinoma arises in a previous chronic gastric ulcer. It is estimated that about 1 per cent of malignant ulcers arise in a previously benign lesion.

Macroscopic pathology

One-third diffusely involve the stomach, one-quarter arise in the pyloric region, and the remainder are distributed fairly evenly throughout the rest of the organ.

There are four macroscopic appearances:

1 *A malignant ulcer* with raised, everted edges.
2 *A polypoid tumour* proliferating into the stomach lumen.
3 *A colloid tumour:* a massive, gelatinous growth.
4 *The leather-bottle stomach (linitis plastica)* caused by submucous infiltration of tumour with marked fibrous reaction. This produces a small, thickened, contracted stomach without, or with only superficial ulceration, hence occult bleeding is rare in this group.

Microscopic appearances

These tumours are all adenocarcinomas with varying degrees of differentiation. The leather-bottle stomach consists of anaplastic cells arranged in clumps with surrounding fibrosis.

An ulcer-cancer (malignant change in a benign ulcer) is suggested when a chronic ulcer, with characteristic complete destruction of the whole muscle coat and its replacement by fibrous tissue and chronic inflammatory cells, has a carcinoma developing in its edge.

Spread

1 *Local:* spread is often well beyond the naked-eye limits of the tumour and the oesophagus or the first part of the duodenum may be infiltrated. Adjacent organs

(pancreas, abdominal wall, liver, transverse mesocolon and transverse colon) may be directly invaded. A gastro-colic fistula may develop.

2 *Lymphatic spread:* the nodes along the lesser and greater curves are commonly involved. Lymph drainage from the cardiac end of the stomach may invade the mediastinal nodes and thence the supraclavicular nodes of Virchow on the left side (Troissier's sign). At the pyloric end involvement of the subpyloric and hepatic nodes may occur.

3 *Blood stream* dissemination occurs via the portal vein to the liver and thence occasionally to the lungs and the skeletal system.

4 *Transcoelomic spread* may produce peritoneal seedlings and bilateral Krukenberg tumours due to implantation in both ovaries.

Clinical features

Symptoms may be produced by the local effects of the tumour, by secondary deposits, or by the general features of malignant disease.

1 *Local symptoms* are epigastric pain and discomfort, pain radiating into the back (suggesting pancreatic involvement), vomiting, especially with a pyloric or antral tumour producing pyloric obstruction (see page 159); or dysphagia in tumours of the cardia. Occasionally carcinoma of the stomach may present with perforation or haemorrhage.

2 *Secondaries:* the patient may first report with jaundice due to liver involvement or abdominal distension due to ascites.

3 *General features:* anorexia (an extremely common presenting symptom), loss of weight or anaemia.

4 *Examination* may reveal features corresponding to these three headings. Local examination may reveal a mass in the upper abdomen; a search for secondaries may show enlargement of the liver with or without jaundice, ascites, enlarged, hard left supraclavicular nodes, or a palpable mass on pelvic examination due to secondary deposits in the pouch of Douglas; there may be obvious signs of loss of weight or anaemia.

Special investigations

The barium meal is usually the first special investigation to carry out in any patient with a suspected gastric neoplasm; accuracy is high and in expert hands is in the region of 95 per cent. The following are important radiological features:

1 A space-occupying lesion, e.g. an irregular stricture at the pylorus or at the cardia, or evidence of complete involvement of the stomach (leather-bottle stomach).

2 The presence of an ulcer with raised edges and surrounding infiltration.

3 The size of the lesion; any ulcer over 2 cm in diameter is suspect, although giant benign ulcers of 5 cm or more are found, especially in old people.

It is important to know that considerable 'healing' may occur when a gastric carcinoma is submitted to medical treatment in hospital and then re-X-rayed. This is due to diminution in the adjacent oedema and may lead to a false diagnosis of benign ulcer.

Fibre-optic gastroscopy is performed if the barium meal reveals a suspicious lesion; it enables direct inspection and biopsy of the lesion.

Gastric cytology using gastric washings is now only rarely used, although the cytology of smears taken through the gastroscope give a high yield of malignant cells.

The occult blood test is frequently positive but is of no help in differentiation from a benign gastric ulcer.

Acid secretion studies using pentagastrin stimulation often shows hypo- or achlorhydria, but this is of little diagnostic value.

Differential diagnosis

There are five common diseases which give a very similar clinical picture, of a patient with slight lemon yellow tinge, anaemia and loss of weight. These are carcinoma of stomach, carcinoma of caecum, carcinoma of the pancreas, pernicious anaemia and uraemia. They form an important quintet which should always be considered together.

The principal differential diagnosis of gastric carcinoma is a benign gastric ulcer. If in doubt, resection should be advised, but it may be difficult, even at operation, to decide between the two, and a frozen section microscopic examination is then useful in planning treatment.

Treatment

May be:

1 *Curative:* partial or total gastrectomy, depending on the extent of the tumour.

2 *Palliative:* palliative gastrectomy may be carried out even in the presence of small secondary deposits elsewhere.

A gastro-enterostomy may be performed for an irremovable obstructuve lesion of the pylorus. A carcinoma of the cardiac end which is irremovable and producing dysphagia can be intubated by means of a plastic Mousseau–Barbin tube. Irradiation and cytotoxic drugs are of limited value.

Prognosis

Depends on the extent of spread and the microscopic nature of the tumour. In addition, the general condition of the patient will affect whether or not he is fit for major curative surgery. The overall prognosis is poor; only 5 per cent of all cases survive for 5 years. However, 20 per cent of patients surviving radical 'curative' surgery are alive at the end of a 5-year period.

Chapter 23
Mechanical Intestinal Obstruction

Classification

Intestinal obstruction may be divided into two main groups, the paralytic and mechanical. Paralytic obstruction (paralytic or adynamic ileus) is dealt with in Chapter 30.

Mechanical intestinal obstruction is further classified according to:

1 Its speed of onset.
2 Its site.
3 Its nature.
4 Its aetiology.

Speed of onset

The speed of onset determines whether the obstruction is acute, chronic or acute on chronic. In acute obstruction the onset is sudden and the symptoms severe. In chronic obstruction the symptoms are insidious and slowly progressive (as, for example, in most cases of carcinoma of the large bowel). A chronic obstruction may develop acute symptoms as the obstruction suddenly becomes complete when a narrowed lumen becomes totally occluded by inspissated bowel contents — this is termed acute on chronic obstruction.

Site

The site of the obstruction is classified into high or low, which is roughly synonymous with small or large bowel obstruction.

Nature

The nature of the obstruction is divided into simple or strangulated. Simple obstruction occurs when the bowel is occluded without damage to its blood supply: in strangulation obstruction the blood supply of the involved segment of intestine is cut off (as may occur, for example, in strangulated hernia, volvulus, intussusception or where a loop of intestine is occluded by a band).

Aetiology

Whenever one considers obstruction of a tube anywhere in the body, this should be classified into:

1 *Causes in the lumen.*
2 *Causes in the wall.*
3 *Causes outside the wall.*

Applying this to the intestinal obstruction:

1 *In the lumen*: faecal impaction, gallstone ileus, food bolus, pedunculated tumour, etc.

2 *In the wall*: congenital atresia, Crohn's disease, tumours, diverticulitis of the colon, etc.

3 *Outside the wall*: strangulated hernia (external or internal), volvulus, obstruction due to adhesions or bands and intussusception.

It is also useful to think of the common intestinal obstructions which may occur at each age group:

Neonatal

Congenital atresia and stenosis, imperforate anus, volvulus neonatorum, Hirschsprung's disease and meconium ileus.

Infants

Intussusception, Hirschsprung's disease, strangulated hernia and obstructions due to Meckel's diverticulum.

Young adults and middle age

Strangulated hernia, adhesions and bands, Crohn's disease.

The elderly

Strangulated hernia, carcinoma of the bowel, colonic diverticulitis, impacted faeces.

A strangulated hernia is an important cause of intestinal obstruction from infancy to old age. The hernial orifices must therefore be carefully examined in every case.

Pathology

When the bowel is obstructed by a simple occlusion the intestine distal to the obstruction rapidly empties and becomes collapsed. The bowel above the obstruction becomes dilated, partly with gas (most of which is swallowed air), and partly by fluid poured out by the intestinal wall together with the gastric, biliary and pancreatic secretions. There is increased peristalsis in an attempt to overcome the obstruction, which results in intestinal colic. As the bowel distends, the blood supply to the tensely distended intestinal wall becomes impaired and in extreme cases there may be mucosal ulceration and eventually perforation. Perforation may also occur from the pressure of a band or the edge of the hernia neck on the bowel wall, producing local ischaemic necrosis, or from pressure from within the gut lumen, for example, by a faecal mass (stercoral ulceration).

In strangulation obstruction the ischaemic bowel is unable to contain its bacteria and their toxins within the lumen, so that a transudation of organisms into the peritoneal cavity rapidly takes place with secondary peritonitis. Unrelieved strangulation is followed by gangrene of the ischaemic bowel with perforation.

The lethal effects of intestinal obstruction result from fluid and electrolyte depletion due to the copious vomiting and loss into the bowel lumen, protein loss into the gut and toxaemia due to migration of toxins and intestinal bacteria into the peritoneal cavity, either through the intact but ischaemic bowel wall or through a perforation.

Clinical features

The cardinal symptoms of intestinal obstruction are four:
1 *Pain.*
2 *Distension.*
3 *Absolute constipation.*
4 *Vomiting.*

It is important to note that not all of these four features need necessarily be present in a case of intestinal obstruction.

Pain

This is usually the first symptom of intestinal obstruction and is colicky in nature. In post-operative obstruction it may be disguised by the general discomfort of the operation and by opiates which the patient may be receiving.

Distension

This is particularly marked in chronic large bowel obstruction and also in volvulus of the sigmoid colon. In a high intestinal obstruction there may, however, only be a short segment of bowel proximal to the obstruction and distension will not then be marked.

Absolute constipation

(i.e. failure to pass flatus in addition to stool)

Although this is a usual feature of acute obstruction, a partial or chronic obstruction may be accompanied by the passage of small amounts of flatus. Even in complete obstruction the patient may pass one or two normal stools as the lower bowel empties after the onset of the obstruction.

Vomiting

This usually occurs early in high obstruction, but is often late or even entirely absent in chronic or in low (large bowel) obstruction. In the late stages of intestinal obstruction the vomiting becomes *faeculent* but not *faecal*. The faeculent vomiting is due to bacterial decomposition of the stagnant contents of the obstructed small intestine and of the altered blood which may transude into the bowel lumen. True vomiting of faeces only occurs in patients with gastro-colic fistula, (e.g. due to a carcinoma of the stomach, carcinoma of the colon or ulceration of a stomal ulcer into the colon), or in coprophagists.

Clinical examination

The patient may be obviously dehydrated if vomiting has been copious. He is in pain and may be rolling about with colic. The pulse is usually elevated, but the temperature frequently is normal. A raised temperature and a very rapid pulse suggest strangulation. The abdomen is distended and visible peristalsis may be present. Visible peristalsis itself is not diagnostic of intestinal obstruction since it may be seen in the normal subject if the abdominal wall is very thin. During inspection it is important to look carefully for two features: the presence of a strangulated external hernia, which may require a careful search in the case of a small strangulated femoral hernia in a very obese and distended patient, and the presence of an abdominal scar. Intestinal obstruction in the presence of this evidence of a previous operation immediately suggests adhesions or a band as the cause.

Palpation reveals generalized abdominal tenderness. A mass may be present (for example, in intussusception or carcinoma of the bowel).

Bowel sounds are usually accentuated and tinkling. Rectal examination must, of course, never be omitted. It may reveal an obstructing mass in the pouch of Douglas, the apex of an intussusception or faecal impaction.

Clinically it is extremely difficult to distinguish with any certainty between simple obstruction and strangulation; no experienced surgeon would hazard more than a guess. In trying to assess the possibility of strangulation the following factors are taken into account:

1 Strangulation usually has an acute onset.
2 Tenderness and abdominal rigidity are more marked.
3 The patient tends to be toxic with a rapid pulse and some elevation of temperature.
4 A raised white cell count with neutrophil predominance is usual with infarcted bowel.

Special investigations

Plain X-rays of the abdomen (erect and supine) are valuable in diagnosis of intestinal obstruction and in attempting to localize the site of the obstruction. A loop or loops of distended bowel are usually seen, together with fluid levels. Small bowel is suggested by a ladder pattern of dilated loops, their central position and by striations which pass completely across the width of the distended loop produced by the circular mucosal folds. Distended large bowel tends to lie peripherally and to show the haustrations of the taenia coli, which do not extend across the whole width of the bowel. A small percentage, perhaps 5 per cent of intestinal obstructions, show no abnormality on plain X-rays. This is due to the bowel being completely distended with fluid in a closed loop and without the fluid levels produced by coexistent gas.

A dilated caecum is a dangerous radiological sign in large bowel obstruction. It means that the ileo-caecal valve is competent, allowing the caecum, the most distensible part of the large bowel, to blow up like a balloon. Perforation of the caecum with faecal peritonitis may occur if the obstruction is not rapidly relieved.

Follow-through X-rays after ingestion of a micropaque barium sulphate suspension may be used in suspected cases of small bowel obstruction. Because of the considerable fluid accumulation above the block, the barium is rapidly diluted and there is little danger of impaction.

An emergency contrast enema, using a water-soluble contrast medium, is helpful in the demonstration of a suspected large bowel obstruction due to carcinoma or diverticular disease.

Treatment

Although the treatment of specific causes of intestinal obstruction is considered under the appropriate headings, certain general principles can be enunciated here.

Chronic large bowel obstruction, slowly progressive and incomplete, can be investigated at some leisure (including sigmoidoscopy and barium enema) and treated electively.

Acute obstruction, of sudden onset, complete and with risk of strangulation, is invariably an urgent problem requiring emergency surgical intervention.

Pre-operative preparation in acute obstruction comprises:

1 Gastric aspiration by means of naso-gastric suction; this helps to decompress the bowel and to remove the risk of inhalation of gastric contents during induction of anaesthesia.

2 Intravenous replacement of fluid and electrolytes together with blood or plasma if the patient is shocked.

3 If there is the possibility of intestinal strangulation (or if this is found at operation) antibiotic therapy is commenced.

At operation the affected bowel is carefully inspected to determine its viability, either at the site of the obstruction (e.g. where a band or the margins of a hernial orifice has pressed against the bowel) or of the whole segment of bowel involved in a closed loop obstruction. Non-viability is determined by four signs:

1 Loss of peristalsis.

2 Loss of normal sheen.

3 Colour (greenish or black bowel is non-viable, purple bowel may still recover).

4 Loss of pulsation of vessels in the supplying mesentery.

Doubtful bowel may recover after relieving the obstruction if wrapped up in a wet pack and left for a few minutes.

The general principle is that small bowel in intestinal obstruction can be resected and primary anastomosis performed with safety because of its excellent blood supply. Large bowel obstruction must first be relieved, either by caecostomy or proximal colostomy, and a later resection performed. If resection is essential (as in strangulation) then the affected segment is excised and the two loops of colon brought out as a temporary colostomy. This is because the blood supply of the large bowel is much less efficient and a colonic primary anastomosis is very liable to leak in the presence of obstruction.

Conservative treatment

There was a phase of treating intestinal obstruction conservatively by decompression via a Miller–Abbott tube passed into the small bowel. This is now very rarely attempted, both because of the considerable difficulty of passing such a tube through the duodenum in the presence of intestinal obstruction, and also because of the impossibility, mentioned above, of being certain that strangulation is not present. Conservative treatment of obstruction by means of nasogastric aspiration and intravenous fluid is now only indicated under certain conditions:

1 Where diagnosis from post-operative paralytic ileus is not certain (see page 222) and where a period of careful observation is indicated.

2 Where the obstruction is one of repeated episodes due to massive intra-abdominal adhesions, rendering surgery hazardous, and where once again a short period of observation with conservative treatment is indicated.

Any increase in distension, aggravation of pain, increase in abdominal tenderness or rise in pulse are indications to abandon conservative treatment and to re-explore the abdomen.

3 Where chronic obstruction of the large bowel has occurred. Here is it reasonable to attempt to remove the obturating faeces by enemata, prepare the bowel with antibiotics and to carry out a subsequent elective operation.

Chapter 24
Specific and Special Forms of Obstruction

NEONATAL INTESTINAL OBSTRUCTION

Classification
1 Intestinal atresia.
2 Volvulus neonatorum.
3 Meconium ileus.
4 Hirschsprung's disease.
5 Ano-rectal atresias.

Continuous vomiting in the newborn suggests intracranial injury, infection or obstruction. Bile vomiting in the neonate indicates, almost without exception, intestinal obstruction.

In addition to vomiting there may be constipation, abdominal distension and visible peristalsis.

Plain X-ray of the abdomen shows distended loops of intestine with fluid levels.

CONGENITAL ATRESIA

This may be a septum, complete or partial, or a complete gap, which may be associated with a corresponding defect in the mesentery. Multiple segments may be involved.

Treatment

Resection of the stricture and anastomosis. The operation is difficult and the mortality is high.

VOLVULUS NEONATORUM

This is due to a defect of normal rotation of the bowel. The caecum remains high, often with a congenital band, (Ladd's band), passing from it across the duodenum, which may thus also be obstructed. The caecum and the midgut are suspended on a narrow attachment of mesentery which readily undergoes volvulus. Untreated, the whole of the midgut becomes gangrenous.

Treatment

Comprises untwisting the volvulus, dividing the transduodenal band and attaching the ascending colon to the lateral abdominal wall.

MECONIUM ILEUS

This is a neonatal manifestation of 10 to 15 per cent of infants with cystic fibrosis (mucoviscidosis), which is a generalised defect of mucus secretion of the intestine, pancreas (fibrocystic pancreatic disease), and the bronchial tree. Because of the loss of intestinal mucus and a blockage of pancreatic ducts with loss of tryptic digestion, the lower ileum of the fetus becomes blocked with inspissated, sticky meconium. Perforation of the bowel may occur in intra-uterine life (meconium peritonitis).

Clinical features

The infant presents with acute obstruction in the first days of life. The loop of ileum impacted with meconium may be palpable. X-ray of the abdomen shows, in addition to distended coils of bowel, the typical mottled 'ground glass' appearance of meconium.

Treatment

It may be possible to clear the meconium by installation of Gastrografin per rectum under X-ray control. This material is radio-opaque, hyper-osmolar (drawing fluid into the bowel lumen) and contains an emulsifying agent, which facilitates evacuation of the meconium. If this fails, or if the bowel has perforated, surgery is indicated. This comprises enterotomy and removal of the inspissated meconium by lavage. Occasionally the impacted segment of ileum may show areas of gangrene and requires resection. Post-operatively the infant is given pancreatin by mouth.

The prognosis is poor since, due to the lack of mucus secretion of the bronchi, recurrent chest infection is almost inevitable.

NECROTISING ENTEROCOLITIS

In recent years, this new entity has emerged in premature infants, particularly those with respiratory distress syndrome. It probably results from invasion of ischaemic mucosa of the small and large bowel by the bacteria of the gut lumen.

Clinical features

The infant shows signs of generalized sepsis. The abdomen is distended and tense. Blood and mucus are passed per rectum in over half the cases. The affected bowel may perforate or undergo stricture formation.

X-rays of the abdomen show distended loops of intestine and gas bubbles may be seen in the bowel wall. Pneumoperitoneum signifies intestinal perforation.

Treatment

Initially this is medical: total parenteral nutrition and wide spectrum antibiotics. Indications for surgery are failure to respond, profuse intestinal haemmorrhage, evidence of perforation or obstruction due to stricture formation. It comprises resection of the frankly gangrenous or perforated segment or segments of intestine.

HIRSCHSPRUNG'S DISEASE

This may present as acute obstruction in the neonate.

Pathology

This condition, also termed congenital or aganglionic megacolon, is produced by

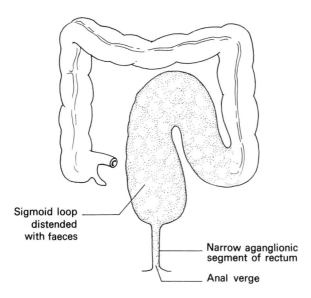

Sigmoid loop
distended
with faeces

Narrow aganglionic
segment of rectum

Anal verge

Fig. 24.1. Hirschsprung's disease.

faulty development of the parasympathetic innervation of the distal bowel. There is an absence of ganglion cells in the plexuses of Auerbach and Meissner in the rectum which sometimes extends into the lower colon and, rarely, affects the whole of the large bowel. The involved segment is spastic with gross proximal distension of the colon (Fig. 24.1).

Until the true nature of the disease was determined surgical treatment was directed, quite fruitlessly, to resection of the dilated portion of the colon.

Clinical features

Eighty per cent of the patients are male. In the most severe cases obstructive symptoms commence in the first few days of life and death results if untreated. Less marked examples present with extraordinarily stubborn constipation in infancy and these children survive into adult life with gross abdominal distension and stunted growth.

Rectal examination reveals a narrow, empty rectum above which faecal impaction may be felt; this examination is usually followed by a gush of flatus and faeces.

Special investigations

1 *Barium enema* demonstrates the characteristic narrow rectal segment above which the colon is dilated and full of faeces.
2 *Biopsy of the rectal wall* shows complete absence of ganglion cells.

Differential diagnosis

This is from acquired megacolon, a condition of severe constipation commencing usually at the age of 1 to 2 years, often in a mentally defective child. Rectal examination in these cases is typical, impacted faeces being present right up to the anal verge. Biopsy of the rectal wall shows normal ganglion cells.

This condition is relieved by regular enemas and aperients.

Treatment

If the child is obstructed in the neonatal period colostomy is performed. Elective surgery is carried out when the infant is 6 to 9 months old, or until at least 3 months have elapsed after a colostomy has been established. The aganglionic segment is resected and an abdomino-perineal pull-through anastomosis performed between normal colon and the anal canal.

It is important at operation to ensure by frozen section histological examination that ganglion cells are present in the remaining colon.

ANO-RECTAL ATRESIAS

Any degree of severity of this condition may occur from imperforate anus to complete absence of anus and rectum. Fifty per cent are associated with fistula; in the female into the vagina, in the male into the bladder or urethra. Twenty-five per cent are associated with congenital anomalies elsewhere.

Clinical features

The anus may be entirely absent or represented by a dimple or by a blind canal. The extent of the defect is judged by X-raying the child, held upside down, with a metal marker at the site of the anus: the distance between the gas bubble in the lower bowel and the marker can then be measured.

Treatment

1 If the septum is thin — division with suture of the edges of the defect to the skin.

2 If there is an extensive gap between the blind end and the anal verge, a colostomy is fashioned with later attempt at a pull-through operation at about 2 years of age. Some surgeons perform an immediate pull-through procedure in the neonate.

3 If a vaginal fistula is present operation is not urgent, since the bowel decompresses through the vagina — elective surgery is performed when the girl is older.

4 If a recto-urethral or vesical fistula is present (meconium escaping in the urine) the fistula must be closed urgently, either with colostomy or reconstruction of the anus in order to prevent ascending infection of the urinary tract.

INTUSSUSCEPTION

Definition

The investigation of one portion of the intestine into the lumen of the immediately adjoining bowel.

Aetiology

Ninety-five per cent occur in infants or young children, where there is usually no obvious cause. The mesenteric lymph nodes in these cases are invariably enlarged. It is postulated that the lymphoid tissue in the bowel wall undergoes hyperplasia due to an adeno-virus; the swollen lymph follicle protrudes into the lumen of the bowel and acts as a 'foreign body' which is then forced distally along the gut.

In adults and in some children a polyp, carcinoma or an inverted Meckel's diverticulum may form the apex of the intussusception.

The inner layer of the intussusception has its blood supply cut off by direct pressure of the outer layer and by stretching of its supplying mesentery, so that, untreated, gangrene of the intussusception may occur.

Terminology

1 *Ileo-ileal:* the ileum is invaginated into the adjacent ileum.
2 *Ileo-colic:* the ileo-ileal intussusception extends through the ileo-caecal valve into the colon.
3 *Ileo-caecal:* the ileo-caecal valve is the apex of the intussusception.
4 *Colo-colic:* the colon invaginates into adjacent colon (usually due to a protruding tumour of the bowel wall).

Clinical features of intussusception in infants

Usually occurs in previously healthy children commonly aged between 3 and 12 months. Boys are affected twice as often as girls.

The history is of paroxysms of abdominal colic typified by screaming and pallor. There is vomiting and usually the passage of blood and/or slime per rectum. On examination the child is pale and anxious, and a typical attack of screaming may be observed. Palpation of the abdomen, after sedation if necessary, reveals a sausage-shaped tumour anywhere except in the right iliac fossa. Occasionally the tumour cannot be felt because it is hidden under the costal margin. Rectal examination nearly always reveals 'red currant jelly' (a mixture of bright blood and slime) on the examining finger and, rarely, the tip of the intussusception can be felt.

If neglected, after 24 hours the abdomen becomes distended, faeculent vomiting occurs and the child becomes intensely toxic, due to gangrene of the intussusception and associated peritonitis.

Treatment

Non-operative

Barium is run in per rectum and X-ray confirmation of the diagnosis is established. If the intussusception is recent it may be completely reduced hydrostatically by the pressure of the column of barium and this is confirmed radiologically.

Operative

The intussusception is reduced at laparotomy by squeezing its apex backwards out of the containing bowel. In late cases reduction may be impossible or the bowel may be gangrenous; resection may then be necessary.

Mortality is very low in the first 24 hours but is naturally very high in the irreducible or gangrenous cases. An intussusception may recur in a small percentage of children.

VOLVULUS

Definition

A twisting of a loop of bowel around its mesenteric axis, which results in a combination of obstruction together with occlusion of the main vessels at the base of the involved mesentery.

Most commonly it affects the sigmoid, caecum and small intestine, but volvulus of the gall bladder and stomach may also occur.

Aetiology

Precipitating factors include:

1 An abnormally mobile loop of intestine, e.g. congenital failure of rotation of small intestine, or a particularly long sigmoid loop.
2 An abnormally loaded loop — as in the pelvic colon of chronic constipation.
3 A loop fixed at its apex by adhesions.
4 A loop of bowel with a narrow base.

Sigmoid volvulus

This occurs usually in elderly, constipated patients, four times more often in men than in women. It is relatively rare in Great Britain (about 2 per cent of intestinal obstructions) but is much more common in Russia, Scandinavia and Central Africa. The loop of sigmoid colon usually twists anti-clockwise from one-half to three turns.

Clinical features

There is a sudden onset of colicky pain with characteristic gross and rapid dilatation of the sigmoid loop.

A plain X-ray of the abdomen shows an enormously dilated oval gas shadow on the left side, which may be looped on itself to give the typical 'bent inner-tube' sign. If left untreated the strangulated bowel undergoes gangrene resulting in death from peritonitis.

Treatment

A rectal tube is passed through a sigmoidscope; this often untwists an early volvulus and is accompanied by the passage of vast amounts of flatus. If this method fails, the volvulus is untwisted at laparotomy and the bowel is decompressed via a rectal tube threaded upwards from the anus. Subsequently an elective resection of the redundant sigmoid loop is performed to prevent recurrent volvulus.

If gangrene has occurred, the affected segment is excised and the two open ends are brought out as a double-barrelled colostomy, which is later closed (Paul-Mikulicz procedure).

Volvulus of the caecum

Usually associated with a congenital defect in rotation so that instead of being fixed in the RIF the caecum has a persistent mesentery. Clinically there is an acute onset of pain in the RIF with rapid abdominal distension. X-ray of the abdomen shows a grossly dilated caecum which is often ectopically placed and is frequently located in the left upper quadrant of the abdomen.

Treatment

Operative untwisting of the volvulus is performed with decompression by means of a temporary caecostomy, which also effects fixation of the caecum by means of adhesions.

Small intestine volvulus in adults

This may occur where a loop of small intestine is fixed at its apex by adhesions or by a Meckel's diverticulum remnant. Occasionally the apex of the volvulus bears a tumour. In Africa primary volvulus of the small bowel is relatively common, and may be due to the loading of a loop of gut with large quantities of vegetable foodstuffs. The clinical picture is one of acute intestinal obstruction.

Treatment

Early operation with simple untwisting and treatment of the underlying cause. If gangrene is present resection must be carried out.

Volvulus neonatorum

This is considered on page 173.

MESENTERIC VASCULAR OCCLUSIONS

Embolism or thrombosis of the mesenteric vessels constitutes a special variety of intestinal strangulation without occlusion of the bowel.

Aetiology

1   Mesenteric embolus: may arise from the left atrium in atrial fibrillation, a mural thrombus secondary to myocardial infarction, a vegetation on a heart valve, or from an atheromatous plaque on the aorta.
2   Mesenteric arterial thrombosis: usually secondary to atheroma.
3   Mesenteric venous thrombosis: associated with portal hypertension, or may follow splenectomy for thrombocytopenic purpura, pressure of a tumour on the superior mesenteric vessels, or septic thrombophlebitis. Both mesenteric arterial and venous thrombosis are well documented in previously healthy young women on oral contraceptives.
4   Non-occlusive infarction of the intestine: may occur in patients with grossly diminished cardiac output and mesenteric blood flow consequent upon myocardial infarction or congestive cardiac failure.

Pathology

Mesenteric vascular occlusion results in infarction of the affected bowel with bleeding into the gut wall, lumen and peritoneal cavity; gangrene and subsequent perforation of the ischaemic bowel occurs. Impaired arterial blood flow to the gut without infarction may produce the symptoms of 'intestinal angina' in which severe abdominal pain follows meals; indeed, fear of eating and thus inducing pain produces rapid loss of weight. There may be an associated steatorrhoea. Minor degrees of occlusion may be overcome by development of a collateral circulation, particularly if the block develops slowly. One or even two of the main branches (coeliac, superior and inferior mesenteric) may be occluded in such cases without symptoms.

Clinical features

There may be some pre-existing factor such as a heart lesion or liver disease. The classical triad is acute colicky abdominal pain, rectal bleeding and shock (due to associated blood loss) in an elderly patient who has atrial fibrillation.

The abdomen is generally tender and a vague, tender mass may be felt which is the infarcted bowel.

Treatment

The shock is treated by blood transfusion. Occasionally successes have been reported from embolectomy in very early cases before frank gangrene has occurred. Resection of the gangrenous bowel is carried out, but this is obviously impossible where the whole mesenteric supply (small intestine and right side of the colon) is affected, usually a fatal situation. In young patients extensive resection of the small bowel can be managed by total parenteral nutrition on a permanent basis. Intestinal transplantation may be available for these cases in the future.

Chapter 25
The Small Intestine

MECKEL'S DIVERTICULUM

This is the remnant of the vitello-intestinal duct of the embryo. It lies on the ante-mesenteric border of the ileum and, as an approximation, occurs in 2 per cent of the population, 2 feet from the caecum and averages 2 inches in length.

Clinical features

It may present in numerous ways:

1   A symptomless finding at operation or autopsy.
2   Acute inflammation, clinically identical with acute appendicitis.
3   Perforation by a foreign body, presenting as peritonitis.
4   Intussusception (ileo-ileal), often gangrenous by the time the patient comes to operation.
5   Peptic ulceration due to the contained heterotopic gastric epithelium which bears HCl-secreting oxyntic cells. This particularly occurs in children and characteristically is the cause of melaena about the age of 10 years. Rarely the peptic ulcer perforates or gives rise to post-cibal pain.
6   Patent vitello-intestinal duct, presenting as an umbilical fistula which discharges intestinal contents.
7   Raspberry tumour at the umbilicus — due to a persistent umbilical extremity of the duct.
8   Vitello-intestinal band stretching from the tip of the Meckel to the umbilicus, which may snare a loop of intestine to produce obstruction or act as the apex of an ileal volvulus.

CROHN'S DISEASE

A non-specific inflammatory disease of the alimentary canal. The term 'regional ileitis' is sometimes used, but is inaccurate since Crohn's disease may affect any part of the alimentary tract from the mouth to the anus. Indeed, in recent years more and more examples of Crohn's disease affecting the large bowel, alone or with small intestine involvement, are being encountered (see page 197).

Aetiology

The aetiology is unknown. Suggestions include a viral or non-specific bacterial infection, atypical tuberculosis, sarcoidosis, ingestion of toothpaste or an auto-immune reaction. Acute regional ileitis can be caused by the bacterium *Yersinia enterocolitica*.

Pathology

The lower ileum is the commonest site, although the disease may affect any part of the alimentary canal from the buccal mucosa to the anal verge. First, the bowel is bright red and swollen in the acute stage; this proceeds to mucosal ulceration with a 'cobble-stone' appearance of the mucous membrane. The wall of the intestine is greatly thickened, as is the adjacent mesentery, and the regional lymph nodes are enlarged. There may be skip areas of normal intestine between involved segments. Fistulae may occur into adjacent viscera. Microscopically, there is fibrosis, lymphoedema and chronic inflammatory infiltration through the whole thickness of the bowel with non-caseating foci of epithelioid and giant cells.

Clinical features

Crohn's disease occurs especially in young adults although it may affect children and the elderly. There is no sex difference. As the disease progresses the clinical features may pass through a number of phases:

1st Acute: an appendicitis-like picture of acute abdominal pains, usually in the RIF; rarely there is perforation of the bowel or acute haemorrhage in this phase.

2nd Mucosal ulceration leads to diarrhoea, positive occult blood and anaemia.

3rd Fibrosis of the wall of the intestine progresses to obstructive symptoms and a palpable mass may be present.

4th Extensive involvement of the bowel produces malabsorption with steatorrhoea and multiple vitamin deficiencies.

5th Fistulae may develop which may be perianal or internal (through bladder or other loops of gut); external faecal fistulae usually follow operative intervention.

The typical clinical picture is a young adult with abdominal pain, diarrhoea and a palpable mass in the RIF.

Special investigations

Crohn's disease is associated with anaemia, positive occult blood and occasionally steatorrhoea. A barium meal and follow through shows a typical stricture in the affected segment, usually the terminal ileum (the string sign of Kantor). In some cases the ulcerated small bowel may show a 'cobble-stone' appearance.

Treatment

Initially conservative; steroids and azathioprine are prescribed for acute episodes. If found at laparotomy in the acute stage the condition should be left undisturbed since in a high proportion the acute phase may subside completely without further episodes. In the chronic stage of the disease surgery is indicated only for severe obstructive symptoms and then the affected segment is either short-circuited or resected. Surgery on the whole is avoided where possible because of the malabsorption which may follow extensive resections of the bowel or the production of blind loops of intestine.

Prognosis

Recurrence of the disease after resection occurs in some 50 per cent of cases within 10 years and repeated operations may be required over the years.

TUMOURS OF THE SMALL INTESTINE

One of the many mysteries of tumour formation is the rarity of growths from beyond the pylorus to the ileo-caecal valve.

Classification

Benign

> (a) adenoma
> (b) leiomyoma
> (c) lipoma
> (d) multiple polyposis (with skin pigmentation; the Peutz–Jeghers syndrome)

Malignant

> 1 *Primary:*
> (a) adenocarcinoma
> (b) lymphoma
> (c) carcinoid
> (d) leiomysarcoma
>
> 2 *Secondary invasion:* (e.g. from stomach, colon or bladder or from a lymphoma)

Clinical features

Tumours of the small intestine may present with intestinal bleeding, obstruction, intussusception or volvulus.

THE CARCINOID SYNDROME

Carcinoid tumours occur most commonly in the appendix, but may be found anywhere in the alimentary canal and occasionally in lung.

Pathology

Macroscopically the tumour consists of a yellowish plaque with intact overlying mucous membrane which later ulcerates. Usually the tumour encircles the bowel at the time of diagnosis.

Microscopically the tumour is made up of Kulchitsky cells, which take up silver stains and arise in the crypts of the intestinal mucosa.

The tumour is very slowly growing; those of the appendix are relatively benign but 4 per cent eventually metastasize. Those arising in the ileum and large bowel spread to the regional lymph nodes and the liver.

Where there is an extensive mass of tumour, symptoms are produced (the so-called carcinoid syndrome) because of the serotonin (5 hydroxytryptamine or 5 HT) secreted by the carcinoid cells.

Clinical features

The carcinoid syndrome comprises one or more of the following features:

1 Enlarged liver or abdominal mass produced by the tumour and its secondaries.

2 Flushing with attacks of cyanosis and a chronic red-faced appearance.
3 Diarrhoea with noisy borborygmi.
4 Bronchospasm.
5 Pulmonary stenosis.

Special investigation

5 Hydroxy-tryptamine is excreted in the urine as 5 hydroxyindole acetic acid (5-HIAA) which can be estimated by paper chromatography. The level is raised in this syndrome.

Treatment

Resection of the tumour in early cases. Local deposits in the liver are also occasionally resectable. More extensive deposits can be treated by embolizing the hepatic arterial supply via a Seldinger catheter passed through the femoral artery. Cytotoxic therapy may induce worth while remission. Symptoms maybe controlled by using 5 HT antagonists e.g. methysergide.

Even if widespread deposits are present, the tumour is slow growing and the patient may survive for many years.

Chapter 26
Acute Appendicitis

This is the commonest abdominal emergency and is estimated to affect one-sixth of the British population. It is, however, prevalent only in civilized communities or in primitive peoples who change to Western diet.

Pathology

Acute appendicitis usually occurs when the appendix is obstructed, either by a faecolith or foreign body in the lumen, by a kink from inflammatory adhesions or by enlargement of lymphoid follicles in its wall secondary to a catarrhal inflammation of its mucosa. Occasionally acute appendicitis occurs proximal to an obstructing lesion (usually carcinoma) in the caecum or ascending colon. Since the appendix of the infant is wide-mouthed and well drained, and since the lumen of the appendix is almost obliterated in old age, appendicitis in the two extremes of life is relatively rare.

The obstructed appendix acts as a closed loop; bacteria proliferate in the lumen and invade the appendix wall, which is damaged by pressure necrosis. The vascular supply to the appendix is made up of end-arteries which are branches of the appendicular branch of the ileo-colic artery; once these are thrombosed gangrene is inevitable and is followed by perforation.

There is no strict time relationship for this chain of events. An appendix may perforate occasionally in under 12 hours; however, it is not rare to see an acutely inflamed but not perforated appendix after 3 or 4 days.

The effects of appendicular obstruction depend on the content of the appendix lumen. If bacteria are present, acute inflammation occurs; if, as sometimes happens, the appendix is empty, then a *mucocele* of the appendix results, due to continued secretion of mucus from the goblet cells in the mucosal wall.

Occasionally appendicitis occurs in the non-obstructed appendix; here there may be a direct infection of the lymphoid follicles from the appendix lumen or in some cases the infection may be haematogenous (the rare streptococcal appendicitis, for example).

The non-obstructed acutely inflamed appendix is more likely to resolve than the obstructed form.

Pathological course

The acutely inflamed appendix may resolve, but if so, a further attack is likely. It is not uncommon for a patient with acute appendicitis to confess to one or more previous milder episodes of pain. More often the inflamed appendix undergoes gangrene and then perforates, either with general peritonitis or, more fortunately, with a localized appendix abscess. These possibilities can be summarized thus:

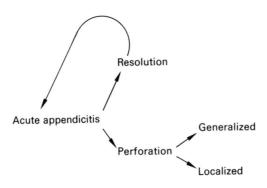

Clinical features

History

The vast majority of patients with acute appendicitis present with marked localized pain and tenderness in the right iliac fossa.

Typically the *pain* commences as a central peri-umbilical colic which shifts after approximately 6 hours to the right iliac fossa, or, more accurately, to the site of the inflamed appendix; thus if the appendix is in the pelvic position the pain may then become suprapubic, or if it is in the high retrocolic position, the symptoms may become localized in the right loin. Occasionally the tip of the inflamed appendix extends over to the left iliac fossa and pain may localize there. The central abdominal pain is visceral in origin; the shift of pain is due to involvement of the sensitive parietal peritoneum by the inflammatory process. Typically the pain is aggravated by movement and the patient prefers to lie still with the knees flexed.

Nausea and vomiting are usually present and follow the onset of pain; Murphy described as a diagnostic sequence — central pain; vomiting; pain moves to the right iliac fossa.

Anorexia is almost invariable.

Constipation is usual, but occasionally diarrhoea may occur (particularly where the ileum is irritated by the inflamed appendix in the retro-ileal position).

There may be a history of previous milder attacks of similar pain.

With perforation of the appendix there may be temporary remission or even cessation of pain as tension in the distended organ is relieved; this is followed by more severe and more generalized pain with profuse vomiting as general peritonitis develops.

Examination

1   The temperature and pulse are usually raised.

2   The patient is flushed, may appear toxic and is obviously in pain.

3   It is unusual for the tongue to be clean and for there not to be fetor oris.

4   The abdomen shows localized tenderness in the region of the inflamed appendix. There is usually guarding of the abdominal muscles over this site with release tenderness.

5 Rectal examination reveals tenderness when the appendix is in the pelvic position or when there is pus in the recto-vesical or Douglas pouch.

6 There is usually a polymorph leucocytosis.

7 In late cases with generalized peritonitis the abdomen becomes diffusely tender and rigid, bowel sounds are absent and the patient is obviously very ill. Later still the abdomen is distended and tympanitic, and the patient exhibits the Hippocratic facies of advanced peritonitis.

Differential diagnosis

This should be considered systematically under the following headings:

1 Other intra-abdominal causes of acute pain.

2 The urinary tract.

3 The chest.

4 The CNS.

5 In the case of female patients, acute pain of gynaecological origin.

1. Intra-abdominal disease

Those which commonly simulate appendicitis are perforated peptic ulcer, acute cholecystitis, acute intestinal obstruction, gastro-enteritis, non-specific mesenteric adenitis, acute regional ileitis (Crohn's disease), Meckel's diverticulitis and acute diverticulitis.

2. The urinary tract

Renal colic and acute pyelonephritis. The urine must be tested for blood and pus cells in every case of acute abdominal pain. Remember, however, that an inflamed appendix adherent to the ureter or bladder may produce dysuria and microscopic haematuria or pyuria; if reasonable doubt exists, it is safer to remove the appendix.

3. The chest

Basal pneumonia and pleurisy may give referred abdominal pain which may be surprisingly difficult to differentiate, especially in children.

4. The CNS

The lightning pains of tabes dorsalis, the pain which precedes the eruption of herpes zoster affecting the 11th and 12th dorsal segments and the irritation of these posterior nerve roots in spinal disease (tuberculosis or invasive tumour) all occasionally mimic appendicitis.

5. Gynaecological causes

The commonest pitfalls are acute salpingitis, ectopic pregnancy ('every lady is pregnant until proved otherwise'), and ruptured cyst of the corpus luteum. Laparoscopy may be helpful in the differential diagnosis.

Nothing can be so easy, nor anything so difficult, as the diagnosis of acute appendicitis. The tiro may smile indulgently at the long list of differential diagnoses given in the text books but, as year follows year, he will experience the chagrin of making most, if not all, of these errors.

Treatment

The treatment of acute appendicitis is appendicectomy, except under the following circumstances:

1 The patient is moribund with advanced peritonitis: here the only hope is to improve his condition by drip and suction, antibiotics and blood transfusion.

2 The attack has already resolved; in such a case appendicectomy can be advised as an elective procedure, but there is no immediate emergency.

3 An appendix mass has formed without evidence of general peritonitis (see below).

4 Where circumstances make operation difficult or impossible, e.g. at sea. Here reliance must be placed on conservative regime and the hope that resolution or local abscess will form, rather than on one's surgical skill with a razor blade and a bent spoon.

When at operation peritonitis is discovered, antibiotic therapy is commenced; metronidazole and gentamicin or a cephalosporin deal with both the anaerobic and aerobic bowel organisms, but this may require to be supplemented or changed when the bacteriological sensitivities of the cultured pus become available after 24 to 48 hours. After appendicectomy, a drain is inserted when there is severe inflammation of the appendix bed, when a local abscess is present, or where closure of the appendix stump is not perfectly sound. Very occasionally the inflamed and adherent appendix cannot be safely removed and in such circumstances the area of the appendix requires adequate drainage and subsequent 'interval appendicectomy' advised in about 3 months.

The appendix mass

Not uncommonly the patient will present with a history of 4 or 5 days of abdominal pain and with a localized mass in the RIF. The rest of the abdomen is soft, bowel sounds are present and the patient obviously has no evidence of general peritonitis. In these circumstances the inflamed appendix is walled off by adhesions to adjacent viscera, with or without the presence of a local abscess. Immediate surgery in such circumstances is meddlesome.

Treatment

Initial treatment is conservative. The outlines of the mass are marked on the skin, the patient is put to bed on a fluid diet and a careful watch kept on his general condition, temperature and pulse. Metronidazole is commenced, but prolonged antibiotics are *not* given since these may merely produce a chronic inflammatory mass honeycombed with abscesses (the so-called 'antibioticoma').

On this regime 80 per cent of appendix masses resolve; in the remaining cases the abscess obviously enlarges over the next day or two and the temperature fails to subside. In these circumstances drainage of the abscess is instituted. In neglected cases an appendix abscess may burst spontaneously through the abdominal wall, into the rectum, or into the general peritoneal cavity.

If resolution occurs, then appendicectomy is carried out after an interval of 3 months to allow the inflammatory condition to settle completely. Unless interval appendicectomy is performed there is considerable risk of a further attack of acute appendicitis.

Differential diagnosis of a mass in the right iliac fossa

The causes of a mass in the right iliac fossa are best thought of by considering the possible anatomical structures in this region:

1   Appendix abscess or appendix mass.

2   Carcinoma of caecum (differentiated from the above by usually an older age group, a longer history, often the presence of diarrhoea, positive occult blood with anaemia and finally the barium enema examination).

3   Crohn's disease (always to be thought of when there is a local mass in a young patient with diarrhoea).

4   Ileo-caecal tuberculosis (rare in the UK, common in India).

5   Psoas abscess — now rare.

6   Pelvic kidney.

7   A distended gall bladder (which may quite often extend down as far as the RIF).

8   Ovarian or tubal mass.

9   Aneurysm of the common or external iliac artery.

10   Retroperitoneal tumour arising in the soft tissues or lymph nodes of the posterior abdominal wall or from the pelvis.

Appendicitis in pregnancy

Appendicitis in pregnancy is no rarer or commoner than appendicitis in the general community, but it has a higher mortality and morbidity because it is confused with other complications of pregnancy. Differentiation must be made from pyelitis, vomiting of pregnancy, red degeneration of a fibroid or torsion of an overian cyst.

Because the appendix is displaced by the enlarging uterus, pain and tenderness are higher and more lateral than in the usual circumstances. There is considerable danger of abortion, particularly in the first trimester.

Chapter 27
The Colon

Constipation and diarrhoea

Constipation and diarrhoea are two symptoms frequently attributable to diseases of the large bowel. There are, of course, many causes of these common complaints, due not only to lesions of the large intestine but also to affection of other parts of the alimentary canal or to general diseases. It is useful here to consider the commoner causes of these two symptoms:

Constipation

Organic obstruction, e.g.
1 Carcinoma of the colon
2 Diverticular disease

Painful anal conditions, e.g.
1 Fissure in ano
2 Prolapsed piles

Adynamic bowel
1 Hirschsprung's disease
2 Senility
3 Spinal cord injuries and disease
4 Myxoedema

Drugs, e.g.
1 Aspirin
2 Opiate analgesics
3 Anticholinergics
4 Ganglion blockers

Habit and diet
1 Dyschezia (rectal stasis due to faulty bowel habit)
2 Dehydration
3 Starvation
4 Lack of bulk in diet.

Diarrhoea

Specific infections
1 Food poisoning (salmonella, gastro-enteritis)

2 Dysentery (amoebic and bacillary)
3 Cholera
4 Viral enterocolitis

Inflammation or irritation of the intestine
1 Ulcerative colitis
2 Tumours of the large bowel
3 Diverticular disease
4 Crohn's disease

Drugs
1 Antibiotics
2 Purgatives
3 Digitalis

Loss of absorptive surface
1 Bowel resections and short-circuits
2 Sprue and coeliac disease
3 Idiopathic steatorrhoea

Pancreatic dysfunction
Steatorrhoea due to lipase deficiency

Post-gastrectomy and vagotomy
Cause unknown

Anxiety states

General diseases
1 Thyrotoxicosis.
2 Uraemia.
3 Carcinoid syndrome (page 183).
4 Zollinger–Ellison syndrome (page 264).

DIVERTICULOSIS AND DIVERTICULITIS

Pathology

Diverticula of the colon consist of out-pouchings of mucous membrane alongside the taenia coli, often overlapped by the appendices epiploicae. They are found most commonly in the sigmoid and descending colon, and become increasingly rare in passing from the left to right side of the colon. They are unusual before the age of 40, but in the elderly they are found in about 30 per cent of all post-mortems. The sex distribution is roughly equal.

Aetiology

Hypertrophy of the muscle of the sigmoid colon produces out-pouchings of mucosa at the sites of potential weakness in the bowel wall, which correspond to the points of entry of the supplying vessels to the bowel (Fig. 27.1). Although colonic diverticula are so common in Western civilized communities they are extremely rare among primitive peoples. It may be that the modern, refined, low roughage diet may be responsible for the muscle thickening which is the primary lesion in this condition.

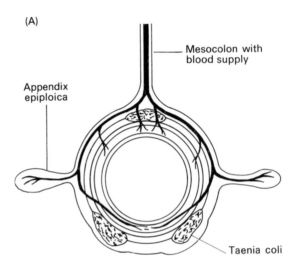

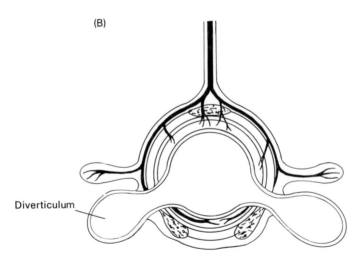

Fig. 27.1. The relationship of diverticula of the colon to the taenia coli and to the penetrating blood vessels. (A) normal colon, (B) colon with diverticula; both shown in transverse section.

Diverticulitis

This results from infection of one or more diverticula.

An inflamed diverticulum may:

1 *Perforate:*

(a) into the general peritoneal cavity

(b) with formation of pericolic abscess

(c) into adjacent structures; bladder, small bowel and vagina

2 *Produce chronic infection with inflammatory fibrosis* resulting in obstructive symptoms — acute, chronic, or acute on chronic.

3 *Haemorrhage,* as a result of erosion of a vessel in the bowel wall. The bleeding varies from acute to a chronic occult loss.

Clinical features

Acute diverticulitis is well nicknamed 'left-sided appendicitis'; an acute onset of central abdominal pain which shifts to the left iliac fossa accompanied by fever, vomiting and local tenderness and guarding. A vague mass may be felt in the LIF and also on rectal examination. Perforation into the general peritoneal cavity produces the signs of general peritonitis. A pericolic abscess is comparable to an appendix abscess but on the left side; a tender mass accompanied by a swinging fever and leucocytosis.

Chronic diverticular disease exactly mimics the local clinical features of carcinoma of the colon (page 199); there may be diarrhoea alternating with constipation which progresses to a large bowel obstruction with vomiting, distension, colicky abdominal pain and constipation: (note that small bowel obstruction from adhesion of a loop of small intestine to the inflammatory mass is not uncommon). There may be episodes of pain in the LIF, passage of mucus or bright red blood per rectum or of melaena, or there may be anaemia due to chronic occult bleeding. Examination reveals tenderness in the LIF and there is often a thickened mass in the region of the sigmoid colon, which may also be felt PR.

More unusual presentations are:

1 A sudden severe rectal haemorrhage. Bleeding from a diverticulum is the most likely cause of a sudden, severe, bright red bleed in an elderly, often hypertensive, patient.

2 Fistula into the bladder with the passage of faeces and gas bubbles (*pneumaturia*) in the urine. Diverticulitis is the commonest cause of vesico-colic fistula, others being carcinoma of the colon, carcinoma of the bladder and trauma.

Investigations

1 *Sigmoidoscopy:* if the affected segment is low in the colon there may be an oedematous block to the passage of the instrument beyond about 15 cm.

2 *A barium enema* demonstrates diverticula as globular outpouchings which often show a signet-ring appearance because of the filling defect produced by contained pellets of faeces. Diverticular disease is characterized by stricture formation which may closely simulate an annular carcinoma. More often the oedema and thickening produce a 'saw tooth' narrowed segment in the sigmoid.

3 *Colonoscopy* may allow the affected segment to be inspected, but often the

rigid and narrow sigmoid in this condition makes onward passage of the instrument impossible.

Differential diagnosis

The important differential diagnosis is from neoplasm of the colon. It is impossible to be certain of this differentiation clinically or even on special investigations unless a positive biopsy is obtained sigmoidoscopically or via the colonoscope to establish definitely the diagnosis of carcinoma. Even at laparotomy it is difficult to be sure whether one is dealing with carcinoma or diverticular disease; indeed these two common conditions may coexist.

Treatment

Acute diverticulitis

This is managed conservatively; a fluid diet is given and the patient placed on antibiotics (metronidazole and gentamicin or a cephalosporin is the combination of choice). The great majority settle on this regime.

A *pericolic abscess* is treated initially conservatively in a similar way to an appendix abscess (page 188), but if the abscess is enlarging drainage is indicated. This is often followed by the formation of a faecal fistula and is therefore best combined with a defunctioning transverse colostomy.

General peritonitis from rupture of an acute diverticulitis is a dangerous condition. Laparotomy is performed, the affected segment of colon resected, and a defunctioning colostomy fashioned. Full antibiotic therapy is given.

Acute obstruction due to diverticulitis requires laparotomy to establish the diagnosis and a transverse colostomy to relieve the obstruction. It is important to determine whether or not the obstruction is caused by an adherent loop of small intestine, which is by no means uncommon. Following this emergency procedure elective resection of the affected segment of colon can be then be carried out and the colostomy subsequently closed.

Chronic diverticular disease

If the diagnosis is made with considerable certainty and symptoms are mild, this can be treated conservatively. The bowels are regulated by means of Milpar or some other lubricant laxative. A high roughage diet, (fruit, vegetables, wholemeal bread and bran),is prescribed. If, however, symptoms are severe or if carcinoma cannot be excluded, then laparotomy and resection of the sigmoid colon is performed.

Vesico-colic fistula is treated by preliminary defunctioning colostomy. The affected segment of the colon is then resected and the fistula into the bladder is sutured; the colostomy is subsequently closed.

ANGIODYSPLASIA

This term is applied to one or multiple small (less than 5mm) mucosal or sub-mucosal telangiectases. Since they occur most commonly in the elderly, they are considered to be degenerative vascular anomalies. The caecum and ascending colon are the sites most usually involved, although they may be found anywhere in the small or large bowel.

Diagnosis

These lesions were unknown before the development of visceral angiography and, more recently, colonoscopy, when asymptomatic lesions may be revealed. Their only clinical manifestation is bleeding, which may take the form of continuous chronic intestinal blood loss, presenting with anaemia, or recurrent acute dark or bright red rectal haemorrhage, which may be severe and life-threatening. They account for some 5 percent of such emergency cases.

Treatment

Blood transfusion is necessary if haemorrhage is severe. Endoscopic electrocoagulation is often curative.

ULCERATIVE COLITIS

Ulcerative colitis is a disease of the colon and rectum of unknown aetiology; among numerous suggestions as to cause are psychosomatic factors, allergy or auto-immune disease.

Pathology

Females are more often affected than males. It is found in any age from infancy to the elderly, but the maximum incidence is between the ages of 20 and 40. The sigmoid colon and rectum are especially affected, but the whole colon may be involved. (Note that the sigmoid is the site of election for all the major diseases of the colon; colitis, volvulus, carcinoma, polyposis and diverticulitis. Why it deserves this notoriety is unknown.)

Initially there is oedema of the mucosa, with contact bleeding and petechial haemorrhage, proceeding to ulceration; the ulcers are shallow and irregular. Oedematous tags of mucosa between the ulcers form pseudopolyps. The wall of the colon is oedematous and fibrotic and is therefore rigid with loss of its normal haustrations. Surprisingly the inflamed colon does not become adherent to its neighbouring intra-abdominal viscera.

Histologically, the principle locus of the disease is mucosal; small abscesses form within the mucosal crypts ('crypt abscesses'). These abscesses break down into ulcers whose base is lined with granulation tissue. The walls of the colon are infiltrated with polymorphs and round cells; there is oedema and submucosal fibrosis. In the chronic, burnt-out disease the mucosa is smooth and atrophic; the bowel wall is thinned.

Clinical features

Manifestations of ulcerative colitis may be fulminant, intermittent or chronic. There is diarrhoea with blood, mucus and pus, and there may be accompanying cramp-like abdominal pains. In severe attacks there is fever, toxaemia, severe bleeding and risk of perforation. Anorexia and loss of weight occur in the acute episodes.

Investigations

1 *Sigmoidoscopy* reveals oedema of the mucosa with contact bleeding in the early mild cases, proceeding to granularity of the mucosa and then frank ulceration with pus and blood in the bowel lumen. Biopsy will give confirming histological evidence of the diagnosis.

2 *Colonoscopy* enables the whole of the large bowel to be inspected and biopsy material to be obtained.

3 *A barium enema* shows a ragged surface, indicating ulceration. Oedema and fibrosis produce loss of haustration and in the chronic case the typical 'drain pipe' colon.

4 *Examination of the stools* reveals pus and blood either to the naked eye or under the microscope, but no specific organism has ever been grown.

Differential diagnosis

From other causes of diarrhoea (page 190) especially the dysenteries and carcinoma or Crohn's disease of the large bowel. Differentiation from colonic Crohn's disease may be difficult, even when the resected colon is examined by an expert pathologist. Indeed, about 10 per cent of cases have to be labelled 'non-specific colitis'.

Complications

Local

Toxic dilatation, leading to perforation, haemorrhage (acute, or chronic with progressive anaemia), stricture, malignant change (see below), fistula-in-ano or fistula into the vagina, and perianal abscesses.

General

Toxaemia, loss of weight, anaemia, arthritis, pyoderma, gangrenosum, iritis, skin rashes and ulceration of the legs.

Malignant change in the ulcerative colitis

There is no doubt that the colitic is at far greater risk of developing carcinoma of the large bowel than a normal individual. Moreover, the tumours occuring in the colitics are more likely to affect a younger age group, be anaplastic and be multiple than those arising in previously healthy bowel.

Often the condition is only diagnosed late, since both the patient and his doctor attribute the symptoms (bleeding, diarrhoea and pus) to the colitis.

The risk is greatest in long standing and continuous colitis which affects the whole large bowel, especially if symptoms commence in childhood or adolescence. Statistics of incidence vary widely, but an actuarial study indicates that 12 per cent of patients with colitis of 20 years duration are likely to develop malignant change.

Treatment

Initially this is medical in the uncomplicated case, but surgery is required when medical treatment fails or when complications supervene.

Medical treatment

A high protein diet is prescribed with vitamin supplements, iron and potassium (the last to replace electrolyte loss in the stools). Blood transfusion is given if the patient is severely anaemic. Diarrhoea may be controlled with codeine or Isogel. Corticosteroids given systemically, by rectal infusion or in combination will often produce remission in an acute attack. Sulphasalazine (salazopyrin), a sulphonamide/salicylate compound, is also of value.

Patients with ulcerative colitis are often highly intelligent, tense and anxious, and treatment should be supplemented with simple psychotherapy in the form of sympathy and reassurance.

Surgery

This usually comprises total removal of the colon and rectum with either a permanent ileostomy or an ileo-anal anastomosis with an interposed pouch of ileum. Occasionally the disease of the rectum is relatively mild and the anal sphincter can be preserved with anastomosis between the ileum and rectum (colectomy with ileorectal anastomosis).

The indications for surgery are:
1 Fulminating disease not responding to medical treatment.
2 Chronic disease not responding to medical treatment.
3 In long standing disease as prophylactic against malignant change.
4 The complications of colitis already listed.

Most patients requiring surgery for ulcerative colitis are either on corticosteroids or have recently received them; surgical procedures must be covered by increased dosage of corticosteroids which can then be tailed off gradually in the post-operative period.

CROHN'S DISEASE

Crohn's disease, although most commonly found in the terminal ileum (see page 181) may occur anywhere in the alimentary tract from the mouth to the anus. It may be confined to the large bowel, or there may be involvement of both the small and large intestine.

Clinical features

Colonic Crohn's disease closely mimics ulcerative colitis in its clinical manifestations. However, unlike ulcerative colitis, the affected segment of colon commonly becomes adherent to adjacent structures with abscess formation and fistulation. Perianal inflammation with abscesses and multiple fistulae in ano is also common and indeed, may be the first manifestation of the disease.

Treatment

This is similar to that of Crohn's disease of the small intestine (see page 182). Resection of extensively involved large bowel may require total excision with a permanent ileostomy since the risk of recurrence in anal sphincter-preserving surgery is high.

TUMOURS OF THE COLON

Classification

Benign

      (a) adenomatous polyp
      (b) papilloma
      (c) lipoma
      (d) neurofibroma
      (e) haemangioma

Malignant

    1 *Primary:*
      (a) carcinoma
      (b) lymphoma
      (c) carcinoid tumour (see page 183)
    2 *Secondary:* invasion from adjacent tumours, e.g. stomach, bladder, uterus and ovary.

CARCINOMA OF THE COLON

Pathology

Carcinomas affecting the large bowel are common; they are next in frequency to cancers of the lung and are thus the second commonest cause of death from malignant disease in this country.

Tumours may occur at any age. Females are affected more often than males (although interestingly enough the incidence of rectal cancer is roughly equal in the two sexes). The sigmoid is the commonest site in the colon, although the rectum accounts for one-third of all the large bowel cancers. Five per cent of tumours of the large bowel are multiple.

Predisposing factors

Pre-existing polyps, familial polyposis coli and ulcerative colitis (see above) all predispose to carcinoma of the large bowel.

Familial polyposis coli

This is a rare disease, but it is important because it invariably proceeds to carcinoma of the colon unless treated. Inheritance is by a Mendelian dominant gene, therefore a patient without polyposis will not transmit the disease. The polyps first appear in adolescence, symptoms of bleeding and diarrhoea commence about the age of 21 and malignant change occurs between 20 and 40 years of age.

Treatment comprises a total colectomy with excision of the rectum. If the polyps are not profuse in the lower rectum it is possible to resect the colon, leave a stump of rectum to which an ileo-rectal anastomosis is performed, and then carry out regular diathermy of the polyps in the rectal stump through a sigmoido-scope.

Classification
The tumours can be classified into the following macroscopic groups:
1 Papilliferous;
2 Malignant ulcer;
3 Annular;
4 Diffuse infiltrating growth;
5 Colloid tumour.
Microscopically these are all adenocarcinomas.

Spread
1 *Local:* encircling the wall of the bowel and invading the coats of the colon, eventually involving adjacent viscera (small intestine, stomach, duodenum, ureter, bladder, uterus, abdominal wall, etc.).
2 *Lymphatic:* to the regional lymph nodes, eventually spreading via the thoracic duct, and may involve supraclavicular nodes in late cases.
3 *Blood stream:* to the liver via the portal vein, thence to the lung.
4 *Trans-coelomic spread:* producing deposits of malignant nodules throughout the peritoneal cavity.

Clinical features
The manifestations of carcinoma of the colon can be divided, as with any tumour, into those produced by the tumour itself, by the presence of secondaries, and by the general effects of the tumour.

1. Local effects
The most common symptom is a change in bowel habit, either constipation, diarrhoea or the two alternating with each other. The diarrhoea may be accompa-nied by mucus (produced by the excessive secretion of mucus from the tumour), or bleeding, which may be bright, melaena or occult.

A constricting neoplasm may present with the features of intestinal obstruc-tion, either acute, chronic or acute on chronic (see page 167). Rarely the tumour may present with perforation, either into the general peritoneal cavity or locally with the formation of a pericolic abscess, or by fistulae into adjacent viscera, e.g. a gastrocolic fistula or vesico-colic fistula.

2. The effects of secondary deposits
The patient may present with jaundice, or abdominal distension due to ascites, or with hepatomegaly.

3. The general effects of malignant disease
Presenting features may be anaemia, anorexia or loss of weight.

Typically, tumours of the left side of the colon are constricting growths;

moreover the contained stool is solid, therefore obstructive features predominate. In contrast, tumours of the right side tend to be proliferative and here the stools are semi-liquid, therefore obstructive symptoms are relatively uncommon and the patient with a carcinoma of the caecum or ascending colon often presents with anaemia and loss of weight.

Examination of the patient suspected of carcinoma of the colon should be directed to four main headings:

1 The presence of a mass palpable either per abdomen or per rectum (a sigmoid tumour may prolapse into the pouch of Douglas).

2 Clinical evidence of intestinal obstruction.

3 Evidence of spread (hepatomegaly, ascites, jaundice or supraclavicular nodes).

4 Clinical evidence of anaemia or loss of weight suggesting malignant disease.

Special investigations

1 *Occult blood in the stool* is frequently present.

2 *Sigmoidoscopy* will reveal tumours in the recto-sigmoid region and allow positive evidence by biopsy to be obtained. Even if the tumour is not reached directly, the presence of blood or slime coming down from above is strongly suspicious of malignant disease.

3 *Colonoscopy*, using the fibre-optic colonoscope, enables the higher reaches of the colon to be inspected and a biopsy to be obtained.

4 *A barium enema* will usually reveal the growth, either as a stricture or filling defect ('apple core' deformity). It is important to remember that a negative barium enema does not exclude definitely the presence of a small tumour, moreover false positive X-rays may result from the presence of faecal material in the bowel lumen. It is by no means easy to differentiate radiologically between a carcinomatous stricture and one produced by diverticular disease.

If there is reasonable doubt as to the diagnosis laparotomy is indicated.

Differential diagnosis

1 From diseases producing local symptoms — diverticular disease, ulcerative colitis, the dysenteries and other causes of diarrhoea and constipation (see page 190).

2 From diseases producing similar general manifestations — a useful quintet characterized by anaemia, a rather lemon yellow tinge of the skin, loss of weight and general malaise are: carcinoma of the large bowel, carcinoma of the stomach, carcinoma of the pancreas, uraemia and pernicious anaemia. These five common conditions are often misdiagnosed one for the other (see page 166).

Treatment

The unobstructed operable case

Pre-operative treatment: the bowel is cleared by enemas and oral Picolax. Metronidazole and gentamicin (or a cephalosporin) are given at the time of surgery. The haemoglobin level is checked and blood transfusion given if necessary.

The principle of operative treatment is wide resection of the growth together with its regional lymphatics:

1 Carcinomas of the caecum, ascending colon and hepatic flexure: right hemicolectomy.

2 Carcinoma of the transverse colon: transverse colectomy.

3 Carcinoma of the splenic flexure or descending colon: left hemicolectomy.

4 Carcinoma of the sigmoid colon: sigmoid colectomy.

The obstructed case

The principle here is preliminary relief of the obstruction followed by elective surgery.

1 Carcinoma of the caecum, ascending colon and hepatic flexure: often a primary resection can be performed by means of a right hemicolectomy, since the small intestine above the ileo-caecal valve is usually not distended. (Occasionally a carcinoma of the ascending colon or hepatic flexure is dealt with by a preliminary caecostomy.)

2 Carcinoma of the transverse colon: preliminary caecostomy with later resection of the tumour; occasionally immediate removal of the tumour with double-barrelled colostomy (Paul-Mikulicz procedure).

3 Carcinomas of the splenic flexure, descending or sigmoid colon: preliminary transverse colostomy followed by subsequent resection of the tumour and then closure of the colostomy.

The incurable case

Even if liver secondaries are present, the best palliation is achieved by resection of the primary tumour. If this is impossible, palliative short-circuit or colostomy is performed to relieve the obstruction. Irradiation and cytotoxic therapy may give temporary alleviation.

Chapter 28
The Rectum and Anal Canal

Bright red rectal bleeding

The passage of bright red blood per rectum is a common symptom which the patient usually attributes to 'piles'; indeed haemorrhoids are by far the commonest cause of rectal bleeding. It is important, however, to bear in mind a list of possible causes of this symptom:

General causes

Bleeding diatheses (rare).

Local causes

1 Haemorrhoids.
2 Fissure in ano.
3 Tumours of the colon and rectum
(a) benign
(b) malignant
4 Diverticular disease.
5 Ulcerative colitis.
6 Trauma.
7 Angiodysplasia of the colon.
8 Rarely, massive haemorrhage from higher up the alimentary canal; even a bleeding duodenal ulcer may produce bright red blood PR instead of the usual melaena.

HAEMORRHOIDS

Haemorrhoids, or piles, may be classified according to their relationship to the anal orifice into internal, external and intero-external. Internal haemorrhoids are congested vascular cushions with dilated venous components draining into the superior rectal veins. External haemorrhoids is a term which should be abandoned since it is applied to a conglomeration of quite different entities including perianal haematoma ('thrombosed external pile') the 'sentinel pile' of fissure-in-ano and perianal skin tags. Strictly speaking, internal piles which prolapse should be termed intero-external haemorrhoids, but this term is seldom employed except by literary perfectionists.

In this chapter, which aims at being neither archaic nor pedantic, the terms 'external' and intero-external' haemorrhoids will not be further employed.

Anal continence depends in part on apposition of subepithelial vascular cushions. Internal haemorrhoids are varices of the superior rectal veins which drain into the inferior mesenteric vein. They are thus the nethermost part of the portal system. The swollen tissue consists of the oedematous vascular cushions. In addition to the dilated veins there are prominent small arteries, hence the bright red blood passed in piles.

With the patient in the lithotomy position the usual arrangement is that three major piles occur at 3, 7 and 11 o'clock.

Classification

1 *First degree haemorrhoids* are confined to the anal canal — they bleed but do not prolapse.

2 *Second degree haemorrhoids* prolapse on defaecation, then reduce spontaneously or are replaced digitally by the patient.

3 *Third degree haemorrhoids* remain persistently prolapsed outside the anal margin.

Predisposing factors

Most haemorrhoids are idiopathic, but they may be precipitated or aggravated by factors which produce congestion of the superior rectal veins. These include compression by any pelvic tumour (of which the commonest is the pregnant uterus), cardiac failure, excessive use of purgatives and chronic constipation. Rarely, they may complicate portal hypertension since the pile-bearing area is at the site of portal-systemic anastomosis between the superior and inferior rectal veins. In such cases the piles are often thin walled veins as are the varices in the oesophagus.

Clinical features

Rectal bleeding is almost invariable; this is bright red and usually occurs at defaecation.

In the case of first degree piles this is the only symptom. More extensive piles prolapse and may produced a mucous discharge and pruritus ani.

Note that pain is not a feature of internal haemorrhoids except when these undergo thrombosis (see below). When a patient complains of 'an attack of piles' he often means that he has developed some acute painful condition at the anal margin. Apart from thrombosed internal piles the common causes of such anal pain to be considered are:

1 Fissure-in-ano.

2 Perianal haematoma.

3 Perianal or ischiorectal abscess.

4 Tumour of the anal margin.

5 Proctalgia fugax.

Every patient presenting with the story suggestive of internal haemorrhoids is submitted to the following procedure:

1 Examination of the abdomen to exclude palpable lesions of the colon or aggravating factors for haemorrhoids, e.g. an enlarged liver or a pelvic mass.

2 Rectal examination. Internal haemorrhoids are not palpable but prolapsing piles are immediately obvious. The presence of prolapsing piles does not exclude a lesion higher in the bowel.

3 Protoscopy, which will visualize the internal haemorrhoids.

4   Sigmoidoscopy is performed routinely, again to eliminate a lesion higher in the rectum — proctitis, polyp or carcinoma.

5   A barium enema is carried out in any case where symptoms such as alteration in bowel habit point to some more sinister condition than internal haemorrhoids.

6   Colonoscopy may be indicated to visualize and biopsy any lesion thus revealed.

Complications

1   Anaemia — following severe or continued bleeding.

2   Thrombosis: this occurs when prolapsing piles are gripped by the anal sphincter ('strangulated piles'); the venous return is occluded and thrombosis of the pile occurs. The prolapsed haemorrhoids are swollen often to the size of large plums, purplish black and tense, and are accompanied by considerable pain. Suppuration or ulceration may occur. After 2 or 3 weeks the thrombosed piles become fibrosed, often with spontaneous cure.

Treatment

Before commencing treatment it is essential to exclude either any predisposing cause or an associated and more important lesion, e.g. carcinoma of the rectum.

Injection treatment

This is suitable for first and second degree piles. 2 to 3 ml of 5 per cent phenol in almond oil is injected above each pile as a sclerosing submucous perivenous injection (The phenol sterilizes the oil which is the main sclerosant). Since the injection is placed high in the anal canal it is painless. One or more repeat injections may be required at monthly intervals. Occasionally, injection treatment is used for more extensive haemorrhoids in elderly patients or those unfit for operative treatment, purely as a palliative measure.

Lord's procedure

Digital dilatation to four fingers of the anal sphincter under general anaesthesia often results in marked improvement of second and third degree piles but can impair continence.

Surgery

Haemorrhoidectomy is performed for extensive third degree piles.

Conservative management

Is instituted for thrombosed strangulated piles. The patient is placed in bed with the foot of the bed elevated. Morphia is given for the severe pain which is also eased by local cold compresses. Often the thrombosed piles fibrose completely with spontaneous cure. At other times residual piles or fibrous tags may require excision 2 or 3 months later. Operation is said to be contraindicated in the acute and infected stage because of the possible risk of portal pyaemia but many surgeons now carry out haemorrhoidectomy at once in these patients.

Specific complications of haemorrhoidectomy

Acute retention of urine
> Due to the acute anal discomfort post-operatively.

Stricture
> This only occurs when excessive amounts of mucosa and skin are excised. It is important to leave a bridge of epithelium between each excised haemorrhoid.

Post-operative haemorrhage
> This may be reactionary, usually on the night of the operation, or secondary, about the seventh or eight day. The bleeding may not be apparent externally since the source of haemorrhage may be above the anal sphincter; blood may fill the large bowel with only a little escaping to the exterior.
>
> *General treatment* comprises blood transfusion if haemorrhage is severe as evidenced by the general appearance of the patient, a pulse raised above 100 and a blood pressure below 100.
>
> *Local treatment* is carried out under general anaesthetic in the operating theatre. The blood is washed out of the rectum with warm saline. Occasionally in reactionary haemorrhage a bleeding point is seen and can be tied. More often there is a general oozing from the operation field and the anal canal requires packing with gauze round a wide-bored rubber tube which allows evacuation of flatus and escape of any blood from the bowel. The tube and gauze are removed after 48 hours.

PERIANAL HAEMATOMA
> This lesion, which is also termed a thrombosed external pile, is produced by thrombosis within the inferior rectal venous plexus. Unlike internal haemorrhoids, it is covered by squamous epithelium supplied by somatic nerves and is therefore painful. The onset is acute, often after straining at stools, with sudden pain and the appearance of a lump at the anal verge. Local examination shows a tense, smooth, dark blue, cherry-sized lump at the anal margin.
>
> Untreated, this perianal haematoma either subsides over a few days, eventually leaving a fibrous tag, or ruptures, discharging some clotted blood.

Treatment
> In the acute phase immediate relief is produced by evacuating the haematoma through a small incision; this can be done conveniently under local anaesthetic. If seen when the haematoma is already discharging or becoming absorbed, hot baths are prescribed and the patient reassured that all will soon be well.

ANAL FISSURE
> A tear at the anal margin which usually follows the passage of a constipated stool. The site is usually posterior in the mid-line (90 per cent of males, 70 per cent of females), occasionally anterior in the mid-line, and rarely multiple. The posterior

position of the majority of fissures is explained by the anatomical arrangement of the external anal sphincter; its superficial fibres pass forward to the anal canal from the coccyx, leaving a relatively unsupported V posteriorly. The anterior fissures of females may be associated with weakening of the perineal floor following tears at childbirth. Multiple fissures may complicate Crohn's disease of the colon.

Clinical features

Acute anal pain is characteristic; fissure is the commonest cause of pain at the anal verge (see list page 203). There is often slight bleeding, and, because of the pain, the patient is usually constipated. On examination the anal sphincter is in spasm, and there may be a 'sentinel pile' protruding from the anus which represents the torn tag of anal epithelium. The fissure can usually be seen by gently pulling open the anal verge. It may be impossible to do a rectal examination without first inserting a pledget of wool soaked in local anaesthetic; the fissure may then be palpable as a crack in the anal canal.

Treatment

Early small fissures may heal spontaneously. A local anaesthetic ointment is prescribed together with a lubricant aperient. A lubricated plastic dilator inserted twice a day for 5 minutes may give relief.

More intractable cases usually respond to stretching the anal sphincter or dividing the internal sphincter submucosally under general anaesthetic. This temporarily paralyses the muscle and allows the rested parts to heal.

A chronic recurring fissure-in-ano requires excision.

ANO-RECTAL ABSCESSES

Classification (Fig. 28.1)

1 *Perianal:* resulting from infection of a hair follicle, a sebaceous gland or peri-anal haematoma.
2 *Ischio-rectal:* from infection of an anal gland leading from the anal canal into the submucosa, spread of infection from a peri-anal abscess or penetration of the ischio-rectal fossa by a foreign body. The abscess may track as a horse-shoe behind the rectum to the opposite ischio-rectal fossa.
3 *Submucous:* infected fissure or laceration of the anal canal, infection after injection of a haemorrhoid.
4 *Pelvi-rectal:* spread from pelvic abscess (rare).

Treatment

Early surgical drainage to prevent rupture and the possible formation of a fistula-in-ano.

FISTULA-IN-ANO

Definitions

1 A *fistula* is an abnormal communication between two epithelial surfaces, e.g.

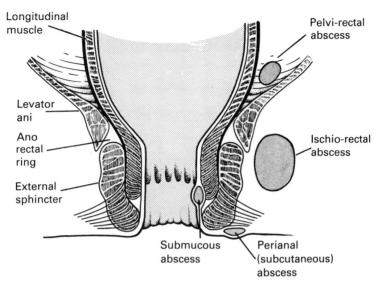

Fig. 28.1. The anatomy of peri-anal abscesses.

between a hollow viscus and the surface of the body or between two hollow viscera.

2 *A sinus* is a granulating track leading from a source of infection to a surface.

Aetiology

The term fistula-in-ano is loosely applied to both fistulae and sinuses in relation to the anal canal. The great majority result from an initial abscess forming in one of the anal glands which pass from the submucosa of the anal canal to open within its lumen. Rarely fistulae are associated with tuberculosis, Crohn's disease, ulcerative colitis and carcinoma of the rectum.

Anatomical classification (Fig. 28.2)

1 Subcutaneous.
2 Submucous.
3 Low anal.
4 High anal.
5 Ano-rectal.

Subcutaneous and submucous fistulae are superficial tracks resulting from rupture respectively of subcutaneous and submucous abscesses. Anal fistulae have their tracks below the ano-rectal ring. Most of these are at a low level, the track passing through the subcutaneous part of the sphincter, but some are high level, opening in close relation to the ano-rectal junction. Ano-rectal fistulae, fortunately rare, extend above the ano-rectal junction. Fistulae with external openings posterior to the meridian in the lithotomy position usually open in the mid-line of the anus, whilst those with anterior external openings usually open directly into the anus — Goodsall's law.

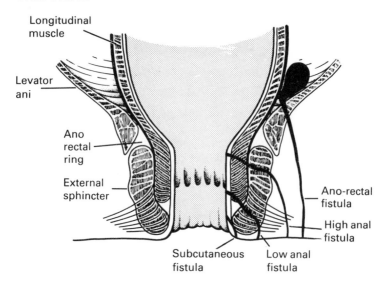

Fig. 28.2. The anatomy of perianal fistulae.

Clinical features

There is usually a story of an initial ano-rectal abscess which discharges. Following this there are recurrent episodes of perianal infection with persistent discharge of pus. Examination reveals the external opening of a fistula. The internal opening may be felt per rectum, but probing of the track is painful and should be deferred until the patient is anaesthetized.

Treatment

Subcutaneous, submucous and low-level anal fistulae are laid open and allowed to heal by granulation. Since either no sphincter or only the subcutaneous part of the external sphincter is divided in this procedure there is no loss of anal continence. High-level fistulae can only be treated in this manner when they quite definitely lie below the level of the ano-rectal ring; if this is divided there is the risk of faecal incontinence. In high fistulae, therefore, only the lower part of the fistula is laid open, a non-absorbable stout ligature is passed through the upper part of the track and left in place for 2 or 3 weeks so that the sphincter is fixed by scar tissue by the time of subsequent division of the upper part of the tract at a second operation.

STRICTURE OF THE ANAL CANAL

Classification

1 Congenital.

2 Traumatic, particularly post-operative, after too radical excision of the skin and mucosa in haemorrhoidectomy.

3 Inflammatory — lymphogranuloma inguinale (mostly female), Crohn's disease, ulcerative colitis.

4 Post-irradiation

5 Infiltrating neoplasm.

Treatment

Depends on the underlying pathology and may call for repeated dilatation, plastic reconstruction, defunctioning colostomy or, in the case of malignant disease, excision of the rectum.

PROLAPSE OF THE RECTUM

This may be partial or complete.

Partial prolapse is confined to the mucosa which prolapses an inch or two from the anal verge. Palpation of the prolapse between the finger and thumb reveals obviously that there is no muscular wall within it. It may occur in infants who, unlike the usual text-book description, are not wasted but often perfectly healthy. Treatment is these babies requires nothing more than reassurance of the parents that the condition is self-curing. In adults it usually accompanies prolapsing piles or sphincter incompetence.

Complete prolapse involves all layers of the rectal wall. It usually occurs in elderly females. Apart from the discomfort of the prolapse there is associated incontinence due to the stretching of the sphincter and mucous discharge from the prolapsed mucosal surface.

Treatment

Treatment of partial prolapse in adults comprises haemorrhoidectomy, excision of the redundant mucosa or a submucosal phenol in oil injection in order to produce sclerosis. In children, as we have already mentioned, self cure without active treatment is the fortunate rule.

Many methods have been described for dealing with complete prolapse. If the patient is particularly feeble and old, the Thiersch wire operation is performed; a wire suture (or preferably one of braided nylon) is passed around the anal orifice to narrow this and keep the prolapse reduced. In fitter patients the rectum is fixed in the pelvis by an abdominal operation; a convenient method is to wrap the mobilized rectum in polyvinyl sponge, which produces a brisk fibrous reaction welding the rectum to the pelvic tissues. Excision of the prolapsed portion of the rectum (rectosigmoidectomy) has a prohibitively high recurrence rate but a modification of mucosal excision and bunching of the bowel muscle to form a doughnut-like ring is becoming popular.

PRURITUS ANI

The clinical varieties of pruritus ani are:

1 Those due to local causes within the anus or rectum; any factor which causes moisture and sogginess of the anal skin, e.g. lack of cleanliness, excessive sweating, leakage of mucus from haemorrhoids, proctitis, colitis, rectal neoplasm or threadworms.

2 Skin diseases: scabies, pediculosis, fungal infections, *Candida albicans*.

3 General diseases associated with pruritus: diabetes mellitus, Hodgkin's disease, obstructive jaundice.

4 Idiopathic: here very often the original cause has disappeared but the pruritus persists because of continued scratching of the anal region by the patient.

Treatment

Directed to the underlying cause. The idiopathic group often responds dramatically to hydrocortisone ointment and attention to local hygiene.

TUMOURS OF THE RECTUM AND ANAL CANAL

Pathology

Benign

    (a) adenoma
    (b) papilloma
    (c) lipoma
    (d) endometrioma

Malignant

1 *Primary:*
    (a) adenocarcinoma
    (b) squamous carcinoma of lower anal canal
    (c) melanoma
    (d) carcinoid tumour
    (e) rodent ulcer of anal verge
    (f) lymphoma
2 *Secondary:* invasion from prostate, uterus or pelvic peritoneal deposits.

CARCINOMA OF THE RECTUM

Pathology

The sexes are equally affected. It occurs in any age group from the twenties onwards, but it particularly common in the age range 50 to 70. Carcinoma of the rectum accounts for approximately one-third of all tumours of the large intestine. Predisposing factors (as with carcinoma of the colon) are pre-existing adenomas, familial polyposis and ulcerative colitis.

Macroscopic appearance

The tumours may be:
1 Papilliferous.
2 Ulcerating (commonest).
3 Stenosing (usually at recto-sigmoid).
4 Colloid.

Microscopic appearance

About 90 per cent are adenocarcinomas. Another 9 per cent are colloid (adenocarcinoma with profuse production of mucus) and the remainder are the highly anaplastic carcinoma simplex. At the anal verge squamous carcinoma may occur, but a malignant tumour protruding through the anal canal is more likely to be an adenocarcinoma of the rectum invading the anal skin.

Spread

1 *Local:*
   (a) circumferentially around the lumen of the bowel
   (b) invasion through the muscular coat
   (c) penetration into adjacent organs, e.g. prostate, bladder, vagina, uterus, sacrum, sacral plexus, ureters, and lateral pelvic wall

2 *Lymphatic:* to regional lymph nodes along the inferior mesenteric vessels. At a late stage there is invasion of the iliac lymph nodes and of the groin lymph nodes (by retrograde spread) and involvement of the supraclavicular nodes via the thoracic duct.

3 *Blood:* via the superior rectal venous plexus, thence the portal vein to the liver and then lungs.

4 *Transcoelomic:* seeding of the peritoneal cavity.

The extent of spread of rectal tumours is conveniently classified by Dukes' method (Fig. 28.3):

   (A) The tumour is confined to the rectal wall, with no spread beyond its muscle layers.
   (B) The growth has completely breached the rectal wall.
   (C) The regional lymph nodes are involved.
   (D) Distant spread has occurred, e.g. to the liver.

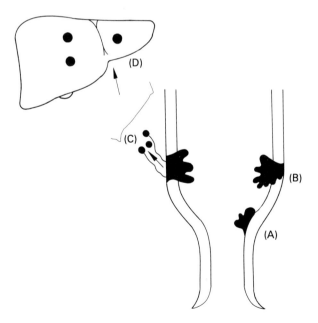

Fig. 28.3. Dukes' classification of tumours of the large bowel: (A) confined to the bowel wall; (B) penetrating wall; (C) involving regional lymph nodes; (D) distal spread.

Prognosis

Depends largely on the stage of progression of the tumour and its histological degree of differentiation. The more advanced its spread and the more anaplastic its cells the worse the prognosis.

Clinical features

The patient may present with:

1 Local disturbances due to the presence of the tumour in the rectum.
2 Manifestations of secondary deposits.
3 The general effects of malignant disease.

Features 2 and 3 need not be repeated since they are similar to those of carcinoma of the colon (page 199) with the addition that rarely carcinoma of the rectum may spread to the groin nodes as a late phenomenon. With carcinoma at the anal verge this commonly occurs.

Local symptoms are: bowel disturbance (constipation and/or diarrhoea occur in 80 per cent of cases), and bleeding, which is almost invariable and is the presenting complaint in about 60 per cent of patients. There may also be mucous discharge, rectal pain and tenesmus.

Abdominal palpation is negative in early cases, but careful attention must be paid to the detection of hepatomegaly, ascites or abdominal distension. Other general features which may be detected in late cases are enlarged supraclavicular nodes, nodes in the groin or jaundice.

Rectal examination reveals the tumour in 90 per cent of cases.

Sigmoidoscopy enables the great majority of tumours to be inspected and a biopsy to be taken.

Barium enema is indicated if the growth is not visualized sigmoidoscopically, if a second tumour is suspected (5 per cent of tumours in the large bowel are multiple), or if there is ulcerative colitis or familial polyposis.

Differential diagnosis

Differential diagnosis of a palpable tumour in the rectum must be made from:

1 Benign tumours.
2 Carcinoma of the sigmoid colon prolapsing into the pouch of Douglas and felt through the mucosal wall.
3 Secondary deposits in the pelvis.
4 Ovarian or uterine tumours.
5 Extension from carcinoma of the prostate or cervix.
6 Endometriosis.
7 Lymphogranuloma inguinale.
8 Amoebic granuloma.
9 Diverticular disease.
10 The rare malignant tumours of the rectum (see page 210).
11 Faeces (these give the classical physical sign of indentation).

The beginner may mistake the normal cervix for a palpable tumour, and should not be caught out by the presence of a ring pessary or tampon in the vagina, which are readily felt per rectum.

Treatment

Curative

Abdomino-perineal excision of the rectum or, if the growth is high enough to allow satisfactory clearance distally, resection of the rectum can be performed with restorative anastomosis between the sigmoid colon and the lower rectum.

Palliative procedures

Even if secondaries are present, palliation is best achieved when possible by excision of the primary tumour. A colostomy may be necessary for intestinal obstruction, but this does not relieve the bleeding, mucous discharge and sacral pain.

In completely inoperable cases deep X-ray therapy or diathermy of the tumour may give temporary relief as may cytotoxic drugs.

Management of a colostomy

In the first few weeks after performing a colostomy the faecal discharge is semi-liquid, but this gradually reverts to normal, solid stools. Thanks to the development of adhesive colostomy appliances, which are both water-proof and wind-proof, the patient can lead a normal life with little risk of leakage or unpleasant odour.

Although there is obviously no sphincteric control of the colostomy opening, most patients find that they pass a single stool a day, usually after breakfast. This can be helped by preparations such as Celevac, which produce a bulky, formed stool. Patients are best advised to avoid large amounts of vegetables or fruit which may produce diarrhoea.

Some surgeons advocate daily colostomy washouts in order to clear the lower bowel. However, these are time consuming, there is risk of perforating the colon the enema tube and patients usually achieve a reasonable colostomy life without their aid.

Complications of colostomy include:

Retraction, perforation (from an enema tube), sloughing (due to inadequate blood supply), lateral space small bowel obstruction (due to failure to obliterate the space between the terminal colon and the lateral abdominal wall), stenosis, prolapse and incisional paracolostomy hernia, which is difficult to repair.

Chapter 29
Peritonitis

Aetiology

Bacteria may enter the peritoneal cavity via four portals:

1 *From the exterior:* penetrating wound or infection at laparotomy.

2 *From intra-abdominal viscera*

(a) gangrene of a viscus, e.g. acute appendicitis, acute cholecystitis, diverticulitis or infarction of the intestine.

(b) perforation of a viscus, e.g. perforated duodenal ulcer, perforated appendicitis, rupture of intestine from trauma

(c) post-operative leakage of an intestinal suture line

3 *Via the blood stream:* as part of a septicaemia (pneumococcal, streptococcal or staphylococcal). This has been badly termed primary peritonitis; in fact it is secondary to some initial source of infection.

4 *Via the female genital tract:* acute salpingitis or puerperal infection.

Approximately 30 per cent of all cases of peritonitis in adults result from post-operative complications, 20 per cent from acute appendicitis and 20 per cent from a perforated peptic ulcer. These are the 3 headliners.

Pathology

Peritonitis of bowel origin usually shows a mixed flora (*Escherichia coli, Streptococcus faecalis, Pseudomonas,* and *Proteus,* together with the anaerobic *Clostridia* and *Bacteroides*). Gynaecological infections may be gonococcal or streptococcal. Blood-borne peritonitis may be streptococcal, pneumococcal, staphylococcal or tuberculous. In young children a rare gynaecological infection is due to the pneumococcus.

The pathological effects of peritonitis are:

1 Widespread absorption of toxins from the large, inflamed surface.

2 The associated paralytic ileus (page 221) with:

(a) loss of fluid

(b) loss of electrolytes

(c) loss of protein

3 Gross abdominal distension with elevation of the diaphragm, which produces a liability to lung collapse and pneumonia.

Clinical features

Peritonitis is inevitably secondary to some precipitating lesion which may itself have definite clinical features, for example the onset may be an attack of acute appendicitis, or a perforated duodenal ulcer, with appropriate symptoms and signs.

Early peritonitis is characterized by severe pain; the patient wishes to lie still because any movement aggravates the agony. Irritation of the diaphragm may be accompanied by pain referred to the shoulder tip. Vomiting is frequent. The temperature is usually elevated and the pulse rises progressively. Examination at this time shows localized or generalized tenderness, depending on the extent of the peritonitis. The abdominal wall is held rigidly and rebound tenderness is present. The abdomen is silent or the transmitted sounds of the heart beat and respiration may be detected. Rectal examination may show tenderness in the pouch of Douglas.

In advanced peritonitis the abdomen becomes distended and tympanitic, signs of free fluid are present, the patient becomes increasingly toxic with a rapid, feeble pulse, vomiting is faeculent and the skin is moist, cold and cyanosed (the Hippocratic facies).

Investigations

These are of only limited value; diagnosis depends on the clinical features. X-ray of the chest and abdomen may reveal free gas in cases of a perforated abdominal viscus (70 per cent of perforated peptic ulcers show gas under the diaphragm). An X-ray of the chest is of aid in excluding pulmonary infection as a differential diagnosis and a serum amylase helps differentiate acute pancreatitis. There is usually a marked leucocytosis.

Differential diagnosis

This is from intestinal obstruction and from ureteric or biliary colic, in all of which the patient tends to be restless. Basal pneumonia, myocardial infarction, intraperitoneal haemorrhage or leakage of an aortic aneurysm are other fairly common misdiagnoses.

Principles of treatment

In this section an outline of treatment only is given, since specific causes of peritonitis may require specific therapy; these are dealt with in their appropriate chapters.

1 *Relieve pain* by means of morphia.

2 *Gastric aspiration* by means of naso-gastric tube; this reduces the risk of inhalation of vomit under anaesthesia and prevents further abdominal distension by removing swallowed air.

3 *Fluid and electrolyte replacement* by intravenous therapy; blood or blood substitutes may be required in the presence of shock.

4 *Antibiotic therapy*, usually to deal with the broad spectrum of bowel organisms, for example gentamicin and metronidazole, but therapy is guided, where possible, by checking the sensitivity of the responsible organisms.

5 *Surgery* is indicated if the source of infection can be removed or closed, for example, the repair of a perforated ulcer or removal of the gangrenous, perforated appendix.

Any localized collection of pus requires drainage and later surgery may be required for the evacuation of residual abscesses, for example, subphrenic or pelvic collections.

Conservative treatment is indicated, at least initially, where the infection has been localized, for example an appendix mass, or where the primary focus is irremoveable, as in pancreatitis or post-partum infection. Where the patient is moribund or where there are lack of surgical facilities, as on board ship, reliance is placed on intravenous therapy, gastric aspiration and antibiotics.

SPECIAL VARIETIES OF PERITONITIS

Pneumococcal peritonitis

This may be secondary to the septicaemia accompanying a pneumococcal lung infection, or, uncommonly these days, may result from an ascending infection from the vagina in girls between the age of 4 and 10.

Clinically there is peritonitis of sudden onset accompanied by severe toxaemia and fever. The white count is elevated above 20 000 per mm^3.

Treatment

Usually laparotomy is performed since a perforated appendicitis is suspected. Clear or turbid fluid containing fibrin flakes is discovered without an obvious primary cause. A slide made of the pus shows the characteristic Gram-positive pneumococci lying in pairs. The condition responds to penicillin therapy.

Haemolytic streptococcal peritonitis

This may occur in children, secondary or streptococcal infection of the tonsil, otitis media, scarlet fever or erysipelas.

Staphylococcal peritonitis

This very rarely complicates staphyloccal septicaemia, which more often produces intra-abdominal or perinephric abscesses.

Tuberculous peritonitis

Tuberculous peritonitis is always secondary to tuberculosis elsewhere although the primary focus may no longer be active. It usually occurs as a result of local spread from the mesenteric lymph nodes or via the female genital tract, although it may complicate generalized miliary tuberculosis.

With the diminution of tuberculosis elsewhere, tuberculous peritonitis is becoming increasingly rare in this country. It may still be seen, however, in immigrants from Third World countries and patients with AIDS.

Pathology

The peritoneum is studded with tubercles in the initial phase, with an accompanying serous effusion. Later the tubercles coalesce, local abscesses may develop and the intra-abdominal viscera become matted together with dense fibrous adhesions.

Clinical features

Three forms are recognized; the acute, the ascitic and the plastic, but the demarcation between them is not sharp.

The *acute* has a sudden onset which mimics general peritonitis; at laparotomy the peritoneum is found to be studded with miliary tubercles and free fluid is present.

The *ascitic type* has a more gradual onset with increasing abdominal distension and signs of free fluid (*note the five main causes of patients presenting with ascites: heart failure, renal failure, liver failure, carcinomatosis and chronic peritonitis*).

The *plastic type* is the stage of gross adhesion formation; the patient may present with intestinal obstruction. The abdomen is swollen, either due to distended loops of intestine, local collections of fluid or to the thickened omentum, which may form a transverse mass across the upper abdomen. Diagnosis is usually made only at operation.

Treatment

Comprises antituberculous chemotherapy. Operation may be required for the relief of intestinal obstruction from adhesions.

Bile peritonitis

May occur as a result of :

1   Traumatic rupture of the gall bladder or its ducts (gunshot wound or closed injury, iatrogenic damage from liver biopsy or percutaneous cholangiography).
2   Leakage from the liver, gall bladder or its ducts after a biliary tract operation.
3   Perforation of the acutely inflamed gall bladder.
4   Transudation of the bile through a gangrenous but non-perforated gall bladder.
5   Spontaneous perforation of the gall bladder.
6   Idiopathic — a rare but well-recognized condition in which bile peritonitis occurs without obvious causes, possibly a small perforation due to a calculus which then becomes sealed.

Bile peritonitis is only a rare accompaniment of acute cholecystitis, because unlike the appendix, which when inflamed rapidly undergoes gangrene, the inflamed gall bladder is usually thickened and walled off by adhesions. In addition, again unlike the appendix, which only receives an end-artery supply from the ileo-colic artery, the gall bladder has an additional blood supply from the liver bed, therefore frank gangrene of the inflamed gall bladder is unusual.

The patient presents with all the features of general peritonitis. Laparotomy is required to deal with the underlying cause, but the mortality is approximately 50 per cent. As with all other causes of peritonitis, not surprisingly it is the elderly patient with late disease who does badly.

LOCALIZED INTRAPERITONEAL COLLECTIONS OF PUS

Following peritonitis, pus may collect in the subphrenic spaces or in the pelvis.

SUBPHRENIC ABSCESS

Anatomy (Fig. 29.1)

The subphrenic region lies between the diaphragm above and the transverse colon

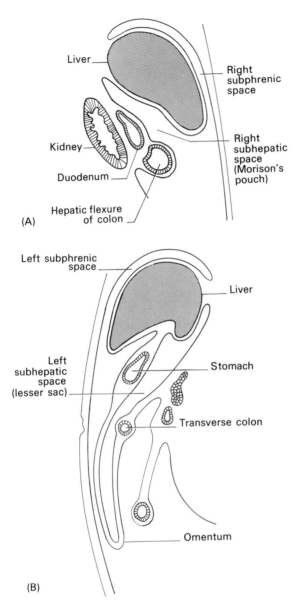

Fig. 29.1. (A) The anatomy of the subphrenic spaces. (A) right; (B) left.

with mesocolon below and is divided further by the liver and its ligaments. The right and left *subphrenic spaces* lie between the diaphragm and the liver and are separated from each other by the falciform ligament. The right and left *subheptic spaces* are below the liver, the right forming Morison's pouch and the left being the lesser sac which communicates with the former through the foramen of Winslow. The right *extra-peritoneal space* lies between the bare area of the liver and the diaphragm. About two thirds of subphrenic abscesses occur on the right side. Rarely, they are bilateral.

Aetiology

A localized collection of pus may occur in the subphrenic region following general peritonitis. Usually the underlying cause is a peritonitis involving the upper abdomen — leakage following biliary or gastric surgery or a perforated peptic ulcer. Rarely, infection occurs from haematogenous spread or from direct spread from a primary chest lesion, e.g. empyema.

Clinical features

Subphrenic infection usually follows general peritonitis after 10 to 21 days, although if antibiotics have been given an abscess may be disguised and may only become manifest weeks or even months after the original episode. There may be no localizing symptoms, the patient presenting with malaise, nausea, loss of weight, anaemia and pyrexia; hence the aphorism 'pus somewhere, pus nowhere else, pus under the diaphragm'. At least half the cases have a fever which continues from the original peritonitis, although the standard description is of a swinging temperature which commences some 10 days after the initial illness.

Localizing features are: pain in the upper abdomen, lower chest or referred to the shoulder with localized upper abdominal or chest wall tenderness. There may be signs of fluid or collapse at the lung base. In late cases a swelling may be detected over the lower chest wall or upper abdomen.

Special investigations

The white count is raised in the region of 15 000 to 20 000 with a polymorph leucocytosis.

The important initial investigation is screening of the chest, which reveals an abnormality in nearly all cases. The radiological signs are (Fig. 29.2):
1 Elevation of the diaphragm on the affected side.
2 Diminished or absent mobility of the diaphragm.
3 Pleural effusion and/or collapse of the lung base.
4 Gas and a fluid level below the diaphragm.
Accurate localization may be achieved by ultrasound or a CT scan.

Treatment

In early cases, where there is absence of gas and free fluid on X-ray, the patient is placed on broad spectrum antibiotic therapy. If there is rapid response the diagnosis is one of a spreading cellulitis of the subphrenic space. If there is clinical or radiological evidence of a localized abscess, or if resolution fails to occur on chemotherapy, percutaneous drainage may be carried out under ultrasound or CT control. If this fails, or if the abscess is loculated, surgical drainage is performed. Depending on the localized of the abscess, this is carried out either by a posterior extraperitoneal approach through the bed of, or below, the 12th rib, or an anterior approach via a subcostal incision.

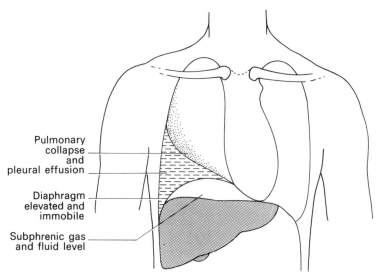

Fig. 29.2. Diagram of the radiological appearance of a right subphrenic abscess. The diaphragm is raised (and fixed on screening), a fluid level is present beneath it and there is a sympathetic pleural effusion with compression — collapse of the lung base.

The image is labelled:

Pulmonary collapse and pleural effusion

Diaphragm elevated and immobile

Subphrenic gas and fluid level

PELVIC ABSCESS

A pelvic abscess may follow any general peritonitis, but it is particularly common after acute appendicitis (75 per cent), or after gynaecological infections. In the male the abscess lies between the bladder and the rectum, in the female between the uterus and posterior fornix of the vagina anteriorly, and the rectum posteriorly (pouch of Douglas).

Left untreated the abscess may burst into the rectum or vagina, or may discharge onto the abdominal wall, particularly if there has been a previous abdominal laparotomy incision at the time of the original episode of peritonitis. Occasionally the abscess may rupture into the peritoneal cavity.

Clinical features

1 *General* — swinging pyrexia, toxaemia, weight loss with leucocytosis.

2 *Local* — diarrhoea, mucous discharge per rectum, the presence of a mass felt on rectal or vaginal examination, which is occasionally large enough to be palpated abdominally.

Treatment

An early pelvic cellulitis may respond rapidly to a short course of chemotherapy, but there is the risk that the prolonged antibiotic treatment of an unresolved infection may produce a chronic inflammatory mass studded with small abscess cavities in the pelvis. It is safer therefore, where there is an established pelvic abscess, to withhold chemotherapy and await pointing into the vagina or rectum through which surgical drainage can be carried out. Very often even this is not required since firm pressure by the finger in the rectum may be followed by rupture of the abscess through the rectal wall.

Chapter 30
Paralytic Ileus

The word ileus comes from the Greek verb 'to roll', from which it became applied to colic and hence to obstruction. Obstructions are sub-divided into mechanical and paralytic, which is produced by lack of intestinal motility. It is therefore a bad habit to say that a patient has 'an ileus' when one really means a 'paralytic ileus', since the word ileus alone implies merely intestinal obstruction.

Paralytic (or adynamic or neurogenic) ileus can be defined as a state of atony of the intestine. Its principal clinical features are:
1   Abdominal distension.
2   Absolute constipation.
3   Vomiting.
4   Absence of intestinal movements.

Aetiology
The state of paralytic ileus may be produced by a large number of factors, sometimes coexisting with each other:

Reflex

Probably as a result of interference with the autonomic nerve supply of the gut; it may complicate fractures of the spine or pelvis, application of a plaster cast, retroperitoneal haemorrhage and retroperitoneal surgery, ureteric colic and occasionally parturition.

Peritonitis

Perhaps as a result of toxic paralysis of intrinsic nerve plexuses, the bowel in peritonitis becomes atonic. There may be an associated mechanical obstruction produced by kinking of loops of bowel by fibrinous adhesions, so that frequently the paralytic ileus is complicated by mechanical obstruction.

Metabolic

Severe potassium depletion, uraemia and diabetic coma.

Drugs

Paralytic ileus is produced by heavy dosage of ganglion blocking drugs (e.g. hexamethonium) and anticholinergic agents (e.g. Pro-Banthine).

Post-operative

Some degree of paralytic ileus occurs after every laparotomy. Its aetiology is complex, including sympathetic overaction, the effects of manipulation of the bowel, potassium depletion (where there has been excessive pre-operative vomiting), peritoneal irritation from blood or associated peritonitis and the atony of stomach and the large bowel which occurs after every abdominal operation for a period of some 24 to 48 hours.

The distension which occurs on the first and second post-operative day is probably produced by swallowed air passing through the small intestine, where peristalsis usually remains fairly normal post-operatively, to the colon, which is atonic and produces a functional hold up. Paralytic ileus which persists for more than 48 hours post-operatively probably has some other aetiological factor present.

The deleterious effects of paralytic ileus are similar to those of a simple mechanical obstruction:

1 There is severe loss of fluid, electrolytes and protein into the gut lumen and in the vomitus or gastric aspirate.

2 Gross gaseous distention of the gut, produced mainly from swallowed air which cannot pass through the bowel, impairs the blood supply of the bowel wall and allows toxic absorption to occur.

Clinical features

Paralytic ileus is most commonly seen in the post-operative stage of peritonitis or of major abdominal surgery. There is abdominal distension, absolute constipation and effortless vomiting. Pain is not present, apart from the discomfort of the laparotomy wound and the abdominal distension. On examination the patient is anxious and uncomfortable. The abdomen is distended, silent and tender. A plain X-ray of the abdomen will show gas distributed throughout the small and large gut and some fluid levels may be present.

The paralytic ileus may merge insidiously into a mechanical obstruction produced by adhesions or bands following abdominal surgery, and an important, often extremely difficult, differential diagnosis lies between these two conditions. The diagnosis is important since paralytic ileus is treated conservatively whereas mechanical obstruction usually calls for urgent operation.

Differential diagnosis

The differential diagnosis from mechanical obstruction (see page 169) is based on the following points:

1 Paralytic ileus rarely lasts more than 3 or 4 days; persistence of symptoms after this time is suspicious of mechanical obstruction.

2 The presence of bowel sounds is important; an absolutely silent abdomen is diagnostic of paralytic ileus, whereas noisy bowel sounds indicate mechanical obstruction.

3 Paralytic ileus is relatively painless, whereas colicky abdominal pain is present in mechanical obstruction.

4 If symptoms commence after the patient has already passed flatus or had a bowel action it is very likely that a mechanical obstruction has supervened. The other possibility to consider is that there has been a leakage from an anastomosis and that peritonitis is now present.

5 A plain X-ray of the abdomen showing a localized loop of distended small

intestine without gas shadows in the colon or rectum is strongly suggestive of mechanical obstruction, in contrast to the diffuse appearance of gas throughout the small and large bowel in paralytic ileus.

Treatment

Prophylaxis: biochemical imbalance is corrected pre-operatively. The bowel is handled gently at operation. Post-operatively gastric distension by air swallowing may require naso-gastric suction.

In the established case naso-gastric suction is employed to remove swallowed air and prevent gaseous distension. The aspiration of fluid also helps to relieve the associated gastric dilatation. The Miller-Abbot tube is so difficult to pass through the atonic bowel that most surgeons have abandoned its use.

Intravenous fluid and electrolyte therapy is instituted with careful biochemical control. Pethidine and chlorpromazine are used to allay discomfort and nausea. Eventually patience is rewarded and recovery from the ileus will occur unless it is secondary to some underlying cause, such as infection.

In the absence of any evidence of mechanical obstruction or infection, prolonged stubborn ileus is occasionally treated pharmacologically by means of guanethidine to block sympathetic inhibition of the intestine, followed by parasympathetic stimulation, either with a cholinergic agent (bethanecol chloride) or an anticholinesterase drug (e.g. prostigmin).

Chapter 31
Hernia

GENERAL CONSIDERATIONS

A hernia is a protrusion of any viscus or part of a viscus through its coverings into an abnormal situation. Most hernias occur as diverticula of the peritoneal cavity and therefore have a sac of parietal peritoneum. The common varieties of hernias through the abdominal wall, in order of frequency, are:

1 Inguinal (indirect or direct)
2 Femoral
3 Umbilical
4 Incisional
5 Ventral and epigastric.

Aetiology

Hernias occur at sites of weakness in the abdominal wall. This weakness may be cogenital, for example persistence of the processus vaginalis of testicular descent giving rise to a congenital inguinal hernia, or failure of complete closure of the umbilical scar. It may occur at the site of penetration of structures through the abdominal wall, e.g. the femoral canal, or the layers of the abdominal wall may be weakened following a surgical incision (incisional hernia), either by poor healing as a result of infection, haematoma formation or poor technique, or by damage to nerves which results in paralysis of the abdominal muscles.

In addition to these primary factors, the formaton of a hernia may be aggravated by anything causing an increase in intra-abdominal pressure, for example chronic cough, constipation, urinary obstruction, pregnancy or distension of the abdomen with ascites, or any factor which weakens the abdominal muscles, for example gross obesity or muscle wasting in cachexia.

Varieties

A hernia at any site may be (Fig. 31.1):

1 Reducible,
2 Irreducible,
3 Strangulated.

The contents of a reducible hernia can be reposed completely into the peritoneal cavity.

A hernia becomes irreducible usually because of adhesions of its contents to the inner wall of the sac, or sometimes as a result of adhesions of its contents to each other to form a mass greater in size than the neck of the sac. Occasionally inspissated faeces within the loops of bowel in the hernia prevent reduction.

When strangulation occurs, the contents of the hernia are constricted by the neck of the sac to such a degree that their circulation is cut off. Unless relieved,

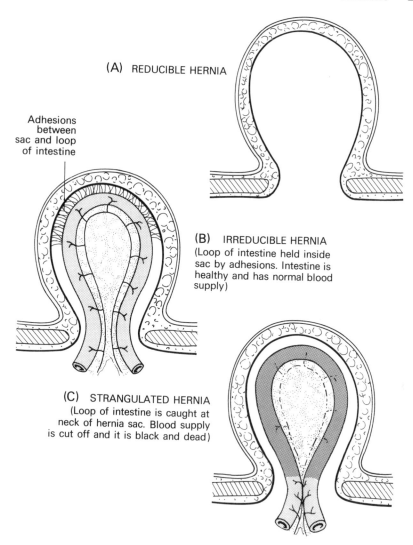

(A) REDUCIBLE HERNIA

Adhesions between sac and loop of intestine

(B) IRREDUCIBLE HERNIA
(Loop of intestine held inside sac by adhesions. Intestine is healthy and has normal blood supply)

(C) STRANGULATED HERNIA
(Loop of intestine is caught at neck of hernia sac. Blood supply is cut off and it is black and dead)

Fig. 31.1. The differences between a reducible, irreducible and strangulated hernia.

gangrene is inevitable and if gut is involved perforation of the gangrenous loop will eventually occur into the sac.

Clinical features

A reducible hernia simply presents as a lump which may disappear on lying down and which is usually not painful, although it may be accompanied by some discomfort. Examination reveals a reducible lump with a cough impulse.

If the hernia will not reduce but is painless and there are no other symptoms, irreducibility is diagnosed. The absence of a cough impulse alone does not indicate strangulation since in an irreducible femoral hernia, for example, the neck is often plugged by omentum which prevents the cough impulse from being felt.

If strangulation supervenes, the patient complains of severe pain in the hernia of sudden onset and also of central abdominal colicky pain. The other symptoms of intestinal obstruction — vomiting, distension and absolute constipation — soon appear. Examination reveals a tender, tense hernia which cannot be reduced and has no cough impulse. The overlying skin becomes inflamed and oedematous and there are the signs of intestinal obstruction with distension, abdominal tenderness and noisy bowel sounds. These features are much less marked when omentum rather than intestine is contained within the sac.

The three common types of hernia to strangulate are, in order of frequency, femoral, indirect inguinal and umbilical.

INGUINAL HERNIA

May be classified into:

1   *Indirect:* entering the internal inguinal ring and traversing the inguinal canal.
2   *Direct:* pushing through the posterior wall of the inguinal canal.

The anatomy of the inguinal canal is the key to the understanding of these hernias.

Anatomy (Fig. 31.2)

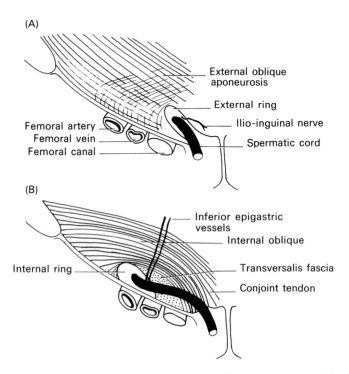

Fig. 31.2. The anatomy of the inguinal canal: (A) with the external oblique aponeurosis intact; (B) aponeurosis laid open.

The inguinal canal represents the oblique passage taken through the lower abdominal wall by the testis and cord (the round ligament in the female). It is 4 cm long and passes downwards and medially, and from deep to superficially, from the internal to the external inguinal rings, lying parallel to, and immediately above the inguinal ligament.

Anteriorly: skin, superficial fascia and external oblique aponeurosis cover the full length of the canal; the internal oblique covers its lateral one-third.

Posteriorly: the conjoint tendon (representing the fused common insertion of the internal oblique and transversus abdominis muscles into the pubic crest) forms the posterior wall of the canal medially, the transversalis fascia lies laterally.

Above: the lowest fibres of the internal oblique and transversus abdominis.

Below: lies the inguinal ligament.

The internal ring represents the point at which the spermatic cord pushes through the transversalis fascia; it is demarcated medially by the inferior epigastric vessels as they pass upwards from the external iliac artery and vein.

The external ring is an inverted V-shaped defect in the external oblique aponeurosis and lies immediately above and medial to the pubic tubercle.

The inguinal canal transmits the spermatic cord (round ligament in the female) and the ilio-inguinal nerve.

INDIRECT INGUINAL HERNIA

This passes through the internal ring, along the canal and, if large enough, emerges through the external ring and descends into the scrotum. If reducible, such a hernia can be completely controlled by pressure with the finger-tip over the internal inguinal ring, which lies 1–2 cm above the point where the femoral artery passes under the inguinal ligament, i.e. 1–2 cm above the femoral pulse. This can be felt at the mid-inguinal point, halfway between the anterior superior iliac spine and the symphysis pubis.

If the hernia protrudes through the external ring, it can be felt to lie above and medial to the pubic tubercle and is thus differentiated from a femoral hernia, which emerges through the femoral canal below and lateral to this landmark (Fig. 31.3).

Indirect hernias may be congenital, due to persistence of the processus vaginalis; these present at or soon after birth or may arise in adolescence. The acquired variety may occur at any age in adult life and here the sac is formed as an outpushing of the abdominal peritoneum.

The narrow internal opening through the internal inguinal ring accounts for two important features of the indirect hernia; the hernia often does not reach its full size until the patient has been up and around for a little time and then does not reduce immediately when the subject lies down, because it takes a little time for the hernial contents to pass in or out of the sac through its narrow neck. Secondly, the indirect hernia has a distinct tendency to strangulate at the site of this narrow orifice.

Direct inguinal hernia

This pushes its way directly forward through the posterior wall of the inguinal canal. Since it lies medial to the internal ring, it is not controlled by digital pressure

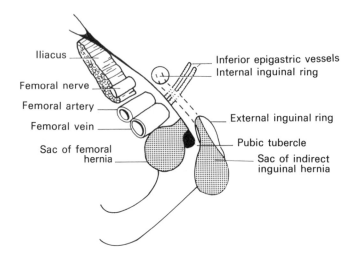

Fig. 31.3. The relationships of an indirect inguinal and a femoral hernia compared; the inguinal hernia emerges above and medial to the pubic tubercle, the femoral hernia lies below and lateral to it.

applied over the ring immediately above the femoral pulse. On inspection the hernia is seen to protrude directly forwards (hence its name) compared with the oblique route downwards towards the scrotum of an indirect inguinal hernia.

Other points which differentiate a direct from an indirect hernia are that the direct is always acquired and is therefore extremely rare in infancy or adolescence; it has a large orifice and therefore appears immediately on standing, disappearing again at once when the patient lies down. Moreover, because of this large opening, strangulation is extremely rare.

Although clinically it is usually quite easy to tell the difference between these two types of inguinal hernia, the ultimate differentiation can only be made at operation; the inferior epigastric vessels demarcate the medial edge of the internal ring, therefore an indirect sac will pass lateral, and a direct hernia medial to these vessels. Quite often both a direct and indirect hernia coexist; they bulge on either side of the inferior epigastric vessels like the legs of a pair of pantaloons.

Sixty per cent of inguinal herniae occur on the right side, 20 per cent on the left and 20 per cent are bilateral.

Treatment

Congenital inguinal herniae in infants do not obliterate spontaneously; the hernial sac is excised at the age of about one year. In adults operation is usually advised; this comprises excision of the sac and repair of the weakened inguinal canal. A truss is only prescribed in patients who are of very poor general condition and are unable to stand operation, although they often have difficulty keeping a truss correctly in place. But even in such cases a painful hernia which threatens strangulation is much better repaired as an elective procedure, if necessary under local anaesthesia, rather than as an emergency should strangulation supervene.

FEMORAL HERNIA

Anatomy

A femoral hernia passes through the femoral canal. This is a gap normally about 1.5 cm in length, which just admits the tip of the little finger and which lies at the medial extremity of the femoral sheath containing the femoral artery and vein. The boundaries of the femoral canal (Fig. 31.4) are:

1 *Anteriorly:* the inguinal ligament.

2 *Medially:* the sharp edge of the lacunar part of the inguinal ligament (Gimbernat's ligament).

3 *Laterally:* the femoral vein.

4 *Posteriorly:* the pectineal ligament (of Astley Cooper) which is the thickened periosteum along the superior pubic ramus.

The canal contains a plug of fat and a lymph node (the node of Cloquet).

Clinical features

Femoral hernias occur more commonly in females than males because of the wider female pelvis, (but note that inguinal hernias are commoner than femoral in females also). They are never due to a congenital sac but are invariably acquired. Although cases do rarely occur in children they are usually seen in the middle-aged and elderly.

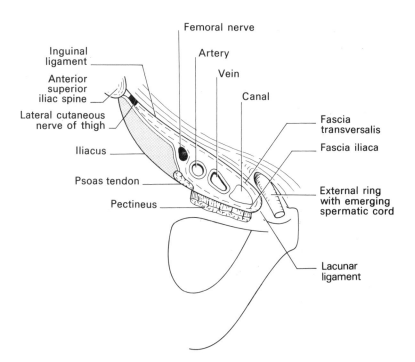

Fig. 31.4. The anatomy of the femoral canal and its surrounds to show the relationships of a femoral hernia.

A non-strangulated hernia presents as a globular swelling below and lateral to the pubic tubercle. It enlarges on standing and on coughing and may disappear when the patient lies down. However, in most cases even when the hernia is completely reduced, a swelling can still be palpated and this is due to extraperitoneal fat around the femoral sac.

As the hernia enlarges it passes through the saphenous opening in the deep fascia (the site of penetration of the great saphenous vein to join the femoral vein) and then turns upwards so that it may project above the inguinal ligament. There should not, however, be any difficulty in differentiating between an irreducible femoral and inguinal hernia; the neck of the former always lies below and lateral to the pubic tubercle, whereas the sac of the latter extends above and medial to this landmark (Fig. 31.3).

The neck of the femoral canal is narrow and has a particularly sharp medial border; for this reason irreducibility and strangulation are extremely common in this type of hernia.

A Richter's hernia (Fig. 31.5) is particularly likely to occur in the femoral sac; here part only of the wall of the small intestine is caught up and strangulated by the femoral ring. Because the lumen of the bowel is not completely encroached upon, symptoms of intestinal obstruction do not occur, although the knuckle of bowel may become completely necrotic and indeed perforate into the hernial sac and thence into the peritoneal cavity.

Treatment

All femoral hernias should be repaired by excision of the sac and closure of the femoral canal because of their great danger of strangulation.

DIFFERENTIAL DIAGNOSIS OF A LUMP IN THE GROIN

A patient presenting with a lump in the groin is a common clinical problem. Whenever one considers the differential diagnosis of a mass situated in a particular area a two-stage mental process is required: first, what are the anatomical

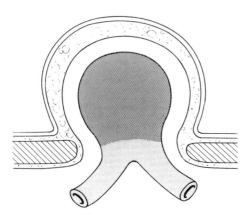

Fig. 31.5. A Richter's hernia. Note that only a part of the wall of the gut is involved.

structures in that particular region, and second, what pathological entities may arise therefrom?

In considering the groin, let these possibilities pass through your mind:

1 *The hernial orifices:*
   (a) inguinal hernia
   (b) femoral hernia
2 *The testicular apparatus:*
   (a) hydrocele of the cord
   (b) ectopic testis
3 *The vein:* saphena varix
4 *The artery:* femoral aneurysm
5 *The lymph nodes:* lymphadenopathy due to infection, neoplasm or lymphoma (see page 77)
6 *The psoas sheath:* psoas abscess
7 *The skin and subcutaneous tissues:* lipoma

UMBILICAL HERNIA

Exomphalos

A rare condition in which there is failure of all or part of the midgut to return to the abdominal cavity in fetal life. The bowel is contained within a translucent sac protruding through a defective anterior abdominal wall. Untreated, this ruptures with fatal peritonitis or rupture may occur during delivery.

Treatment

Immediate surgical repair if possible. Where the sac is massive it is protected with dressing soaked in mild antiseptic. Gradual epithelialization takes place and later repair may then be undertaken.

Congenital umbilical hernia

Results from failure of complete closure of the umbilical cicatrix. It is especially common in black children. The vast majority close spontaneously during the first year of life.

Treatment

Surgical repair should not usually be carried out unless the hernia persists after the child is 2 years old. The parents of an infant with a congenital umbilical hernia should be reassured that the majority disappear spontaneously. Strapping the hernia or providing a rubber truss are only required to allay parental anxiety.

Acquired umbilical hernia

Occurs just above or below the umbilicus and is more accurately termed a para-umbilical hernia. It especially occurs in obese, multiparous, middle-aged women. The neck is narrow and, like a femoral hernia, it is particularly prone to become irreducible or strangulated. The contents are nearly always the omentum, and often in addition transverse colon and small intestine.

Treatment

Excision of the sac and overlapping the edges of the rectus sheath above and below the hernia (Mayo's operation).

VENTRAL HERNIA

A midline ventral hernia may exist as an elongated gap between the recti in elderly wasted patients, (divarication of the recti); in the majority of cases no treatment is required.

EPIGASTRIC HERNIA

A particular variety of ventral hernia is the epigastric hernia, which consists of one or more small protrusions through defects in the linea alba above the umbilicus. These usually contain only extra-peritoneal fat but are often surprisingly painful.

Treatment

A simple matter of suturing the defect.

INCISIONAL HERNIA

An incisional hernia occurs through a defect in the scar of a previous abdominal operation. The causes, which are the same as those of a burst abdomen, are given on page 23.

There is usually a wide neck and strangulation is in consequence rare.

Treatment

If the general condition of the patient is good, the hernia is repaired by dissecting out and suturing the individual layers of the abdominal wall. Large hernias are repaired with a sheet of synthetic polymer plastic mesh. If operation is considered inadvisable an abdominal belt is prescribed.

UNUSUAL HERNIAS

1 *Obturator hernia* (found particularly in thin, elderly females) develops through the obturator canal where the obturator nerve and vessels traverse the membrane covering the obturator foramen. Pressure of a strangulated obturator hernia upon the nerve causes referred pain in its area of cutaneous distribution, so that intestinal obstruction associated with pain along the medial side of the thigh in a thin old lady should suggest this diagnosis.

2 *Spigelian hernia* passes upwards through the arcuate line into the lateral border of the lower part of the posterior rectus sheath; it presents as a tender mass to one side of the lower abdominal wall.

3 *Gluteal hernia* traverses the greater sciatic foramen.

4 *Sciatic hernia* passes through the lesser sciatic foramen.

5 *Lumbar hernia* most commonly is an incisional hernia following an operation on the kidney, but may, rarely, occur through the inferior lumbar triangle bounded by the crest of the ilium below, the latissimus dorsi medially and the external oblique on the lateral side.

Chapter 32
The Liver

LIVER ENLARGEMENT

Physical signs

The infant's liver is normally palpable two fingers below the right costal margin. It is also felt in thin adults, particularly on deep inspiration. The enlarged liver forms a mass which extends downwards below the right costal margin and may fill the subcostal angle or extend beneath the left costal margin in gross hepatomegaly. The mass moves with respiration, is dull to percussion and is continuous with the liver dullness, which may itself extend above the normal upper level of the fifth right interspace.

Causes

1 *Congenital:*
   (a) Riedel's lobe
   (b) polycystic disease
2 *Inflammatory:*
   (a) infective hepatitis
   (b) portal pyaemia
   (c) leptospirosis (Weil's disease)
   (d) actinomycosis
3 *Parasitic:*
   (a) amoebic hepatitis and abscess
   (b) hydatid
4 *Neoplastic:*
   (a) primary tumour
   (b) secondary deposits
5 *Cirrhosis:*
   (a) portal
   (b) biliary
   (c) cardiac
   (d) haemochromatosis
6 *Haemopoietic diseases and reticuloses:*
   (a) Hodgkin's
   (b) non-Hodgkin's lymphoma
   (c) leukaemia
   (d) polycythaemia
7 *Metabolic diseases:*
   (a) amyloid
   (b) Gaucher's disease

Whenever the liver is felt, automatically the patient must be examined to detect any accompanying splenomegaly or lymphadenopathy. If the spleen is palpable in addition to the liver, consider cirrhosis, polycythaemia, leukaemia or amyloid as possible diagnoses. If, in addition, the lymph nodes are enlarged, the diagnosis is almost certainly a lymphoma (see page 77).

JAUNDICE

The normal serum bilirubin is below 9 µmol/l (0.5 mg per cent). Jaundice becomes clinically detectable when the serum level rises to over 35 µmol/l (2 mg per cent).

Jaundice may result from excessive destruction of red cells (pre-hepatic jaundice), liver damage (hepatic jaundice) or obstruction of the biliary tree (post-hepatic jaundice). Quite frequently the hepatic and post-hepatic forms coexist; for example, a stone in the common bile duct may produce jaundice partly by obstructing the outflow of bile and partly by secondary damage to the liver (biliary cirrhosis), and both tumour deposits in the liver and cirrhosis may result in icterus partly by actual destruction of liver tissue and partly by intrahepatic duct compression.

Classification

Pre-hepatic jaundice:

Haemolytic disorders, e.g. spherocytosis, pernicious anaemia, incompatible blood transfusion

Hepatic jaundice:

1 Hepatitis (viral, leptospirosis, glandular fever)
2 Cirrhosis
3 Cholestasis from drugs, e.g. chlorpromazine
4 Liver poisons, e.g. phosphorus, carbon tetrachloride, chloroform, paracetamol overdosage
5 Liver tumours

Post hepatic jaundice:

1 *Obstruction within the lumen:* Gallstones
2 *In the wall:*
    (a) congenital atresia of common bile duct
    (b) traumatic stricture
    (c) tumour of bile duct
    (d) chronic cholangitis
3 *External compression:*
    (a) tumour of head of pancreas
    (b) tumour of ampulla of Vater
    (c) pancreatitis

Differential diagnosis of jaundice

This is based on history, examination and special investigations.

History

A family history of anaemia, splenectomy or gallstones suggests a congenital red cell defect (acholuric jaundice, etc.). Clay-coloured stools and dark urine accompanying the episodes of jaundice indicate hepatic or post-hepatic causes. Enquire after recent blood transfusions, drugs (chlorpromazine, paracetamol, methyldopa, repeated exposure to halothane), injections and alcohol consumption. Has there been contact with cases of virus hepatitis? What is the patient's occupation? (Farmers and sewer workers are at risk of leptospirosis.)

Usually painless jaundice of sudden onset with liver tenderness in a young person is viral in origin. Attacks of severe colic, rigors and intermittency of jaundice suggest stone. Remorselessly progressive jaundice, often accompanied by continuous pain radiating to the back, is suspicious of malignant disease.

Examination

The colour of the jaundice is important; a lemon yellow tinge suggests haemolytic jaundice (due to combined anaemia and mild icterus). Deep jaundice suggests the hepatic or post-hepatic types.

Look for other signs of cirrhosis: spider naevi, liver palms, gynaecomastia, testicular atrophy, flapping tremor, encephalopathy, splenomegaly and occasionally finger clubbing. There may also be ascites and leg oedema, but these may be associated with intra-abdominal malignant disease as well as cirrhosis.

Examination of the liver itself is helpful; in viral hepatitis the liver is slightly enlarged and tender, in cirrhosis the liver edge is firm, although the liver may be shrunken and impalpable. A grossly enlarged, knobbly liver suggests malignant disease.

If the gallbladder is palpable and distended, it is probable that the cause of the jaundice is not a stone (Courvoisier's law, see page 254). The liver is usually smoothly enlarged in post-hepatic obstructive jaundice.

A pancreatic tumour may be palpable or a primary focus of malignant disease may be obvious, e.g. a melanoma.

Splenomegaly suggests cirrhosis of the liver, blood disease or a lymphoma; in the latter there may also be obvious lymphadenopathy.

Special investigations

It is easy enough to differentiate the prehepatic causes of jaundice from hepatic and post-hepatic, but that the latter two are often very difficult to differentiate one from the other and, as already stated, are often associated with each other. Laboratory tests are of some help but are by no means diagnostic. Imaging techniques are valuable in visualizing the liver, gall bladder and pancreas, while endoscopic cannulation of the bile ducts, or trans-hepatic duct puncture enable the bile duct system to be outlined. However, it is not unusual for the diagnosis to be established finally only at laparotomy.

Bile pigment metabolism and excretion must be clearly understood if many of the laboratory investigations in jaundice are to be comprehensible.

Red cells are destroyed in the reticulo-endothelial system. The porphyrin ring of the haemoglobin molecule is disrupted and a bilirubin-iron-globin complex produced. The iron is released and used for further haemoglobin synthesis in the red marrow. The bilirubin-globin fraction reaches the liver as a lipid-soluble, water insoluble substance. In the liver the bilirubin is conjugated with glucuronic acid and excreted in the bile as the now water-soluble bilirubin-diglucuronide.

In the bowel lumen, bilirubin is reduced by bacterial action to the colourless urobilinogen, most of which is excreted in the faeces, in which it becomes converted to urobilin which is pigmented and which, with the other breakdown products of bilirubin, gives the stool its normal colour.

A small amount of urobilinogen is reabsorbed from the intestine into the portal venous tributaries and passes to the liver, where most of it is excreted once more in the bile back into the gut. Some, however, reaches the systemic circulation and this is excreted by the kidney into the urine. When urine is exposed to air, its contained urobilinogen is oxidized to urobilin.

Bilirubin is not excreted by the kidney except in its water-soluble (conjugated) form. It is therefore absent from the urine in pre-hepatic jaundice (hence the old term 'acholuric jaundice') although present when there is post-hepatic obstruction.

In pre-hepatic jaundice, large amounts of bilirubin are excreted into the gut, therefore the urobilinogen in the faeces is raised, the amount absorbed from the bowel increases and there is therefore greater spillover into the urine.

In hepatic damage the urinary urobilinogen may also be raised because of the inability of the liver to re-excrete the urobilinogen reabsorbed from the bowel.

In post-hepatic obstruction, very little bile can enter the gut, therefore the urobilinogen must be low in both the faeces and the urine.

The important laboratory findings in the various types of jaundice can now be summarized:

Urine

The presence of bilirubin indicates obstructive jaundice, either intra- or post-hepatic.

Excess of urobilinogen indicates pre-hepatic jaundice or sometimes liver damage, whereas an absence of urobilinogen suggests obstructive causes.

Faeces

Absence of bile pigment indicates intra- or post-hepatic causes. The faecal urobilinogen is raised in pre-hepatic jaundice. The occult blood test may be positive, either on account of oozing oesophageal varices secondary to portal hypertension (indicating cirrhosis), or due to an ampullary carcinoma which is occluding the orifice of the common bile duct and also bleeding into the duodenum.

Blood

Full haematological investigations (RBC fragility, Coombs' test, reticulocyte count) confirm haemolytic causes.

The serum bilirubin is invariably raised. It is rarely higher than 100 μmol/l (5 mg per cent) in pre-hepatic jaundice, but may be considered higher in obstructive cases. In late malignant disease it may exceed 1000 μmol/l (50 mg per cent).

In pre-hepatic jaundice bilirubin is present in the unconjugated form. In the pure post-hepatic obstructive jaundice the bilirubin is mainly in the conjugated form, whereas in hepatic jaundice it is present in the mixed conjugated and unconjugated forms due to a combination of liver destruction and intra-hepatic duct blockage.

The alkaline phosphatase is normal in pre-hepatic jaundice (90 to 330 iu/l), raised in hepatic jaundice, and considerably raised (above 600 iu/l) in post-hepatic jaundice and in primary biliary cirrhosis.

Serum proteins are normal in pre-hepatic jaundice, have a reversed A:G ratio with depressed albumin in hepatic jaundice and are usually normal in post-hepatic jaundice, unless associated with liver damage.

Serum transaminases are raised in acute viral hepatitis and in the active phase of cirrhosis.

The prothrombin time is normal in pre-hepatic jaundice, prolonged but correctable with Vitamin K in post-hepatic jaundice (where functioning liver tissue is still present) and prolonged but not correctable in advanced hepatic jaundice, where not only is absorption of fat-soluble Vitamin K impaired but also the damaged liver is unable to synthesize prothrombin.

Ultrasound and CT scanning

These are extremely useful as well as non-invasive. Gall stones within the gall bladder can be demonstrated with a high degree of accuracy. Unfortunately, stones within the bile ducts often fail to visualize. Dilatation of the duct system within the liver is a good indication of duct obstruction, so that if the ducts are not dilated, an obstructive cause for the jaundice is unlikely. Both techniques are valuable in the demonstration of intrahepatic lesions (e.g. tumour deposits, abscess, cyst), which may then be accurately needled for biopsy material under scan control. A mass in the pancreas can usually be demonstrated, but differentiation between carcinoma and chronic pancreatitis is difficult.

X-rays

A plain X-ray of the abdomen may show gallstones (10 per cent are radio opaque). *Cholecystography* is useless when the patient is jaundiced since the dye is not excreted by the damaged liver. A *barium swallow* may confirm the presence of oesophageal varices in jaundice due to cirrhosis, or the subsequent barium meal may reveal a distorted duodenum (suggesting a pancreatic tumour) or the presence of a primary neoplasm of the stomach. In some instances of obstructive jaundice a pre-operative *trans-hepatic cholangiogram* is performed by direct puncture of a dilated biliary radicle in order to locate the exact site of the obstruction. This should be undertaken immediately prior to surgery since bile leakage is common when the needle is withdrawn in obstructed cases. A useful investigation is *retrograde cholangiography* via a catheter introduced into the ampulla of Vater under direct vision via a fibre-optic duodenoscope. A periampullary tumour is also directly visualized at this examination.

Both transhepatic and retrograde cholangiography may be used to introduce dilators and stents into the biliary duct system.

Liver isotope scanning

A gamma-emitting isotope which is excreted in the bile is injected, either I^{131} labelled Rose Bengal, or HIDA, which is taken up by the hepatocytes and excreted in the bile, or colloidal technetium, which is incorporated into the macrophage Kupffer cells. Lesions which do not contain functioning liver tissue, such as tumour deposits, abscesses or cysts, appear as defects on the scan.

Needle biopsy

If the ultrasound scan reveal no dilatation of the duct system, an obstructive lesion is unlikely and needle biopsy of the liver will give valuable information regarding hepatic pathology (e.g. hepatitis or cirrhosis). If the ultrasound demonstrates focal lesions in the liver, a biopsy can be obtained under scanning control. Needle biopsy is potentially dangerous in the presence of jaundice. The prothrombin time, if prolonged, should first be corrected by administration of vitamin K. Should bleeding occur following biopsy, an immediate laparotomy may be necessary.

Laparotomy

Since most causes of post-hepatic obstructive jaundice can be relieved surgically, it may be necessary to submit a doubtful case to laparotomy even though it is suspected that the aetiology is entirely hepatic, lest an easily remediable condition (e.g. stones in the common bile duct) is overlooked.

CONGENITAL ABNORMALITIES

Riedel's lobe is a projection downwards from the right lobe of the liver of normally functioning liver tissue. It may present as a puzzling and symptomless abdominal mass.

Polycystic liver may reach a very large size but the remaining liver functions normally. It may be associated with polycystic disease of the kidneys and pancreas.

LIVER TRAUMA

This may be due to penetrating wounds (gunshot or stab), or closed crush injuries, often associated with fractures of the ribs and injuries to other intra-abdominal viscera, especially the spleen. Severe abdominal trauma is becoming increasingly common and accurate pre-operative diagnosis of the source of the haemorrhage may be impossible.

Clinical features

Following injury, the patient complains of abdominal pain. Examination reveals generalized abdominal tenderness together with the signs of progressive bleeding. CT scanning, if available, can be very helpful in showing the lesion and differentiation from a ruptured spleen. Occasionally there is delayed rupture of a subcapsular haematoma, so that abdominal pain and shock may not be in evidence until some hours after the initial injury.

Treatment

If the patient's vital observations are stable, the condition can be managed conservatively with blood transfusion and careful observation. However, bleeding often continues and there is the risk of overlooking damage to other viscera. In such cases, laparotomy is performed. Minor liver tears can be sutured. If bleeding continues, the relevant main hepatic arterial branch should be tied. If this does not control bleeding, major hepatic lobar resection may be necessary. Temporary packing of the injury with a gauze pack, removed after 48 hours, may be life-saving in severe trauma when the patient's condition is deteriorating. Antibiotic cover must be given because of the danger of infection of the devitalized liver. Liver transplantation may be needed to manage gross trauma to both lobes.

ACUTE INFECTIONS OF THE LIVER

Possible sources of infection are:
1 Arterial, as part of a general septicaemia — this is unusual.
2 Portal, from an area of suppuration drained by the portal vein.
3 Biliary, resulting from an ascending cholangitis.
4 Spread from adjacent infection, e.g. subphrenic abscess or acute cholecystitis.

PORTAL INFECTIONS

Portal pyaemia (pyelophlebitis)

Infection may reach the liver via the portal tributaries from a focus of intra-abdominal sepsis, particularly acute appendicitis or diverticulitis. Multiple abscesses may permeate the liver; in addition there may be septic thrombi in the intra-hepatic radicles of the portal vein, and infected clot in the portal vein itself. The condition has become very rare since the advent of antibiotics.

Clinical features

The condition should be suspected in patients who develop rigors, high swinging temperature, a tender palpable liver and jaundice after any acute infective abdominal condition.

Special investigations

A blood culture should be carried out before treatment is commenced; it is often positive.

Whenever a space occupying lesion of the liver is suspected, ultrasound or CT scanning should give confirmation and localization (see page 237).

Treatment

Comprises antibiotic therapy. Occasionally a large, single abscess may require drainage. This may be carried out percutaneously under ultrasound control.

Actinomycosis

Actinomycosis of the liver is a rare variety of portal infection; spread via the portal blood stream from ileo-caecal actinomycosis (see page 6).

Amoebic hepatitis

Another special variety of portal infection, secondary to an *Entamoeba histolytica* infection of the large intestine. In severe infection the cytolytic enzyme produced by the amoebae destroys the liver tissue producing an amoebic abscess, which is sterile, although amoebae may be found in the abscess wall.

A liver CT scan and ultrasound are the most valuable special investigations.

Treatment

The majority respond to medical treatment with metronidazole, which has replaced emetine as the drug of choice. Ultrasonographically directed percutaneous drainage is required infrequently in non-responding cases.

BILIARY INFECTION

Multiple abscesses in the liver may occur in association with severe suppurative cholangitis secondary to impaction of gallstones in the common bile duct. Clinically the features are those of Charcot's intermittent hepatic fever — pyrexia, rigors and jaundice. Renal failure may occur (the hepato-renal syndrome).

Treatment

Antibiotic therapy is commenced (checked, where possible, against the bacteriology of the bile). Urgent drainage of the bile ducts is performed, either by open operation or, more usually, by endoscopic sphincterotomy. Fluid replacement and mannitol given intravenously guard against renal failure.

HYDATID DISEASE OF THE LIVER

The liver is the site of 75 per cent of hydatid cysts in man.

Pathology

Dogs are infected with the ova of *Echinococcus granulosus (Taenia echinococcus)* as a result of eating sheep offal. The tapeworms develop in the dog's intestine from whence ova are discharged in the faeces. Man (as well as sheep) ingests the ova from contaminated vegetables, etc.; the ova penetrate the stomach wall to invade the portal tributaries and thence pass to the liver. Hydatid disease is therefore common in sheep rearing communities, e.g. Australia, Iceland, Cyprus, Southern Europe, Africa and Wales. Public health measures, e.g. destruction of stray dogs, has resulted in a marked drop in incidence.

The cyst consists of:

1   An adventitia: comprising the fibrous coat of the host's reaction.
2   A laminated membrane: white elastic material derived from the cyst itself.
3   Germinal epithelium: upon which brood capsules develop.
4   Cyst fluid: which is clear unless secondarily infected and which contains hooklets and scolices derived from the daughter cysts.

Clinical features

A cyst may present as a symptomless mass. The contents may die and the walls become calcified so that this inactive structure may be a harmless post-mortem finding.

The active cyst may, however:

1 Rupture into the peritoneal cavity, pleural cavity, alimentary canal or biliary tree.

2 Become infected.

3 Press on intra-hepatic bile ducts and produce obstructive jaundice, although jaundice is much more often due to intrabiliary rupture and release of cysts into the bile ducts.

Investigations

1 *Plain X-ray* of the liver may show a clear zone produced by the cyst, or may show flecks of calcification in the cyst wall.

2 *Ultrasound and CT scan* are invaluable in localizing the cyst.

3 *Serological tests* depend on the sensitization of the patient to hydatid fluid, which contains a specific antigen, leakage of which induces the production of antibodies. Among the various test now available, hydatid immuno-electrophoresis is the one of choice. This depends on the formation of a specific arc of precipitation produced by the interaction of the serum from the hydatid patient with the antigen as compared to a control.

4 There may be *eosinophilia*, which is not specific but should at least arouse clinical suspicion.

Treatment

A calcified cyst should be left alone. Other cysts should be treated to prevent complications. Treatment with albendazole may result in shrinkage or even disappearance of the cysts. Failure to respond or the presence of complications are indications for surgery. The cyst is exposed and aspirated. It is then possible to excise the cyst, working in the plane between the fibrous adventitia and the laminated membrane, taking care not to liberate daughter cysts.

VIRAL HEPATITIS

Aetiology

There are several separate viral agents:

1 The infective hepatitis (type A) virus, which has an incubation period of 2 to 6 weeks and is spread by nasal droplets and faeces. Children or young adults are usually affected.

2 The serum hepatitis (type B) virus, with an incubation period of 6 weeks to 6 months and which is transmitted by inoculation with contaminated syringes or a transfusion of blood or plasma from an infected patient. The blood in these subjects contains the Australia antigen and is highly infective. Any age may be infected.

3 Type C. Similar in transmission to type B, both of which can lead to chronic infection, cirrhosis and tumour formation.

Clinical features

There is a prodromal period of a few days with anorexia, aversion to tobacco, fever, malaise, nausea and vomiting. The patient then becomes jaundiced with dark urine and clay coloured stools. There may be upper abdominal pain, although this is usually not marked. The liver is palpable and tender. The great majority recover in up to 4 weeks, treated simply by bed rest and a low fat diet. Alcohol should be avoided for 12 months; not only is the patient unusually susceptible to intoxication but the liver is vulnerable to damage by alcohol.

Complications

1   Hepatic failure, massive necrosis (acute yellow atrophy), with extremely high mortality, is fortunately rare, about 2 per 1000 cases.
2   Relapse, which may occur a few weeks after the initial episode.
3   Post-hepatic cirrhosis.

Patients with positive Australia antigenaemia are a risk to nursing, laboratory and medical staff, especially if multiple venepunctures or surgery are required. All hospital workers should be protected by vaccination. The danger to unprotected non-immunized staff can be lessened by the administration of convalescent gamma globulin given at, or shortly after, the time of exposure. Great care must be taken in handling blood or in operation on these patients, since the virus can gain access via minute and unrecognized cuts or pin pricks and probably also through the intact mucosa of the mouth, genital tract, respiratory tract and conjunctiva.

CIRRHOSIS

Definition

A group of conditions in which there is chronic hepatic injury; healing occurs by regeneration and fibrosis. Fibrosis leads to further cell damage and destruction of hepatic architecture progressing to liver failure and portal hypertension.

Aetiology

A convenient classification of the cirrhoses is:
1   *Portal:*
   (a) alcoholic
   (b) nutritional (deficient protein diet)
   (c) post-hepatic
   (d) idiopathic
2   *Biliary:*
   (a) primary (Hanot's cirrhosis); an auto-immune disease with raised serum anti-mitochondrial antibodies
   (b) secondary to prolonged biliary obstruction
3   *Cardiac:* in severe chronic congestive failure
4   *Other causes:*
   (a) chronic active hepatitis. An auto-immune disease
   (b) haemochromatosis
   (c) hepatolenticular degeneration (Kinnier Wilson's disease)
   (d) schistosomiasis

In countries with a high consumption of alcohol (France and USA), alcohol is the commonest aetiological factor. In the tropics schistosomiasis heads the list (Egyptian splenomegaly). In Great Britain 50 per cent of cirrhosis cases are alcoholic.

PORTAL HYPERTENSION

The normal portal pressure is between 80 and 150 mm of water. In portal hypertension this pressure may be raised to 500 mm or more.

Aetiology

Portal hypertension results from an obstruction in the portal tree. The causes are classified according to the site of the block:

1 *Pre-hepatic (obstruction of the portal venous inflow into the liver):*
   (a) congenital malformation
   (b) spreading portal vein thrombosis in the neo-natal period from an umbilical infection
   (c) occlusion by tumour or pancreatitis
2 *Hepatic (obstruction of the portal flow within the liver):* the cirrhoses.
3 *Post-hepatic (obstruction of the hepatic veins):* Budd–Chiari syndrome:
   (a) idiopathic hepatic venous thrombosis in young adults of both sexes. A possible complication of oral contraceptives in women. In many cases there is an underlying haematological neoplasm for example, polycythemia or mono-clonal gammaglobulinopathy.
   (b) congenital obliteration
   (c) blockage of hepatic vein by tumour invasion

By far the commonest cause of portal hypertension is cirrhosis, yet there is no strict relationship between the severity of the liver disease and the extent of portal hypertension, which is not therefore entirely explained on the basis of mechanical obstruction.

Pathological effects

The four important effects of portal hypertension are:
1 The development of a collateral portal-systemic circulation.
2 Splenomegaly.
3 Ascites (in hepatic and post-hepatic portal hypertension only).
4 The manifestations of hepatic failure (in severe cirrhosis).

Collateral channels

Portal obstruction results in the development of collateral channels between the portal and systemic venous circulations. These are:
1 Between the left gastric vein and the oesophageal veins, forming oesophageal varices; the largest and clinically the most important connections.
2 Between the superior and inferior rectal veins with development of haemor-rhoids, which are true varices.
3 Along the obliterated umbilical vein to the superior and inferior epigastric veins (caput medusae).

4 Retroperitoneal and diaphragmatic anastomoses, which present technical hazards to the surgeon at time of operation.

The oesophageal varices, and to a much lesser extent the haemorrhoids, may result in gastro-intestinal haemorrhage, which is the most serious complication of portal hypertension *per se*.

Splenomegaly

Progressive splenic enlargement occurs as a result of portal congestion together with some degree of hypertrophy of the splenic substance itself. This is often associated with the haematological changes of hypersplenism — leucopenia and thrombocytopenia. Anaemia accompanying splenomegaly can be accounted for entirely by gastro-intestinal bleeding and is not a result of splenic enlargement.

Ascites

This is due to a combination of factors. The raised portal pressure itself increases transudation of fluid into the peritoneal cavity but alone will not produce ascites, which is not therefore seen in the pre-hepatic obstruction. Liver damage results in a low serum albumin, therefore a low plasma osmotic pressure and consequent deficient reabsorption of ascitic fluid. Liver damage is associated with increased aldosterone activity with sodium retention. Increased lymphatic pressure in the cirrhotic liver results in lymph transudation from the liver surface, and this high lymphatic pressure is also a feature in the post-hepatic block.

The effects of liver failure

1 Jaundice.

2 CNS effects — mental changes, flapping tremor and hepatic coma. This portal-systemic encephalopathy is brought about by a shunt of nitrogenous breakdown products from the intestine via the portal tract into the systemic circulation without the interposition of the hepatic detoxicating filter.

3 A group of features of, as yet, uncertain aetiological significance — gynaeco-mastia, testicular atrophy, amenorrhoea, spider naevi, finger clubbing and palmar erythema ('liver palms').

Clinical features

To the surgeon portal hypertension presents as three groups of problems:

1 As a differential diagnosis of jaundice or hepatomegaly.

2 As a cause of gastrointestinal haemorrhage.

3 As one of the causes of ascites.

Investigations

In addition to history and examination (which includes a careful search for the stigmata of liver disease) the following investigations are indicated:

1 *Barium swallow* to demonstrate the presence of oesophageal varices.

2 *Fibre-optic endoscopy* will demonstrate varices and differentiate between bleeding from this source and from a peptic ulcer or multiple gastric erosions, both of which are common in patients with cirrhosis.

3 *Liver function tests,* together with liver biopsy if necessary.

4 *A splenic venogram* or the venous phase of a selective superior mesenteric arteriogram to delineate the exact site of the portal obstruction before elective surgery is undertaken.

Treatment

The mere demonstration of oesophageal varices on a barium swallow is not an indication for surgery. Nothing more is required than treatment of the underlying condition on medical lines, e.g. cirrhosis is managed by a high calorie, well-balanced diet with added protein in malnourished patients (provided liver damage is not severe), and with avoidance of precipitating factors such as alcohol. Surgical intervention is only indicated if haemorrhage occurs.

The management of haemorrhage from oesophageal varices

This is particularly dangerous, especially in patients with liver damage. In these subjects the liver is further injured by the hypotension of blood loss, and portal-systemic encephalopathy may be precipitated due to the absorption of large amounts of nitrogenous breakdown products from the 'meal of blood' within the intestine. Prognosis is better in the small group of patients with normal liver function and a prehepatic block.

An attempt must be made to confirm the diagnosis. The presence of established liver disease, an enlarged spleen and proven varices does not necessarily mean that bleeding is from the varices. Such patients are prone to bleed from gastric erosions and are commonly affected by peptic ulceration. Fibre-optic endoscopy should always be performed in order to visualize the bleeding point and to exclude non-variceal haemorrhage. Bleeding varices are injected directly with sclerosant solution. Active bleeding may, however, prevent a satisfactory view at endoscopy.

The immediate treatment of haemorrhage is blood replacement by transfusion. Nitrogenous absorption from the bowel is reduced by emptying as much as possible of the blood from the colon by means of an enema, giving neomycin by mouth to reduce bacterial decomposition of blood in the gut, withholding protein from the diet and maintaining nourishment by means of glucose given by mouth or intravenously. If bleeding continues, more vigorous methods may be required, but here careful decision must be taken; if the patient is in advanced hepatic failure with jaundice, ascites, a low serum albumin, impaired clotting, thrombocytopenia and precoma or coma, then it is wise practice to refrain from further treatment since the prognosis is hopeless and further procedures merely add to the discomfort of an already dying patient.

In fitter subjects, the haemorrhage is stemmed either by:

1 Direct pressure on the varices using a Sengstaken tube which is introduced through the mouth into the oesophagus and cardia, then distended (Fig. 32.1), or

2 Intravenous Pitressin (20 units by slow intravenous injection) which produces a marked fall in portal venous pressure and temporary cessation of bleeding by mesenteric arteriolar constriction. Therapeutic doses cause intestinal colic.

The emergency surgical procedures are:

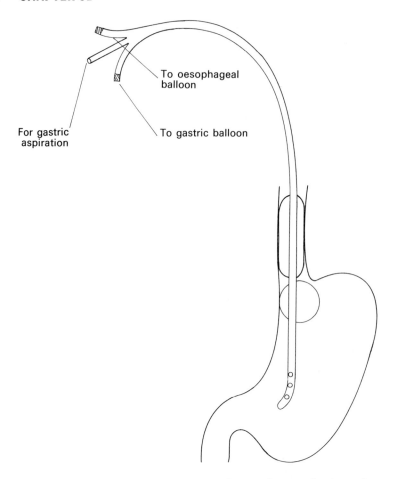

For gastric
aspiration

To oesophageal
balloon

To gastric balloon

Fig. 32.1. The Sengstaken tube. Balloons in the oesophagus and in the cardia compress
the bleeding varices; the gastric tube can be used either for aspirating the stomach or for
feeding purposes.

1   Trans-thoracic ligation of the varices, which is effective for varices limited to
the oesophagus.
2   Porta-caval anastomosis between the portal vein and the inferior vena cava,
which shunts the portal blood directly into the venous systemic circulation and
thus lowers the portal pressure.
3   Injection of the varices via a long needle introduced through a rigid or
fibre-optic oesophagoscope. This technique is analogous to the injection treatment of piles. This procedure can stop bleeding with minimal trauma to the patient
although there are the risks of perforation of the oesophagus and repeated
injections may produce ulceration or fibrosis. Control of the bleeding allows the
surgeon to assess the patient as a candidate for liver transplantation. Laparotomy
should be avoided if possible if a subsequent transplant is planned, since the
resulting vascular adhesions will greatly add to the dangers of the transplant

operation. If the patient is not a candidate for a transplant, then definitive surgery to prevent further bleeding may be contemplated. This may comprise:

4 Porta-azygos disconnection, in which the varices around the lower end of the oesophagus and the upper stomach are divided at the cardio-oesophageal junction using the circular stapling gun, in order to interrupt the communications between the two systems of veins within the wall of the lower oesophagus.

5 If the portal vein itself is occluded by a thrombus or is congenitally abnormal, porta-caval anastomosis is impossible. The portal system can be shunted to the systemic system by a variety of techniques, spleno-renal anastomosis between the splenic vein (after splenectomy) and the left renal vein is that most often performed.

Portal-systemic shunting may be performed in the elective stage when there have been previous episodes of haemorrhage. Such procedures again should only be carried out in patients with reasonable hepatic function. Jaundice, plasma albumin of less than 25 g/l and poor general condition are contra-indications to surgery.

Unfortunately, operative procedures in which an anastomosis is made between the portal and systemic circulations are likely to precipitate portal-systemic encephalopathy and such patients often have to be maintained indefinitely on a low protein diet. However, liver transplantation is now a preferable option except in cases of prehepatic obstruction with good liver function.

Treatment of ascites

1 Paracentesis gives immediate relief if discomfort is intense, but it has the disadvantage that the patient loses protein.

2 Low sodium, high protein diet, intravenous albumin.

3 Diuretics: chlorothiazide (with potassium supplement) and

4 Peritoneo-venous shunt (LeVeen or Denver): a silicone rubber catheter with a pressure-activated valve, which shunts ascitic fluid from the peritoneal cavity back into the venous systems via the internal jugular vein.

5 Surgery: only occasionally indicated; a few patients may be fit enough for porta-caval anastomosis which sometimes relieves ascites.

LIVER NEOPLASMS

Classification

Benign (rare)

(a) cavernous haemangioma
(b) adenoma

Malignant

1 *Primary* (rare in this country):
(a) hepatoma
(b) cholangiocarcinoma
2 *Secondary* (common):

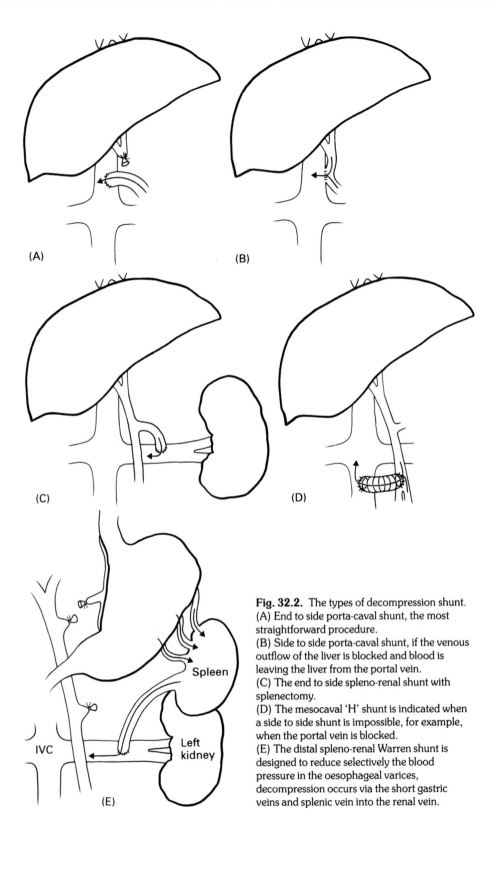

(A)

(B)

(C)

(D)

Spleen

Left
kidney

IVC

(E)

Fig. 32.2. The types of decompression shunt.
(A) End to side porta-caval shunt, the most
straightforward procedure.
(B) Side to side porta-caval shunt, if the venous
outflow of the liver is blocked and blood is
leaving the liver from the portal vein.
(C) The end to side spleno-renal shunt with
splenectomy.
(D) The mesocaval 'H' shunt is indicated when
a side to side shunt is impossible, for example,
when the portal vein is blocked.
(E) The distal spleno-renal Warren shunt is
designed to reduce selectively the blood
pressure in the oesophageal varices,
decompression occurs via the short gastric
veins and splenic vein into the renal vein.

(a) *portal spread* (from alimentary tract)
(b) *systemic blood spread* (from lung, breast, testis, melanoma, etc.)
(c) *direct spread* (from gall bladder, stomach and hepatic flexure of colon)

Hepatoma

About 50 per cent occur in cirrhotics, especially those with nutritional deficiencies, and is common in Central Africa (50 per cent of cancer deaths) and the Far East associated with hepatitis B and C infection.

The tumour forms a large, solitary mass, or there may be multiple foci throughout the liver. Spread occurs through the liver substance and metastasis outside this organ is late.

Clinically there is massive liver swelling which develops in a cirrhotic. Blood-stained ascites collects and there is a rapid downward course.

Cholangiocarcinoma

Much less common (20 per cent of primary tumours); an adenocarcinoma arising from the intrahepatic bile duct system which may complicate chronic sclerosing cholangitis. It usually presents with jaundice. Spread occurs directly through the liver substance with a fatal outcome.

Secondaries

The liver is an extremely common site for secondary deposits, which are found in about one in three post-mortems carried out on patients who have died of advanced malignant disease. Necrosis at the centre of metastases lead to the typical umbilication of these tumours.

The clinical effects of secondary deposits in the liver are:
1   Hepatomegaly: the liver is large, hard and irregular.
2   Jaundice: due to liver destruction and intrahepatic duct compression.
3   Hepatic failure
4   Portal vein obstruction: producting oesophageal varices and ascites.
5   Inferior vena cava obstruction: producing leg oedema.

Treatment

A primary hepatoma, confined to one lobe, can be treated by hepatic lobectomy. It may be possible to relieve the jaundice in cholangiocarcinoma by passing a plastic tube upwards along the common bile duct through the growth into the dilated radicles above the obstruction or downwards by a percutaneous intubation. This relieves the jaundice often for months and occasionally for more than a year.

In young people with a primary hepatic tumour confined to the liver, liver transplantation has proved to be a valuable form of treatment.

Resection of secondary tumours is seldom of value but may be considered when isolated deposits are confined to one lobe. Pain may be relieved by ligation of the hepatic artery and occasionally temporary response follows the use of cyto-toxic drugs.

Chapter 33
The Gall Bladder and Bile Ducts

CONGENITAL ABNORMALITIES

Developmentally, a diverticulum grows out from the ventral wall of the foregut (primitive duodenum) which differentiates into the hepatic ducts and the liver. A lateral bud from this diverticulum becomes the gall bladder and cystic duct.

Anomalies are found in 10 per cent of subjects; obviously these are of importance to the surgeon during cholecystectomy. The principal developmental abnormalities include:

1 A long cystic duct travelling alongside the common hepatic duct to open near the duodenal orifice. This occurs in 10% of cases.

2 Congenital absence of the gall bladder.

3 Reduplication of the gall bladder.

4 Congenital obliteration of the ducts (one of the causes of neonatal jaundice).

5 Absence of the cystic duct, the gall bladder opening directly into the side of the common bile duct.

6 A long mesentery to the gall bladder which allows acute torsion of the gall bladder to occur with consequent gangrene and rupture.

7 Anomalies of the arrangement of the blood vessels supplying the gall bladder are common; for example, the right hepatic artery crosses in front of the common hepatic duct instead of behind it in 25 per cent of subjects.

8 Cystic dilatation of the main bile ducts (choledochal cyst).

CHOLELITHIASIS

Gall stones are rare in children, but then their incidence increases with each decade. In this country they are found in approximately 10 per cent of females in their 40's increasing to 30 per cent after the age of 60. They are about half as common in men. Stones are particularly common in the Mediterranean races, and the highest incidence is found among the Indians of New Mexico.

The aphorism that gall stones occur in fair, fat, fertile females of forty is only an approximation to the truth; patients of either sex, any age, colour, shape or fecundity may have gall stones, but certainly the incidence is higher in fat, middle-aged female patients.

There are three common varieties of stone (Fig. 33.1):

1 *Cholesterol* (approximately 20 per cent): these occur either as a solitary, oval stone (the cholesterol solitaire) or as two stones, one indenting the other, or as multiple mulberry stones associated with a strawberry gall bladder (see below).

A cut section shows crystals radiating from the centre of the stone; the surface is yellow and greasy to the touch.

2 *Bile pigment* (approximately 5 per cent), which are small, black, irregular, multiple, gritty and fragile.

CHOLESTEROL

"Solitaire"
or clusters of "mulberries"

Cut surface –
Radiating crystals

PIGMENT

Multiple, small,
black and brittle

Cut surface –
Amorphous

MIXED

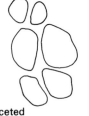

Faceted
May be in "generations"

Cut surface –
Concentric rings

Fig. 33.1. The varieties of gall stones.

3 *Mixed* (approximately 75 per cent): multiple, faceted one against the other, and can often be grouped into two or more series, all of the same size, suggesting 'generations' of stones. The cut surface is laminated with alternate dark and light zones of pigment and cholesterol respectively.

This traditional classification into three groups is an over-simplification; calculi with widely different appearances simply represent different combinations of the same ingredients.

Cholesterol stones

May be associated, although far from invariably, with a high blood cholesterol, which may occur in pregnancy and diabetes. There is also a definite correlation between stones and the contraceptive pill. The mulberry cholesterol stones are often associated with cholesterosis of the gall bladder; here the mucosa is studded with yellow submucous aggregations of cholesterol ('the strawberry gall bladder') which may detach and become the nidus of a cholesterol stone. Cholesterol is virtually insoluble in water but is held in solution in bile as a mixed micelle with bile salts and phospholipids. The bile from patients with gall stones shows a reduction in concentration of both these substances in relation to the cholesterol content, which would favour cholesterol crystallization ('lithogenic bile').

Bile pigment stones

These may occur in the haemolytic anaemias, e.g. acholuric jaundice, where excess of circulating bile pigment is deposited in the biliary tract. If stones are found in the gall bladder of children or adolescents haemolytic anaemia should be suspected, particularly if there is a family history of calculus.

Mixed stones

It is now considered that the majority of mixed stones have the same metabolic origin as cholesterol stones, that is to say, some slight alteration in the composition of bile enabling precipitation of cholesterol together with bile pigment. It may be that an excess of mucus production by the gall bladder wall is an important factor in aggregating these substances into calculi. In other cases clumps of bacteria or desquamated mucosa, perhaps resulting from an episode of infection, may form the nucleus on which crystals may deposit. It may be confessed, however, that a great deal still remains to be discovered about the exact origin of this extremely common condition.

The pathological effects of gall stones

1   Silent: gall stones lying free in the lumen of the gall bladder produce no pathological disturbance of the wall and the patient is symptom-free.

2   Impaction at the exit of the gall bladder or in the cystic duct: water is absorbed from the contained bile which becomes concentrated and produces a chemical cholecystitis. This is usually at first sterile but may then become secondarily infected from organisms secreted from the liver into the bile stream. (Acute cholecystitis can be produced in animals with sterile bile by ligating the cystic duct.)

If the gall bladder happens to be empty when a stone impacts in its outlet, the walls of the organ continue to secrete mucus and the gall bladder distends to form a *mucocele*, a relatively unusual event.

3   Migration into the common bile duct; this may be silent, or produce an intermittent or complete obstruction of the common bile duct with pain and jaundice.

4   Ulceration through the wall of the gall bladder into the duodenum or colon. The gall stone may pass per rectum or produce a gall stone ileus — impaction in the distal ileum with resulting intestinal obstruction.

In addition, the presence of gall stones in the biliary tree is associated with:

5   Acute and chronic pancreatitis.

6   Carcinoma of the gall bladder.

Clinical features

The following syndromes can be recognized:

1   Biliary colic.

2   Acute cholecystitis.

3 Chronic cholecystitis.

4 Obstruction and/or infection of the common bile duct.

Two or more of these syndromes may occur in the same patient.

Biliary Colic

This is produced by impaction of the stone in the gall bladder outlet or duct system for a short period, following which the calculus either falls back or is passed along the duct.

Countractions of the smooth muscle in the wall of the gall bladder and the cystic duct produce severe pain, usually rising to a plateau which lasts for many hours. It is situated usually in the right subcostal region but may be epigastric, or spread as a band across the upper abdomen. Radiation of the pain to the lower pole of the right scapula is common and is accompanied by vomiting and sweating. Characteristically the patient is restless and rolls about in agony, but an intermittent pain is extremely rare.

Differential diagnosis is from the other acute colics, especially ureteric colic.

Acute cholecystitis

If the stone remains impacted in the gall bladder outlet, the gall bladder wall becomes inflamed due to the irritation of the concentrated bile contained within it producing a chemical cholecystitis. The gall bladder fills with pus, which is frequently sterile on culture. In these instances the pain persists and becomes ever more severe. There is a fever in the range of 38–39°C with marked toxaemia and leucocytosis. The upper abdomen is extremely tender and often a palpable mass develops in the region of the gall bladder. This represents the distended, inflamed gall bladder wrapped in inflammatory adhesions to adjacent organs, especially the omentum. Occasionally an empyema of the gall bladder develops or, rarely, perforation takes place into the general peritoneal cavity (see page 217). The swollen gall bladder may press against the adjacent common bile duct and may produce a tinge of jaundice, even through stones may be absent from the duct system.

Ninety-five per cent of cases of acute cholecystitis are associated with gall stones; occasionally fulminating non-calculous cholecystitis may occur and this may be associated with typhoid fever or gas-gangrene infection.

Differential diagnosis is from acute appendicitis, perforated duodenal ulcer, acute pancreatitis, right-sided basal pneumonia and coronary thrombosis.

Chronic cholecystitis

This is almost invariably associated with the presence of gall stones. Repeated episodes of inflammation result in chronic fibrosis and thickening of the entire gall bladder wall, which may contain thick, sometimes infected, bile.

There are recurrent bouts of abdominal pain due to mild cholecystitis which may or may not be accompanied by fever. Discomfort is experienced after fatty meals and there is often flatulence. The picture may be complicated by episodes of acute cholecystitis or symptoms produced by stones passing into the common bile duct.

Differential diagnosis is from other causes of chronic dyspepsia, including peptic ulceration and hiatus hernia. Occasionally the symptoms closely mimic coronary insufficiency. It is well to remain clinically suspicious — any or all of these common diseases may well occur in association with gall stones.

Stones in the common bile duct

May be symptomless. More often they produce attacks of biliary colic accompanied by obstructive jaundice with clay-coloured stools and dark urine, these attacks lasting for hours or for several days. The attack ceases either when a small stone is passed through the sphincter of Oddi or when it disimpacts and falls back into the dilated common duct. Above the impacted stone other stones or bilary mud may deposit. Occasionally the jaundice is progressive and rarely it is painless.

If the obstruction is not relieved either spontaneously or by operation back-pressure liver failure may occur (biliary cirrhosis).

If infection of the common bile duct supervenes (suppurative cholangitis) the jaundice and pain are complicated by rigors, a high intermittent fever and severe toxaemia (the intermittent hepatic fever of Charcot). In these instances the duct system is severely inflamed and filled with pus and the liver may be dotted with multiple small abscesses.

Differential diagnosis of stone in common bile duct

1 With jaundice (75 per cent of cases):
   (a) carcinoma of the pancreas or other malignant obstructions of common bile duct
   (b) acute hepatitis
   (c) other causes of jaundice (page 234)
2 Without jaundice (25 per cent of cases):
   (a) renal colic
   (b) intestinal obstruction
   (c) angina pectoris

Courvoisier's law (Fig. 33.2)

'If in the presence of jaundice the gall bladder is palpable, then the jaundice is unlikely to be due to stone.' This is an extremely useful rule provided that it is enunciated correctly. The principle on which it is based is that if the obstruction is due to stone, the gall bladder is usually thickened and fibrotic and therefore does not distend. Moreover, unlike obstruction due to malignant disease, calculus obstruction is not usually complete. This allows some escape of bile into the duodenum, with decompression of the gall bladder. Obstruction of the common bile duct due to other causes (carcinoma of the head of the pancreas, for example) is usually associated with a normal gall bladder which can dilate. However, in carcinoma of the bile ducts arising above the origin of the cystic duct, the gall bladder, distal to the obstruction, will be collapsed and empty.

Note that the law is not phrased the other way round — 'If the gall bladder is *not* palpable the jaundice is due to stone' — since 50 per cent of dilated gall bladders cannot be palpated on clinical examination, due to either the patient's

COURVOISIER'S LAW

The rule

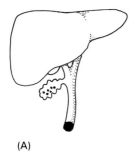

(A)

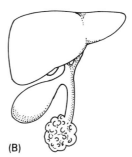

(B)

The exceptions to the rule

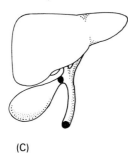

(C)

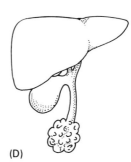

(D)

Fig. 33.2. Obstructive jaundice due to stone is usually associated with a small contracted gall bladder (A). Therefore, 'in the presence of jaundice, a palpable gall bladder indicates that the obstruction is probably due to some other cause — the commonest being carcinoma of the pancreas (B). Exceptions are a palpable gall bladder produced by one stone impacted in Hartmann's pouch resulting in a mucocele, another in the common duct causing obstruction (C), which is very rare or, much more commonly, the gall bladder is indeed distended but is clinically impalpable (D).

obesity or because of overlap by the liver, which itself is usually enlarged as a result of bile engorgement.

Only rarely is the gall bladder dilated when the jaundice is due to stone. These circumstances occur where a stone impacts in Hartmann's pouch to produce a mucocele while at the same time jaundice is produced by a second stone in the common duct, or where a stone forms *in situ* in the common bile duct, the gall bladder itself being normal and therefore distensible; these situations are encountered only rarely in one surgeon's lifetime.

Special investigations

1   *Plain X-ray* of the abdomen reveals radio-opaque gall stones in 10 per cent of cases. These usually appear as rings due to calcium deposited on a central translucent organic core.

2   *An oral cholecystogram* depends on giving an iodine-containing preparation

by mouth which is excreted by the liver into the bile and then concentrated in the gall bladder. The gall bladder may fill but the contained stones are outlined as defects. A diseased gall bladder, being unable to concentrate the dye, will give no shadow on X-ray. Non-filling of the gall bladder in a cholecystogram may not only represent failure of the diseased gall bladder to concentrate, but may also be accounted for either by the patient having vomited the preparation, passed it through the bowel because of diarrhoea which it sometimes induces, or because of associated liver disease which results in failure of secretion of the compound into the bile; the gall bladder is therefore never visualized in any form of hepatic or post-hepatic jaundice.

3 *Ultrasound.* This non-invasive technique is invaluable for the demonstration of stones within the gall bladder. If present, these will usually be revealed as intensely echogenic foci which cast a clear acoustic shadow beyond them. The thickened wall of the gall bladder in chronic inflammation can also be delineated. Unfortunately, ultrasound is unreliable in detecting stones in the bile ducts, especially at the lower end (as is the more expensive CT scan). However, it does demonstration dilatation of the duct system which suggest distal duct obstruction.

4 *Intravenous cholangiography.* Biligrafin given intravenously is excreted in high concentration in the bile, providing liver function is adequate. Often the bile ducts, as well as the gall bladder, can be visualized.

5 *HIDA scanning* gives similar information to a cholecystogram but, in addition, will usually outline the bile ducts.

6 *A barium meal* is always advisable in cases of chronic cholecystitis to exclude an associated peptic ulcer or hiatus hernia.

7 *Liver function tests* are performed whenever jaundice, present or past, is a feature.

8 Endoscopic intubation of the bile ducts through the ampulla of Vater enables the ducts to be visualized radiographically and contained calculi detected.

Treatment

Non-surgical treatment of gall stones

Since cholesterol is held in solution by bile salts, dissolution of small cholesterol stones is possible by administering bile salts orally in the form of chenodeoxycholic or ursodeoxycholic acid. This therapy may be used for small, non-calcified stones in a functioning gall bladder. Treatment must be continued for many months and may be interrupted by attacks of biliary colic as small fragments of calculus pass through the bile ducts. Moreover, recurrences commonly occur after therapy is discontinued. Obviously the indications for this treatment are limited.

Ultrasonic destruction of small stones is also possible, but again there is the problem of the passage of small fragments of stone through the duct system. This may be overcome by aspirating the bile debris from the gall bladder via a catheter placed percutaneously under ultrasound control. Again, this method of treatment has limited indications and disadvantages.

The symptomless gall stone

Gall stones are becoming diagnosed more and more commonly during routine ultrasound examination of the abdomen. Cholecystectomy may be advised, either by open operation or by laparoscopic technique when the patient is young and otherwise well, since symptomless stones may eventually produce the numerous problems listed above. If the patient is elderly or unfit, symptomless stones are left untreated. Alternatively, the non-surgical methods described above might be considered in such cases.

Acute cholecystitis

At least 90 per cent settle on bed rest with pain relief from pethidine and with antibiotics. Elective cholecystectomy is performed about 6 weeks later because of the undoubted danger of further attacks of acute pain. Although classically this operation is carried out by laparotomy, more and more centres perform laparoscopic cholecystectomy. This has the advantage of minimal scarring of the abdominal wall and rapid convalescence, but obviously requires a surgeon well trained in this technique who can also proceed to open operation if technical difficulties are encountered at laparoscopy.

Occasionally an empyema of the gall bladder fails to resolve. Emergency drainage (cholecystotomy) is required, either at open operation or percutaneously under ultrasound control.

Rarely the patient presents with perforation of the acutely inflamed gall bladder and requires urgent surgery.

If diagnosis is in doubt in the early stages of acute cholecystitis, laparotomy is performed. Cholecystectomy is comparatively easy in the first 24–48 hours of the illness; dissection is facilitated by the oedema of adjacent tissues, although after this time operation becomes difficult because of the inflammatory adhesions. Because of the comparative facility of early surgery, many surgeons advise urgent surgical intervention in acute cholecystitis.

Chronic cholecystitis

Cholecystectomy is performed, either by laparotomy or laparoscopy. The cystic duct is intubated and an operative cholangiogram performed by injecting radio-opaque contrast medium into the common duct. If the stones are demonstrated and laparotomy has been performed, the common bile duct is then explored, the stones removed, a T-tube inserted into the common duct and a check X-ray performed. The T-tube is removed 10 days post-operatively,provided that a check cholangiogram taken through the tube confirms that the ducts are clear and that there is free flow into the duodenum. There is still controversy about the best line of treatment if stones within the common duct are demonstrated at laparoscopic cholangiography. Some surgeons will then proceed to immediate laparotomy and removal of the stones while others will perform a subsequent endoscopic sphincterotomy and extraction of the stones with a Dormier basket. The comparative advantages and late results of these two techniques remain to be assessed.

Obstructive jaundice due to stone

The great majority of cases resolve on conservative treatment. Subsequent cholecystectomy and exploration of the common duct is performed. Persistent or progressive jaundice, particularly in the presence of high fever, makes removal of the impacted stones and drainage of the obstructed common bile duct imperitive as an emergency procedure. This can be performed by open operation or, especially in the severely ill patient, by endoscopic sphincterotomy. This is preceded by giving intravenous vitamin K, since depressed absorption of this fat-soluble vitamin lowers the serum prothrombin with consequent bleeding tendency.

Complications of cholecystectomy

There are two special dangers after cholecystectomy, whether performed by laparotomy or laparoscopy:

1 *Leakage of bile* resulting from injury to bile canaliculi in the gall bladder bed of the liver, slipping of the ligature from the cystic duct, or leakage from the suture line after common bile duct exploration.

Providing the common bile duct is patent, the bile fistula will close spontaneously; if this does not occur further exploration may be required.

2 *Jaundice* due to:
(a) missed stones in the common bile duct
(b) inadvertent ligature of the common bile duct
(c) cholangitis or associated pancreatitis

Residual stones in the common duct may require operative removal. However, in the majority of cases they can be removed by endoscopic sphincterotomy or, if a T-tube is still present in the common duct, by means of a Dormier basket passed along the track thus formed under X-ray control.

CARCINOMA OF THE GALL BLADDER

Pathology

This is a relatively unusual tumour, but it is associated in about 95 per cent of cases with the presence of gall stones. It is debatable whether this is due to chronic irritation or to the carcinogenic effect of cholic acid derivatives. Since gall stones are commoner in females, carcinoma of the gall bladder is not surprisingly four times commoner in females than males. Ninety per cent are adenocarcinoma and 10 per cent squamous carcinoma.

There is local invasion of the liver and its ducts and lymphatic spread to the nodes in the porta hepatis; portal vein dissemination, also to the liver, may occur.

Clinical features

Carcinoma of the gall bladder usually presents with a picture closely resembling chronic cholecystitis, progressing to obstructive jaundice. At this stage a palpable mass may be present in the gall bladder region.

Treatment

Occasionally cholecystectomy performed for stone reveals the presence of an unexpected tumour. Under these circumstances, long term survival is likely to follow; but by the time liver invasion has occurred by direct spread, wide local excision is only rarely possible and the prognosis is therefore usually poor.

Chapter 34
The Pancreas

CONGENITAL ANOMALIES

The pancreas develops as a dorsal and a ventral bud from the duodenum. The ventral bud rotates posteriorly, thus enclosing the superior mesenteric vessels; it forms the major part of the head of the pancreas and its duct becomes the main duct of Wirsung, which in the great majority of cases has a common opening with the common bile duct in the ampulla of Vater. The dorsal bud becomes the body and tail and its duct becomes the accessory duct of Santorini.

Annular pancreas

The two developmental buds may envelop the second part of the duodenum, producing this rare form of duodenal extrinsic obstruction.

Heterotopic pancreas

Produced by an accessory budding from the primitive foregut and occurs in 20 per cent of subjects. A nodule of pancreatic tissue may be found in the stomach, duodenum or jejunum. Occasionally this produces obstructive or dyspeptic symptoms.

ACUTE PANCREATITIS

Aetiology

The aetiology of acute pancreatitis is not completely determined, but it appears to be an auto-digestion of the pancreas by its activated pro-enzymes, especially trypsin. This may result from a number of factors, some definite, others only postulated, which include:

1 There is a definite association with the presence of gall stones (found in about 50 per cent). Possibly the gall bladder disease prevents the safety valve effect of the normal distensible gall bladder and allows a rapid rise in biliary pressure with regurgitation along the pancreatic duct. Alternatively, this reflux in the pancreatic duct may be produced by temporary impaction of a stone at the ampulla of Vater.

2 Alcohol: recurrent attacks of pancreatitis are usually associated with chronic alcoholism, which is the chief cause of pancreatitis in North America and France.

3 Trauma — either a crush injury or at operation, e.g. damage to the pancreas during mobilization of the duodenum at partial gastrectomy. It may occur after endoscopic sphincterotomy.

4 Regurgitation of infected bile — normal reflux appears to do no harm and is often seen at cholangiography, but may be a factor if the bile itself is infected or the pancreatic duct already diseased.

5 Infection — acute pancreatitis may complicate mumps, typhoid or Coxsackie infection.

6 Corticosteroids — may precipitate acute pancreatitis.

7 Vascular — pancreatitis may occur in malignant hypertension and polyarteritis nodosa, probably as a result of local infarction.

8 Duodenopancreatic reflux — this is undoubtedly an important factor. Duodenal fluid contains enterokinase which activates the pancreatic pro-enzymes. Duodenal reflux can be shown experimentally to produce pancreatitis. Reflux through the papilla may occur as a result of its injury following endoscopic cannulation or trauma or surgery in this region. Damage to the sphincter may result from alcohol or from the recent passage of a stone. Duodenal reflux may therefore be a common factor which underlies many of the aetiological associations mentioned above.

Macroscopic pathology

At operation, the appearances are quite typical. There is a blood-stained peritoneal effusion. White spots of fat necrosis are scattered throughout the peritoneal cavity; these are produced by lipase released from the pancreas which liberates fatty acids and glycerol from fat; these acids combine with calcium to produce insoluble calcium soaps. The pancreas is swollen, haemorrhagic or, in severe cases, actually necrotic. Occasionally suppurative pancreatitis may occur.

Clinical features

The patient is often obese and middle aged or elderly. Women are more often affected than men. Pain is severe, constant, usually epigastric and often radiates into the back. Vomiting is early and profuse. The patient is usually shocked with a rapid pulse, cyanosis (indicating circulatory collapse) and a temperature which may either be subnormal or be raised up to 39.5°C (103°F). The abdomen reveals generalized tenderness and guarding. About 30 per cent of the cases have a tinge of jaundice due to oedema of the pancreatic head obstructing the common bile duct.

Less common features are glycosuria due to islet cell damage (about 15 per cent of cases) and tetany, which may occur, it is suggested, as a consequence of the destruction of parathormone by circulating proteolytic enzymes and calcium deposits from the plasma into areas of fat necrosis.

A few days after a severe attack the patient may develop a bluish discoloration in the loins from extravasation of bloodstained pancreatic juice into the retroperitoneal tissues (Grey Turner's sign).

Pseudocyst formation may occur as fluid accumulates in the lesser sac.

Differential diagnosis

The less severe episode of acute pancreatitis simulates acute cholecystitis; the more severe attack, with a marked degree of shock, is usually mistaken for a perforated peptic ulcer or coronary thrombosis. Differentiation must also be made from high intestinal obstruction and from other causes of peritonitis.

Special investigations

1 *Serum amylase* — raised from the normal (up to 150 Somogyi units per 100 ml) to 600 units or more in the acute phase, but returns to normal within 2 or

3 days. Occasionally an overwhelming attack of pancreatitis with extensive destruction of the gland is associated with a normal amylase. The level may be raised to 400 units or more in some cases of perforated peptic ulcer, coronary thrombosis or intestinal obstruction, and may also be raised if morphia or codeine have been given (associated with sphincter of Oddi spasm).

2 *Moderate leucocytosis.*

3 *Glycosuria* is present in 15 per cent of cases.

4 *Serum bilirubin* is often raised.

5 *Serum calcium* may be lowered; in these cases the prognosis is bad.

6 *EGG* may show a diminished T wave; the cause of this is not known.

7 *X-rays of the abdomen* often give no direct help. The absence of free gas or of localized fluid levels assist in the differential diagnosis of perforated duodenal ulcer or high intestinal obstruction. In some cases a solitary dilated loop of proximal jejunum may be seen (the 'sentinel loop sign'). Occasionally radio-opaque pancreatic calculi may be present.

8 *Ultrasound and CT scanning* will demonstrate associated gall stones and may show enlargement of the pancreas. At a later stage, necrotic pancreas, abscess or pseudocyst may be visualized. Of the two, the CT scan is more valuable because the ultrasonography may be obscured by gas in the upper gastro-intestinal tract.

9 *Blood gases* — hypoxia occurs in severe cases.

Note that each of the three enzymes liberated by the pancreas plays a part in the overall picture of acute pancreatitis:

1 *Trypsin:* produces the auto-digestion of the pancreas.

2 *Lipase:* results in the typical fat necrosis.

3 *Amylase:* absorbed from the peritoneal cavity produces a rise in the serum level and is thus a helpful test in diagnosis.

Treatment

In the established case treatment is conservative and consists of:

1 Relief of pain with pethidine (avoiding morphia which produces sphincter spasm). If the pain remains unrelieved, a splanchnic nerve block is performed.

2 Shock is treated with blood transfusion and mannitol to maintain a diuresis.

3 Electrolyte and water replacement by intravenous drip.

4 Antibiotics are given to reduce the chance of secondary infection of peritoneal exudate.

5 Pancreatic secretion is reduced by probanthine or atropine.

6 Calcium gluconate is given to replace immobilized calcium.

7 Cortisone is given in severe shock.

Surgery is indicated if the diagnosis is not certain, or occasionally for the drainage of an abscess or pseudocyst.

After recovery from an attack of pancreatitis, the patient is investigated for the presence of gall stones (cholecystogram, ultra-sound) and cholecystectomy advised if these are present.

The mortality rate is in the region of 20 per cent and is directly proportional to the severity of the attack.

Complications
1 Abscess formation with pancreatic necrosis
2 Pseudocyst
3 Further attacks (relapsing pancreatitis)
4 Persistent diabetes mellitus
5 Renal failure associated with shock and pancreatic necrosis
6 Pulmonary insufficiency, possibly due to loss of surfactant

CHRONIC RELAPSING PANCREATITIS

Occasionally a patient suffers repeated attacks of pancreatitis. Eventually the pancreas undergoes atrophy, calcification and cyst or abscess formation, passing into a stage of chronic pancreatitis; the ducts are dilated and may contain calculi.

Alcoholism is the main cause. The condition is comparatively rare in this country but is prevalent in America and France.

Clinical features

The patient may present with one or more of the following:
1 Asymptomatic (X-ray diagnosis only from pancreatic calcification).
2 Episodes of recurrent abdominal pain radiating through to the upper lumbar region.
3 Steatorrhoea due to pancreatic insufficiency.
4 Diabetes due to islet cell damage.
5 Obstructive jaundice, which is very difficult to differentiate, even at operation, from carcinoma of the head of the pancreas.

Special investigations

Amylase estimations performed during attacks of pain may be elevated and there may be X-ray evidence of calcification or calculi. A CT scan may demonstrate enlargement and irregular consistency of the gland. An ERCP may show dilatation and irregularity of the pancreatic duct. However, the differential diagnosis from a pancreatic carcinoma may only be established by laparotomy.

Treatment

1 Mild cases: low fat diet, pancreatic enzymes by mouth, prohibition of alcohol.
2 Removal of associated factors: cholecystectomy if gallstones are present.
3 In severe cases partial pancreatectomy or drainage of the whole length of the pancreatic duct into a loop of intestine may be required.
4 Painless obstructive jaundice may be relieved by a short-circuit of the gall bladder (cholecyst-jejunostomy).

PANCREATIC CYSTS

Classification

1. True (20 per cent)
    (a) congenital polycystic disease of pancreas

(b) retention
(c) hydatid
(d) neoplastic
  (i) cystadenoma
  (ii) cystadenocarcinoma

2. False

A collection of fluid in the lesser sac (80 per cent):
  (a) after trauma to the pancreas
  (b) following acute pancreatitis
  (c) perforation of a posterior gastric ulcer (rare)

Clinical features

Pancreatic cyst presents as a firm, large, rounded, upper abdominal swelling. Initially the cyst is apparently resonant because of loops of gas-filled bowel in front of it, but as it increases in size the intestine is pushed away and the mass becomes dull to percussion.

Treatment

True cysts require surgical excision; false cysts are drained. This may be performed internally, (by anastomosis either into the stomach or into the small intestine), or percutaneously, under ultrasound control.

PANCREATIC TUMOURS

Classification

Benign

(a) adenoma
(b) cystadenoma
(c) islet cell tumour
  (i) Zollinger — Ellison tumour (non-beta cell tumour)
  (ii) Insulinoma (beta cell tumour. Alpha cells produce glucagon)

Malignant

1 *Primary:*
  (a) carcinoma
  (b) cystadenocarcinoma
  (c) malignant islet cell tumour
2 *Secondary:* invasion from carcinoma of stomach or bile duct

ISLET CELL TUMOURS

These tumours, although rare, are of great interest because of their metabolic effects even from small lesions which may be difficult to localize even with CT or MR scanning and selective angiography.

Occasionally they are associated with multiple endocrine adenomas, affecting the parathyroid and the anterior pituitary gland.

Zollinger–Ellison tumour (non-beta cell islet tumour)

This tumour of non-beta cells may be benign or malignant, the latter being relatively slow growing, although eventually producing hepatic metastases. It secretes a gastrin-like substance into the blood stream which produces an extremely high gastric secretion of HCl. The patient may present with diarrhoea, the cause of which is not yet certain but which may be acid stimulation of the small bowel. The majority of cases develop fulminating peptic ulceration, which rapidly recurs after gastrectomy or vagotomy and drainage.

Treatment

Treatment comprises excision of the tumour or, if this is not possible, control of the high acid secretion by means of the histamine H_2 receptor antagonists (cimetidine, ranitidine) or, if these fail, omeprazole, which is a direct gastric anti-secretory drug. Failure of medical treatment may require total gastrectomy.

Insulinoma (beta cell islet tumour)

Ninety per cent are benign, 10 per cent malignant and about 10 per cent are multiple tumours. Because of the high production of insulin by the growth two groups of hypoglycaemic symptoms may be produced:

1   *CNS phenomena:* weakness, sweating, trembling, epilepsy, confusion, hemiplegia and eventually coma, which may be fatal.

2   *Gastro-intestinal phenomena:* hunger, abdominal pain and diarrhoea. These symptoms appear particularly when the patient is hungry; they are often present early in the morning before breakfast and are relieved by eating. Often there is excessive appetite with gross weight gain.

Whipple's triad, typical of this condition, states that:

1   The attacks are induced by starvation.

2   During the attack hypoglycaemia is present.

3   The episode is relieved by sugar given orally or intravenously.

Diagnosis is confirmed by a glucose tolerance test which shows hypoglycaemia; the test should be continued for several hours since it may require 8 or 10 hours of starvation to induce the hypoglycaemia.

Treatment

Excision of the tumour.

CARCINOMA OF THE PANCREAS

Pathology

Sixty per cent are situated in the head of the pancreas, 25 per cent in the body and 15 per cent in the tail.

Of the tumours of the head of the pancreas, one-third are periampullary, arising from the ampulla of Vater, the duodenal mucosa or the lower end of the common bile duct.

Males are affected twice as commonly as females and the age distribution is middle-aged and elderly. The incidence of this tumour is increasing, particularly in the USA, where deaths from this cause are now commoner than from carcinoma of the stomach.

Macroscopically the growth is infiltrating, hard and irregular.

Microscopically the tumours may be:

1 Mucus-secreting (of duct origin).
2 Non-mucus secreting (of acinar origin).
3 Undifferentiated.
4 Cystadenocarcinoma (rare).

Spread

1 *Direct:* invading the common bile duct, with obstructive jaundice, the duodenum, producing occult or obvious intestinal bleeding, the portal vein, producing portal hypertension and ascites, and the inferior vena cava, resulting in bilateral leg oedema.
2 *Lymphatic:* to adjacent lymph nodes and nodes in the porta hepatis.
3 *Blood stream:* to the liver and then to the lungs.
4 *Trans-coelomic:* with peritoneal seeding and ascites.

Clinical features

Carcinoma of the pancreas may present in a variety of ways:

1 The classical text-book story is of *painless progressive jaundice* but this form is, in fact, rather uncommon and, when it does occur, is usually found in the peri-ampullary type of tumour. Obviously this is because the bile duct is compressed at an early stage, before extensive painful invasion of surrounding tissues.
2 *Pain:* at least 50 per cent present with epigastric pain of a dull, continuous aching nature which frequently radiates into the upper lumbar region. This pain often precedes:
3 *Jaundice,* which is usually progressive, but which may temporarily remit or even disappear as necrosis of the tumour occurs, allowing a transient escape of bile into the duodenum.
4 *Diabetes:* glycosuria of recent onset in the elderly is suspicious.
5 *Thrombophlebitis migrans* (the pathogenesis of this is unknown).
6 *The general features of malignant disease:* anorexia and loss of weight.

On examination, the patient is frequently jaundiced. Fifty per cent have a palpable gall bladder (Courvoisier's Law, see page 254); if the tumour is large, an epigastric mass may be palpable. The liver is frequently enlarged, either from the back-pressure of biliary obstruction (biliary cirrhosis) or because of secondary deposits.

Investigations

It is important to know that these are often completely negative, even in advanced cases, especially carcinoma of the pancreatic body or tail.

A barium meal may show widening of the duodenal loop and a filling defect or irregularity of the duodenum resulting from invasion by the tumour (the 'reversed 3' sign).

Occult blood may be present in the stools, especially from a periampullary tumour ulcerating into the duodenum.

The serum amylase is only rarely elevated.

When jaundice is present the biochemical changes are those of obstructive jaundice (see page 236).

CT scanning and ultrasonography may demonstrate the tumour mass. Fine needle biopsy may be performed under imaging control.

An ampullary growth may be visualized through a fibrescope and a biopsy obtained.

Differential diagnosis

This is from other causes of obstructive jaundice (see page 234) and from other causes of upper abdominal pain. Carcinoma of the body and tail of the pancreas, in which obstructive jaundice does not occur, is notoriously difficult to diagnose. Laboratory and X-ray investigations are usually negative and the patient is frequently labelled 'neurotic'.

Treatment

In the presence of jaundice, vitamin K must be given preoperatively. Laparotomy is performed; open biopsy is avoided because of the risk of pancreatic fistula, but needle biopsy through the wall of the second part of the duodenum may be helpful. If the tumour is operable, excision of the head of the pancreas and the duodenum is performed (pancreaticoduodenectomy).

Small tumours of the peri-ampullary region can occasionally be excised locally through an incision in the duodenum.

The majority of tumours are inoperable because of their advanced nature at the time of diagnosis. The obstructive jaundice (and its associated severe pruritus) can be relieved either by intubation by means of a stent passed through the duodenal papilla at endoscopy or by operation. This comprises a palliative short circuit between the distended gall bladder and a loop of jejunum (cholecystoje-junostomy). The severe pain may be relieved by radiotherapy but usually requires management with opiates.

Occasionally a patient has a surprisingly prolonged survival after a short circuit operation; in such a case one must revise the diagnosis and assume that the obstructive lesion in the head of the pancreas was in fact an example of chronic pancreatitis.

Prognosis

The outlook for patients with carcinoma of the pancreas itself is gloomy; even if the growth is resectable, the operation has a mortality of about 10 per cent and only a small percentage survive for 5 years. Peri-ampullary growths, however, which present relatively early, have a reasonably good prognosis after resection with about 25 per cent 5-year survival.

Chapter 35
The Spleen

SPLENOMEGALY

Physical signs

The spleen must be enlarged to about three times its normal size before it becomes clinically palpable. It then forms a swelling which descends below the left costal margin, moves on respiration, and has a firm lower margin which may or may not be notched. The mass is dull to percussion, the dullness extending above the costal margin.

There are two important differential diagnoses:

1 An enlarged left kidney; unless this is enormous there is resonance over the swelling anteriorly since it is covered by the gas-containing colon.

2 Carcinoma of the cardia or upper part of the body of the stomach; by the time such a tumour reaches palpable proportions there are usually symptoms of gastric obstruction which suggest the site of the lesion.

Classification

It is essential to have a working classification of enlargements of the spleen:

1 *Infections:*
    (a) viruses; glandular fever
    (b) bacterial: typhus, typhoid, septicaemia ('septic spleen')
    (c) protozoal: malaria, kala-azar, Egyptian splenomegaly (schistosomiaais)
    (d) parasitic: hydatid

2 *Haemopoietic diseases:* e.g. leukaemia, Hodgkin's disease, non-Hodgkin's lymphoma, pernicious anaemia, polycythaemia, haemolytic·anaemia, myelosclerosis

3 *Portal hypertension*

4 *Metabolic and collagen disease:* e.g. amyloid, Gaucher's disease, Still's disease, Felty's syndrome

5 *Cysts, abscesses and tumours of the spleen:* all uncommon

Two points of practical clinical value: A massive splenomegaly in this country is likely to be due to one of the following: chronic leukaemia, lymphoma, polycythaemia or portal hypertension.

If the spleen is palpable special attention must be paid to detecting the presence of hepatomegaly and lymphadenopathy (see page 77).

SPLENECTOMY

This is indicated under the following circumstances:

1 Rupture: either from closed or open trauma or accidental damage during abdominal surgery.

2 As a part of some other operative procedure, e.g. radical excision of carcinoma of the stomach, spleno-renal anastomosis.

3 Blood diseases: haemolytic anaemia, thrombocytopenic purpura.

4 Tumours and cysts.

Splenectomy in children is associated with a risk of overwhelming sepsis, particularly from the pneumococcus. Children undergoing splenectomy should be immunized with anti-pneumococcal vaccine and put on oral prophylactic penicillin for an indefinite period.

RUPTURED SPLEEN

This is the commonest internal injury produced by non-penetrating trauma to the abdominal wall. It usually occurs alone, but may coexist with fractures of the ribs and rupture of the liver, the left kidney, the diaphragm or the tail of the pancreas.

Clinical features

Ruptures of the spleen fall into four groups:

1 Massive bleeding with rapid death from shock: this results from a complete shattering of the spleen or its avulsion from the splenic pedicle, and death may occur in a few minutes. Fortunately this is rare.

2 Following injury there are the symptoms and signs of progressive blood loss together with evidence of peritoneal irritation. Over a period of several hours after the accident the patient becomes increasingly more pale, the pulse rises and the blood pressure falls. There is abdominal pain, which is either diffuse or confined to the left flank. The patient may complain of referred pain to the left shoulder or admit to this only on direct questioning. The abdomen is generally tender, particularly on the left side, but rigidity may vary from being generalized and extremely marked to being confined to slight guarding in the left flank. The percussion note is impaired in the left flank due to the local collection of blood; this is a sign on which we have come to rely. Surprisingly enough, bruising of the abdominal wall is often absent or only slight.

3 Delayed rupture, which may occur from hours up to several days after trauma. There is the initial injury with concomitant pain which soon settles, then, following a completely asymptomatic interval, the signs and symptoms described above become manifest. This picture is produced by a subcapsular haematoma of the spleen which increases in size due to haemolysis and which then ruptures the thin overlying peritoneal capsule with a resultant sudden, sharp haemorrhage.

4 Spontaneous: a spleen diseased by malaria, glandular fever, leukaemia etc., may rupture after only trivial trauma.

Investigations

The diagnosis of rupture of the spleen is a clinical one and in the face of massive haemorrhage, the surgeon must proceed at once to laparotomy. In the less acute situation, the following investigations are useful:

1 The *urine* is tested for blood; haematuria will suggest associated renal damage.

2 *Chest x-ray* may reveal associated rib fractures, rupture of the diaphragm or injury to the left lung.

3 *Abdominal x-ray;* the stomach bubble may be displaced to the right and there may be indentation of its gas shadow. The splenic flexure of the colon, if containing gas, may be seen to be displaced downwards by the haematoma.

4 *Ultrasound and CT* will often demonstrate the laceration of the spleen and the presence of intra-abdominal fluid.

Treatment

Blood transfusion is commenced and laparotomy performed. If the spleen is found to be avulsed or hopelessly pulped, emergency splenectomy is required. If there is minor laceration of the spleen, an attempt is made to preserve it, especially in children and young adults where there is a risk of post-splenectomy septicaemia. This may be carried out by using fine sutures and haemostatic absorbable gauze.

Having controlled the bleeding, it is important to carry out a full examination to exclude injury to other organs.

Chapter 36
The Kidney and Ureter

Embryology (Fig. 36.1)

The pronephros disappears in man. The distal part of its duct receives the mesonephros to become the mesonephric (Wolffian) duct. The mesonephros itself then disappears except that, in the male, some of its ducts become the efferent tubules of the testis. A diverticulum then forms in the lower end of the Wolffian duct which grows into the metanephric duct on top of which develops a cap of tissue, the metanephros. The metanephros gives rise to the glomeruli and the proximal part of the renal duct system. The metanephric duct forms the ureter, renal pelvis, calcyces and distal ducts. The mesonephric duct atrophies in the female, the remnant being called the epoöphron, but in the male it gives rise to the epididymis and the vas deferens.

The kidney originally develops in the pelvis of the embryo and then migrates cranially, acquiring successively a more proximal arterial blood supply as it does so.

CONGENITAL ANOMALIES

This complex developmental process explains the high frequency with which congenital anomalies of the kidney, the ureter and the renal blood supply are found. Among the more important of these are:

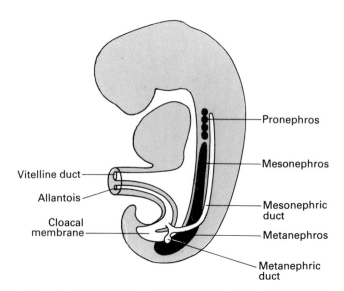

Fig. 36.1. Development of the pro-, meso- and metaphrenic systems (after Langman).

1   Pelvic kidney: due to failure of cranial migration of the developing kidney.

2   Horseshoe kidney: produced by fusion of the two metanephric masses across the midline (see below).

3   Double ureters and/or kidneys (duplex kidney): due to reduplication of the metanephric bud.

4   Congenital absence of one kidney (1 in every 2500 subjects).

5   Polycystic kidneys: possibly due to failure of linkage between the metanephric duct system and the metanephros (see below).

6   Congenital hydronephrosis: produced by neuromuscular inco-ordination at the pelvi-ureteric junction.

7   Both kidneys may lie on the same side.

8   Aberrant renal arteries — one or more arteries supplying the upper or lower pole of the kidneys are very common; they represent the persistence of aortic branches which pass to the kidney in its lower embryonic position.

Congenital absence of a kidney is extremely rare, but should be borne in mind whenever the possibility of nephrectomy arises, for instance, after kidney trauma.

Polycystic disease, the various types of reduplication of the renal pelvis and the abnormal fusions are all associated with an increased incidence of infection when compared with kidneys that are anatomically normal.

POLYCYSTIC DISEASE

Pathology

This is believed to arise from failure of fusion of the metanephros with its duct; the result is multiple cysts throughout the renal substance, nearly always in both kidneys. These cysts are surrounded by attenuated renal tissue. The condition is frequently familial, present in each generation due to dominant inheritance, 50 per cent of siblings being affected.

There may be associated multiple cysts in other viscera — the liver in 30 per cent, the lungs, spleen or pancreas in 10 per cent.

Clinical modes of presentation

Polycystic kidneys may present at birth as a cause of obstructed labour. The infant may be born dead as a result of multiple congenital anomalies.

The condition may be detected because symptomless, bilateral, lobulated renal swellings are found on routine examination.

Haematuria, aching pain in the loin or renal infection may occur, although these symptoms pointing to some renal anomaly are relatively unusual.

Much more often the patient presents with one or other of the two lethal terminations of this disease: renal failure or hypertension. The first may produce headache, lassitude, vomiting and a refractory anaemia; the second cardiac failure or cerebral haemorrhage. Subarachnoid haemorrhage is especially likely as there is an increased incidence of circle of Willis 'berry' aneurysm.

On examination the enlarged lobulated kidneys are usually readily palpable. There may be the clinical features of chronic uraemia and the blood pressure is often considerably elevated.

Special investigations

Ultrasonography is very accurate in detecting the multiple cysts in adults, but is less so in children because of the smaller size of the cysts.

If the blood urea is not raised, an intravenous urogram demonstrates the typical elongated spidery calyces stretched out, and indented by the cysts.

Treatment

Left untreated, many patients may survive in reasonable health well passed middle age. Medical treatment is required in the management of the complicating hypertension and renal failure. In advanced cases, renal transplantation, often combined with bilateral nephrectomy, gives excellent long-term results.

Renal cysts

A unilocular cyst of the kidney is quite common. It may be small or may reach a very large size. Several cysts may be present and both kidneys may be affected. The cause is unknown.

Clinical features

The cyst may be symptomless and may be found as a mass on routine clinical examination. If very large, it may present as an aching pain in the loin. Haematuria is absent, and this is an important point in differentiation from a renal carcinoma.

Special investigations

The urine is clear, even on microscopic examination.

The intravenous urogram demonstrates a round filling defect which displaces but does not invade the calyces.

Ultrasonography confirms a cystic mass.

Selective renal arteriography will show a smooth, avascular filling defect, in contrast to the rich tumour circulation typical of a renal tumour.

Treatment

The cyst can be aspirated under ultrasound control. Clear serous fluid is obtained. Occasionally surgical exploration is indicated if a firm differential diagnosis cannot be made between cyst and tumour. Simple decapping of the cyst is all that is required, leaving the base of the cyst attached to the kidney.

HORSESHOE KIDNEY

The two kidneys may be joined together in a variety of ways, but the commonest is the horseshoe kidney, in which the fusion occurs across the midline. The linked lower ends of the kidneys usually lie in front of the aorta in the region of the fourth or fifth lumbar vertebra and the ureters descend from the front of the fused kidneys. This disorder may present as a firm mass in the pelvis or as attacks of renal tract infection. An intravenous pyelogram will show rotation of the two renal pelvises with the ureters arising close to the midline. Usually the renal pelvises are directed laterally.

The main surgical importance of horseshoe kidneys is the differential diagnosis of a lump in the pelvis and the importance of not removing such renal tissue as an undiagnosed 'mass' — the consequences are disastrous.

HAEMATURIA

Classification (Fig. 36.2)

Two useful rules:

    1 When considering the causes of bleeding from any orifice in the body, always remember the general causes due to bleeding diatheses.

    2 When considering any local cause of symptoms in the genitourinary tract, always think of the whole tract — from the kidneys to the urethra.

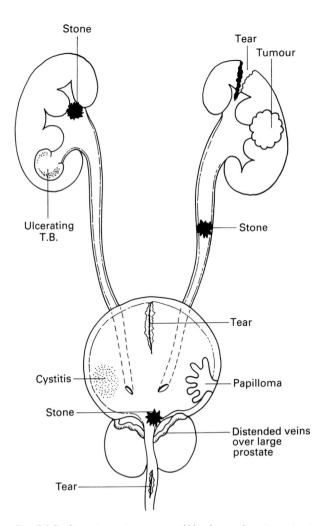

Fig. 36.2. Some important causes of bleeding in the urinary tract.

Haematuria is an excellent example of these two general rules and the causes can be classified as follows:

General

Bleeding diatheses, e.g. anticoagulant drugs, thrombocytopenic purpura.

Local

1 Kidney: trauma, polycystic disease, glomerulonephritis, TB, infarction (from mitral stenosis or subacute bacterial endocarditis), stone and tumour.
2 Ureter: stone and tumour.
3 Bladder: trauma, cystitis, stone, tumour and bilharzia.
4 Prostate: 'varices'.
5 Urethra: trauma, stone and tumour.

Management of haematuria

Blood in the urine is an alarming symptom and usually brings the patient rapidly to the doctor. It should always be taken seriously and requires full elucidation — history, examination and special investigations.

History

Completely painless and otherwise symptomless haematuria is suggestive of a tumour in the urinary tract. Pain in one or other loin suggests renal origin and typical colic indicates a stone in the renal pelvis or ureter or partial ureteric obstruction by clot. Terminal bleeding with severe pain and frequency indicates bladder calculus. Dribbling of blood from the urethra independent of micturition is typical of urethral origin.

A history of recent sore throat, especially in a child, would make a diagonsis of acute nephritis a possibility. Enquiries are made as to whether the patient is on anticoagulant therapy or if there is a history of bleeding tendencies.

Examination

One or other kidneys may be palpable, a carcinoma of the bladder may be felt on bimanual examination. An enlarged prostate, particularly if the patient is hypertensive, suggests prostatic 'varices' although other causes must be excluded before this diagnosis is finally made.

Special investigations

The urine is examined both naked eye and microscopically; the presence of red cells will exclude haemoglobinuria and beeturia. The presence of casts will indicate nephritis; pus cells and organisms suggests an infective process.

An intravenous urogram may reveal a localized renal lesion or may show a filling defect in the ureter or bladder. Stones in the urinary tract will be displayed on this investigation; look for them carefully on the preliminary plain films — they may be obscured by contrast in the urogram.

Cystoscopy will show any intravesical lesion; bleeding from the prostate will be visible or blood may be seen to emerge from one or other ureter. Cystoscopy is therefore a valuable investigation to perform immediately if the patient is seen at the time that haematuria is obvious.

Selective renal angiography may demonstrate a small bleeding tumour of the kidney or pelvis.

At the end of these investigations the cause for the haematuria may still not have been determined. It is occasionally seen in hypertensive patients ('renal epistaxis'), but in such cases the patient should be kept under close observation and the investigations repeated if haematuria persists.

INJURIES OF THE KIDNEY

The kidney may be injured by a direct blow in the loin or occasionally by a penetrating wound; the degree of damage varies from slight subcapsular bruising to complete rupture and fragmentation of the kidney or its avulsion from its vascular pedicle.

Clinical features

Clinically there is usually local pain and tenderness and haematuria is a common finding. Retro-peritoneal haematoma may cause abdominal distension due to ileus. There may be associated injury to other viscera, especially the spleen.

Special investigations

The urine usually demonstrates macroscopic haematuria.

Intravenous urography is a valuable help in management; damage to the kidney may be shown by extravasation of dye outside the renal outline or distortion or rupture of the renal calyces. This examination will also determine the very important fact whether or not there is a normal kidney on the other side.

Ultrasound examination of the abdomen can delineate a renal tear as well as indicating injury to other solid viscera, the liver and spleen. Views may be obscured, however, if there is considerable intra-abdominal gas.

CT scanning is particularly useful in defining solid viscera injuries and is not affected by distended loops of bowel.

Treatment

Associated injuries and shock will require appropriate treatment.

In practice most cases fortunately resolve with conservative management, namely bed rest, serial observations of the urine to determine whether or not the haematuria is clearing, and careful clinical charting of blood pressure and pulse rate.

Nephrectomy is required in renal trauma in the following circumstances:

1 Continued bleeding which threatens life.
2 Severe hypertension persisting after renal injury.
3 Evidence of lack of function in the affected kidney after several months have elapsed in which recovery should have occurred.

HYDRONEPHROSIS

Pathology

Hydronephrosis is a dilatation of the renal pelvis and calyces. It may result from congenital neuromuscular incoordination at the pelvi-ureteric junction or from obstruction of the urinary outflow. This obstruction may be unilateral, for example due to a stone in the ureter, or the block may involve the urethra, e.g. prostatic hypertrophy or urethral stricture, with resultant bilateral hydronephrosis.

Aberrant renal vessels were considered to be a common cause of hydronephrosis since they frequently cross the dilated renal pelvis at its junction with the ureter. It is probably unusual for these aberrant vessels actually to initiate the hydronephrosis; more likely they snare the congenitally dilated pelvis and merely act as a secondary constrictive factor.

Complications

1 Infection: resulting in pyonephrosis (page 281).
2 Stone formation: phosphatic calculi readily deposit in the infected stagnant urine.
3 Hypertension: secondary to renal ischaemia.
4 Uraemia: where there is extensive bilateral destruction of renal tissue.
5 Traumatic rupture of the hydronephrotic bag.

Clinical features

An uncomplicated hydronephrosis on one side may be symptomless or may produce a dull, aching pain in the loin often mistaken for 'lumbago' or 'rheumatism'. Occasionally there may be acute attacks of pain resembling ureteric colic. Associated infection may present with fever, pyuria, rigors and sever loin pain. Bilateral hydronephrosis may present with the clinical features of uraemia. Very often it is the underlying cause, e.g. the ureteric calculus, the enlarged prostate or the urethral stricture which manifests itself clinically.

On examination the enlarged kidney may be palpable. The size of this may vary according to the state of distension of the renal pelvis.

Special investigations

Diagnosis is confirmed by an intravenous urogram which demonstrates the enlarged renal pelvis and the swollen, dilated club-like calyces. If renal function is severely impaired, the kidney may not secrete contrast at all, but can be demonstrated by ultrasonography or a CT scan. A retrograde pyelogram may be required to show the exact anatomy of the hydronephrosis and to demonstrate any obstructive cause in the ureter.

Treatment

This is directed to removal of any underlying obstructive cause of the hydronephrosis. Where the cause is a neuromuscular incoordination, a plastic operation at the pelvi-ureteric junction may save the kidney from progressive damage. A completely useless (particularly an infected) kidney is an indication for nephrectomy — provided the other kidney has reasonable function.

URINARY TRACT CALCULI

Aetiology

It must be admitted that our knowledge of stone formation within the urinary tract is still inadequate and many stones form without apparent explanation. Predisposing factors may be classified under three main groupings; inadequate drainage, excess of normal constituents in the urine, and the presence of abnormal constituents.

Inadequate drainage

Wherever urine stagnates, there calculi may deposit. Thus stones may form within a hydronephrosis or in a diverticulum of the bladder. They may develop in the retroprostatic pouch in chronic urinary obstruction due to an enlarged prostate. Immobilization of the whole patient, for example a long-standing orthopaedic case or paraplegic confined to bed, is also associated with stone formation. In these cases, mobilization of calcium from the skeleton is an additional factor.

Excess of normal constituents

Renal stones are particularly common in people from temperate climates who go to live in the tropics where dehydration produces extremely concentrated urine. Hyperparathyroidism (see page 333) and prolonged immobilization are both associated with an increase of serum calcium and with an increased tendency to stone formation. An excess of serum uric acid in gout, or following chemotherapy for leukaemia and polycythaemia, may be accompanied by uric acid stone formation.

Presence of abnormal constituents

Urinary infection, particularly in the presence of obstruction, e.g. hydronephrosis or chronic retention, produces epithelial sloughs upon which calculi may deposit. This is true of any foreign body introduced into the renal tract; thus stones may form on unabsorbable sutures inserted at operation or on a fragment of broken off catheter tip. Vitamin A deficiency, which may occur in primitive communities, results in hyperkeratosis of the urinary epithelium which again provides the debris upon which stones may form. Cystinuria (an inborn error of amino-acid metabolism) may result in cystine stone deposition.

Composition of urinary calculi

The three common stones are oxalate, phosphate and urate.

Calcium oxalate calculi (60 per cent) are hard with a sharp, spiky surface which traumatizes the urinary epithelium; the resultant bleeding usually colours the stone a dark brown or black.

Phosphatic calculi (33 per cent) are composed of a mixture of calcium, ammonium and magnesium phosphate ('triple phosphate stone'). These are hard, white and chalky. They are nearly always found in an infected urine and produce the large 'staghorn' calculus deposited within a pyonephrosis.

Uric acid and urate calculi (5 per cent) are moderately hard and brown in colour with a smooth surface. Pure uric acid stones are radiotranslucent but, fortunately for diagnosis, most contain enough calcium to render them opaque to X-rays.

Cystine stones account for about 1 per cent of urinary calculi.

Note that a stone found in the lower urinary tract may have arisen there primarily or it may have migrated there from a primary source within the kidney.

Clinical features (Fig. 36.3)

Pain is the presenting feature of the great majority of kidney stones, but if the calculus is embedded within the solid substance of the kidney it may be entirely symptom-free. Within the minor or major calyx system the stone produces a dull loin pain. Impaction of the stone at the pelvi-ureteric junction, or migration down the ureter itself produces the dreadful agony of ureteric colic; the pain radiates from loin to groin, is of great severity and is accompanied by typical restlessness of the patient, who is quite unable to lie still in bed. Unlike the usual text-book description, the pain is not usually intermittent, but is continuous, though quite often with sharp exacerbations on a background of continued pain. There is often accompanying vomiting and sweating.

Haematuria, which may be microscopic or macroscopic, is frequently present so that detection of blood in the urine is an extremely helpful means of confirming the clinical diagnosis.

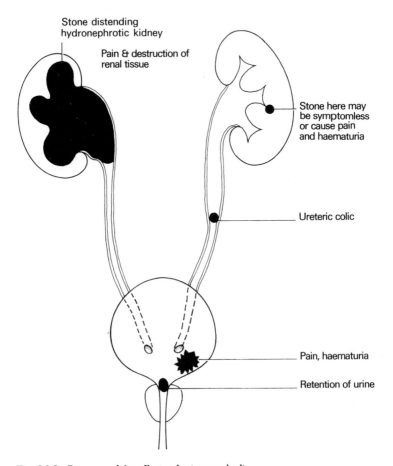

Fig. 36.3. Diagram of the effects of urinary calculi.

Special investigations

1 *The urine* is tested for the presence of blood.

2 *A plain abdominal X-ray* will show the presence of stone in 90 per cent of cases.

3 An *intravenous urogram* will demonstrate the exact anatomy of the renal system, e.g. the presence of associated hydronephrosis, although a completely obstructed kidney may show no function whatsoever.

There is an important catch for the unwary; a small stone within the kidney may be completely obscured by the contrast of the pyelogram. Never state that a kidney is free from stones without first carefully inspecting a plain X-ray of the renal area.

In a search for the aetiology of the stone, the urine is cultured for bacteria and examined microscopically for the presence of cystine crystals. The stone itself, when passed spontaneously or removed surgically, is subjected to chemical analysis.

5 *The serum uric acid* is raised in gout — with its associated uric acid stones.

4 A *serum calcium* estimation is carried out; a value above 2.75 mmol/l (11 mg per cent) is very suspicious of the presence of a parathyroid tumour although the incidence of stones due to this cause is low.

Complications of renal stone

1 *Hydronephrosis.*

2 *Infection* (pyelonephritis, pyonephrosis).

3 *Anuria* due either to impaction of calculi into the ureter on each side, or blockage of the ureter in a remaining solitary kidney.

Treatment

A small calculus lodged in the solid substance of the kidney without symptoms can be left alone but kept under periodic survey. Larger renal stones require removal. This may be performed by passing grasping forceps along a percutaneous track established under X-ray control or using the track to insinuate an ultrasonic probe which is used to disintegrate the stone. Extracorporeal ultrasound lithotripsy can be employed to shatter the stone without any open surgery. Only occasionally now is it necessary to perform open surgery simply to remove the stone either through the kidney substance (*nephrolithotomy*) or, wherever possible, through its pelvis (*pyelolithotomy*). If it is associated with a severe degree of hydronephrosis, removal of the stone alone rarely suffices and may have to be combined with plastic reconstruction of the kidney or removal of the lower pole of the kidney (partial nephrectomy) in order to ensure adequate drainage and thus to prevent early recurrence. Where the kidney is grossly and irreparably damaged, nephrectomy should be performed.

Acute calculous anuria, due to blockage of both ureters by stone, is treated by catheterizing the ureters or, if the ureteric catheter cannot be passed beyond the obstruction, the impacted stone must be removed, and, if necessary, drainage of the renal pelvis is carried out via a nephrostomy. If the patient is uraemic, his general condition is first improved by haemo- or peritoneal dialysis.

Acute ureteric colic is treated by repeated injections of pethidine to relieve the severe pain. The great majority of small stones within the ureter (up to the size and shape of a date-stone) pass spontaneously. These ureteric stones tend to lodge at one of three places; the pelvi-ureteric junction, the point at which the ureter crosses the pelvic brim and the entrance of the ureter into the bladder. The lower the stone, the more likely it is to pass spontaneously.

If the stone cannot or will not pass spontaneously, surgical intervention is necessary. Stones in the upper one-third of the ureter can be removed by percutaneous renal surgery after the stone has been pushed upwards into the renal pelvis with a ureteric catheter. Stones lower in the ureter can be removed with the ureterorenoscope, which allows the full length of the ureter to be inspected by direct vision. The stone can either be disrupted with ultrasound or removed by means of an endoscopic stone basket. A stone lodged at the ureteric orifice may be dislodged by diathermy incision of the mouth of the ureter. If non-invasive methods fail, then the stone may have to be removed by open operation (*uretero-lithotomy*).

In every case of renal stone an attempt is made to determine the underlying cause and then to eliminate this; thus renal infection is dealt with and any obstructive lesion within the urinary tract may require surgical correction. A small percentage of recurrent and bilateral stones are found to be due to parathyroid tumour (see page 333), removal of which will prevent further recurrences. In every case of renal calculous disease the patient should be instructed to drink liberal quantities of fluid in order to encourage the production of a dilute urine.

RENAL TRACT INFECTIONS

The kidney may be infected either via the blood stream or by an ascending infection from the lower urinary tract.

ACUTE PYELONEPHRITIS

Pathology

Macroscopically the lesion may affect one or both kidneys, which are enlarged, hyperaemic and show scattered small abscesses.

Microscopically the kidney is acutely inflamed, infiltrated by polymorphs and later shows necrosis and abscess formation. The calyces and pelvis also demonstrate acute inflammatory changes.

Pathogenic bacteria usually invade the kidney from the lower urinary tract, e.g. after catheterization, secondary to urinary infection associated with a bladder stone, diverticulum or prostatic obstruction, or during pregnancy where there is a combination of urinary obstruction and ureteric relaxation ('pyelitis of pregnancy'). It is especially common where is a congenital abnormality of the kidney, e.g. horseshoe or double kidney, or where an incompetent uretero-vesical valve allows ureteric reflux during micturition.

Clinical features

There is pain in one or both loins, dysuria and frequency, with acute fever and perhaps rigors. Examination reveals tenderness in the loin and upper abdomen and the tender lower pole of the affected kidney may be palpable. The urine is cloudy and may be bloodstained.

Special investigations

1 *Urine:* microscopic examination of the urine reveals many leucocytes and Gram-negative rods are usually apparent on a smear.

Culture of the urine grows *E.coli* in the majority of cases. Other causative organisms include *Proteus, Pseudomonas* and faecal streptococci.

2 *An intravenous urogram* shows blunting of the calyces and dilatation of the ureter. An underlying cause such as calculus, a diverticulum of the bladder or enlarged prostate may also be evident.

Treatment

Once urine has been obtained for culture, appropriate antibiotic treatment is commenced, e.g. Septrin for 2 to 6 weeks. If the bacteriological studies reveal that the organism is insensitive to sulphonamides, then the appropriate antibiotic treatment is instituted. A copious fluid intake is encouraged and the urine, if strongly acid, is alkalinized by prescribing sodium citrate.

Once the infection is controlled any underlying cause should be removed if possible.

PYONEPHROSIS

This is an infected hydronephrosis in which the kidney becomes no more than a bag of pus. If the ureter is obstructed there may be little to find on examining the urine, although more commonly pyuria is a marked feature. Usually the enlarged tender kidney is easily palpable.

An intravenous urogram shows little or no function and the enlarged renal shadow is usually obvious.

Treatment

Nephrectomy.

CARBUNCLE OF THE KIDNEY

This is better termed cortical abscess of the kidney and represents a haematogenous infection, usually *Staphylococcus aureus*, coming from a primary focus such as a cutaneous boil.

Clinical features

There is pyrexia, toxaemia, pain and tenderness in the loin and the kidney may be palpable.

Special investigations

The white count is always elevated but, interestingly enough, the urine is frequently sterile unless the abscess bursts into the calyceal system.

An intravenous urogram shows distortion of the calyces but often the oedematous kidney excretes poorly.

Treatment

Consists of surgical drainage, together with antibiotics.

PERINEPHRIC ABSCESS

Infection of the perinephric space is usually secondary to rupture of a carbuncle of the kidney. Rarely it may complicate a pyonephrosis or infection of a traumatic peri-renal haematoma.

Clinical features

There is the constitutional evidence of acute infection and in addition a diffuse tender bulge in the affected loin. This is particularly well seen when the back is carefully inspected with the patient lying prone.

Special investigations

X-ray of the abdomen shows, typically, loss of the psoas shadow due to retroperitoneal oedema. An intravenous urogram may be normal or may show the features of a renal cortical abscess or a pyonephrosis. CT scan will enable accurate localization of the abscess.

Treatment

Surgical drainage through a flank incision.

RENAL TUBERCULOSIS

Pathology

The kidney may be involved either as part of a generalized miliary spread of tuberculosis or more commonly as a focal lesion representing haematogenous spread from a distant site in the lungs (25 per cent of cases have pulmonary tuberculosis), the bone or gut. The original focus may be quiescent at the time of active renal disease.

It is now no longer considered that ascending infection from bladder or epididymis to the kidney can occur either directly or via peri-ureteric lymphatics.

Early lesions are found near the junction of the cortex and medulla. These enlarge, caseate and then rupture into a calyx, eventually producing extensive destruction of renal substance. The ureter becomes infiltrated and thickened; its obstruction leads to tuberculous pyonephrosis. Rarely a pyonephrosis becomes completely walled off as a symptomless, caseous and calcified mass ('autonephrectomy').

Spread of infected urine down the ureter frequently produces a tuberculous cystitis and may result in infection of the epididymis and seminal vesicles.

Untreated, the contralateral kidney often becomes involved, but this probably represents a separate haematogenous spread.

Since the introduction of antituberculous drugs the pathological process has been modified. Healing occurs with the production of fibrous tissue which in early cases merely produces a small scar. If treatment is only commenced in advanced disease then this fibrous tissue may lead to stricture formation at the neck of a calyx or at the pelvi-ureteric junction with a secondary hydronephrosis. Similar scarring of the heavily involved bladder may produce gross contraction on healing.

Clinical features

The patient is usually a young adult, often with a present or previous history of tuberculosis elsewhere. In this country, the patient is likely to be an immigrant from Asia. Symptoms in the early stages are mild and indeed may be entirely absent. There may be dysuria, frequency, pyuria or haematuria, which may be gross but is more usually slight or only microscopic. There may be loin pain on the affected side.

In more advanced cases the dysuria and frequency become intense because of extensive involvement of the bladder, and then constitutional symptoms of tuberculosis, with fever, night sweats, loss of weight and anaemia, may be present.

In some case a tuberculous epididymitis is the presenting feature. (See page 313.)

Examination is usually negative, but the kidney may be tender and palpable. The epididymis and seminal vesicles may be enlarged and thickened if involved. The epididymis often feels craggy due to calcification.

Special investigations

1 *The urine* is commonly sterile to ordinary culture but contains pus cells, protein and usually red cells. It is acid in reaction — 'sterile acid pyuria'. Acid-fast bacilli may be present on ZN staining of a spun deposit from an early morning specimen of urine. Three early morning specimens of urine are sent for culture on Lowenstein–Jensen's medium and guinea pig inoculations are carried out. The results of these special investigations are not available for 6 weeks.

2 *An intravenous urogram* may show failure of calyceal filling, irregularity of calyces and patchy calcification.

3 *Chest X-ray* may show a primary lung focus.

4 *Cystoscopy* may reveal a decreased capacity of the bladder, an oedematous mucosa on which tubercles may be seen and perhaps a 'golf-hole' ureteric orifice, the ureter being held rigidly open by surrounding fibrosis.

Treatment

Anti-tuberculous therapy should not be commenced until the diagnosis has been confirmed since, once undertaken, treatment must be prolonged. Initially, isoniazid and rifampicin supplemented by pyrazinamide are prescribed. These drugs are continued for 2 months. After this initial phase, the first two drugs are continued for at least 2 more months.

Surgery is only indicated in a minority of patients with advanced disease or where complications occur. Thus, a totally destroyed kidney may require nephrectomy, or a walled off abscess cavity may need drainage. The damage produced by fibrosis may also indicate surgery; thus late hydronephrosis with a totally destroyed kidney secondary to fibrosis of the ureter may require nephrectomy and a contracted bladder may call for either plastic enlargement or transplantation of the ureters into an ileal loop artificial bladder.

RENAL TUMOURS

Tumours of the kidney are divided into those arising from the kidney substance itself and those originating from the renal pelvis.

Classification

Of the kidney itself:

Benign

    (a) adenoma (small and symptomless)
    (b) haemangioma (a rare cause of haematuria)

Malignant

  1 *Primary:*
    (a) nephroblastoma
    (b) adenocarcinoma
  2 *Secondary:* the kidney is an uncommon site for deposits of carcinoma although it may be involved in advanced cases of lymphoma and leukaemia.

Of the renal pelvis:
    (a) papilloma
    (b) transitional carcinoma
    (c) squamous carcinoma

The two principal tumours of the kidney are the nephroblastoma, which usually occurs in children under 4, and adenocarcinoma which usually occurs over the age of 40.

NEPHROBLASTOMA
(Wilms' tumour, embryoma or adenomyosarcoma)

Pathology

This is an extremely anaplastic tumour which usually arises in children under the age of 4, although it occasionally affects older children and adolescents. It probably originates from embryonic mesodermal tissue.

Histologically there is a mixed appearance of spindle cells, epithelial tubules and smooth or striated muscle fibres.

The regional lymph nodes are soon invaded and spread occurs by the blood stream to the lungs and liver.

Clinical features

Rapid growth produces a large mass in the loin, although involvement of the renal pelvis is late and therefore haematuria relatively uncommon.

Treatment

Where possible nephrectomy is performed, followed by radiotherapy and cyto-toxic therapy. This intensive therapy has improved the prognosis of a condition that previously could seldom be cured. Occasionally a massive tumour may be shrunk down sufficiently by pre-operative irradiation to allow subsequent removal.

ADENOCARCINOMA
(hypernephroma, or Grawitz's tumour)

Pathology

This tumour accounts for 80 per cent of all renal growths. Males are affected twice as often as females. The patients are usually 40 years of age or over.

The tumour appears as a large, vascular, golden-yellow mass, usually in one or other pole of the kidney.

Microscopically the tumour cells are typically large with an abundant foamy cytoplasm and a small central densely staining nucleus.

The tumour originates from the renal tubules and not from adrenal rests as was postulated by Grawitz.

Spread

1 *Directly* throughout the renal substance with invasion of the perinephric tissues.

2 *By lymphatics* to the para-aortic lymph nodes.

3 *By blood stream* with growth along the renal vein into the IVC.

Deposits in the lung, bones and brain are common.

The adenocarcinoma of the kidney is a tumour which may occasionally produce a solitary blood-borne deposit, so that removal of the primary together with this deposit has been followed in some instances by prolonged survival.

Clinical features

The patient may present with local symptoms, of which the commonest is haematuria (40 per cent of presenting symptoms). The bleeding may produce clot colic. The patient may notice a mass in the abdomen or complain of an aching pain in the loin; these account for another 40 per cent of presenting symptoms. The remaining 20 per cent of patients manifest either with secondary deposits, e.g. a pathological fracture, or with the general features of malignancy: anaemia, loss of weight and occasionally as a PUO (pyrexia of unknown origin).

On examination the diseased kidney may be palpable.

Special investigations

1 *The urine* nearly always contains either macroscopic or microscopic blood.

2 *The IVU* reveals distortion of the calyces by a polar tumour which may occasionally show flecks of calcification.

3 *Ultrasonography and CT scanning* provide accurate visualization of the tumour and can indicate spread to lymph nodes and caval invasion.

4 *Angiography* is valuable. It demonstrates a typical tumour circulation and differentiates the avascular filling defect of a renal cyst.

Treatment

Nephrectomy followed, if extensive, by radiotherapy. The vascularity of a large tumour may be reduced by pre-operative angiographic embolization of its arterial supply.

The 5-year survival rate after successful resection is about 50 per cent, but metastases may occur many years after nephrectomy.

TUMOURS OF THE RENAL PELVIS

Transitional cell tumours of the renal pelvis vary in malignancy from benign papillomas to highly anaplastic transitional cell carcinomas. A squamous carcinoma of the renal pelvis may occur when there has been squamous metaplasia of the epithelium; one-third of these cases are associated with renal calculus.

Clinical features

Patients present usually either with haematuria or with hydronephrosis due to ureteric obstruction. The tumour may seed down the ureter and even involve the bladder.

Treatment

Treatment is nephro-ureterectomy or, if feasible, local wide excision and plastic reconstruction.

Chapter 37
The Bladder

URACHAL ANOMALIES

Urachal defects may result from anomalies of the primitive urachal connection. There may be a urinary discharge at the umbilicus from persistence of the tract, or a cyst may develop if the urachus persists but is closed above and below; this cyst may subsequently become infected.

Treatment

In all cases treatment is excision.

ECTOPIA VESICAE

A condition in which the bladder fails to develop properly and the ureters together with the trigone open directly onto the anterior abdominal wall below the umbilicus. In the male there is an associated epispadias and in both sexes there is frequently maldevelopment of the pubic bones with a failure of the pubes to meet at the symphysis; typically there is a widened pelvis with a waddling gait.

The infant is, of course, completely incontinent of urine and is a pitiful sight, with excoriation of the abdominal skin and a permanent unpleasant ammoniacal smell of infected urine.

If the condition is untreated the child may die of pyelonephritis or else frequently develops a carcinoma of the bladder rudiment after initial metaplastic change.

Treatment

The most satisfactory treatment is reimplantation of the ureters either into the colon or into an ileal loop (ureteroileostomy) combined with excision of the bladder itself as a prophylaxis against malignant change. Elaborate reconstructive operations in an attempt to refashion a new bladder are usually unsuccessful.

RUPTURE OF THE BLADDER

The bladder may rupture either intraperitoneally or extraperitoneally. Rupture into the peritoneum either follows a penetrating wound (e.g. a bullet wound) or crush injury to the pelvis when the bladder is distended. Occasionally it is consequent upon instrumentation of the bladder and rarely the overdistended bladder of retention may rupture spontaneously. Extraperitoneal rupture is more common; the bladder may be torn by a spicule of bone in a pelvic fracture or occasionally may be wounded during a hernia operation or repair of a cystocele.

Clinical features

Intraperitoneal rupture produces the typical picture of peritonitis with generalized abdominal pain, marked rigidity and a silent abdomen.

Extraperitoneal rupture is associated with extraperitoneal extravasation of blood and urine producing a painful swelling which arises out of the pelvis. In this case, differentiation must be made from rupture of the membranous urethra (see page 302) although this may not be possible until surgical exploration is carried out. Typically, however, a urethral tear is accompanied by anterior displacement of the prostate which can be detected on rectal examination.

Treatment

Invariably surgical. The intraperitoneal rupture is sutured and the bladder drained by means of an indwelling Foley catheter. It may be possible to suture the extraperitoneal rupture, but if this is inaccessible at the base of the bladder suprapubic drainage alone will suffice to allow healing to occur.

In all cases the retropubic space is drained and the patient given antibiotic therapy.

DIVERTICULUM OF THE BLADDER

The vast majority of diverticula of the bladder are secondary to bladder outflow obstruction, although a small number are congenital in origin. Since it is usually the male bladder which becomes obstructed, 95 per cent of diverticula occur in men.

Pathology

As a result of obstruction, the muscle of the bladder wall hypertrophies and becomes trabeculated; outpouches of mucosa occur between the bands of muscle fibres. One or more of these sacs may increase in size to form a fully-developed diverticulum which, since it is devoid of practically all muscle in its wall, is unable to empty and undergoes progressive distension.

Such a diverticulum may:

1 Become infected: because of urinary stagnation.
2 Develop a calculus: because of a combination of infection and stasis.
3 Undergo malignant change in its wall.
4 Press against the adjacent ureter and produce a hydronephrosis of the corresponding kidney.

Clinical features

The majority of diverticula remain silent unless they undergo one of the complications listed above; or their presence may become known only as a result of the investigation of an underlying obstructive lesion, for example a prostatic hypertrophy or urethral stricture. Occasionally a large, uninfected diverticulum gives the strange symptom of double micturition ('pis en deux'). In this circumstance the patient empties his bladder but a good deal of the urine passes into the distensible diverticulum. No sooner does micturition end than the diverticulum passively empties again into the bladder, giving the surprised patient the desire once again to empty his bladder.

Special investigations
Diagnosis is confirmed by intravenous urography, when dye is seen to enter the diverticulum, and at cystoscopy, when the mouth of the diverticulum can be visualized.

Treatment
Although small diverticula can be left alone, larger examples must be excised at the time of definite treatment of the underlying obstructive lesion. Unless excised they become the source of persistent post-operative infection.

BLADDER STONE
The varieties of bladder calculus are the same as renal stones — phosphatic, oxalate, urate and rarely cystine.

Aetiology
The stone may have originated in the kidney and then migrated into the bladder so that any of the aetiological factors of renal calculus (page 277) may have been responsible. Alternatively the stone may have arisen in the bladder itself; here the underlying causes may be:

1 *Stasis and infection,* e.g. diverticulum of bladder, obstruction due to stricture, prostatic enlargement, etc., or the atonic bladder of paraplegia.

2 *Foreign body:* a calculus will deposit on the broken-off end of a catheter or on any foreign body inadvertently admitted into, and left within, the bladder.

Clinical features
The typical triad of symptoms of bladder stone are frequency, pain and haematuria. Frequency is more troublesome during the day than at night, probably because in the upright position the stone lies over, and irritates, the bladder trigone. The pain is felt in the suprapubic region, in the perineum and the tip of the penis; it particularly occurs at the end of micturition when the bladder contracts down upon the calculus. Similarly the haematuria tends to occur as the last few drops of urine are passed.

Sometimes the patient complains of intermittent stopping of the urinary flow as the stone blocks the internal urinary meatus like a ball-valve. Indeed, actual retention of urine may occur if the stone impacts in the urethra.

Special investigations
The majority of bladder stones are radio-opaque and are readily visible on plain abdominal X-ray. They can also be seen easily on cystoscopy.

Treatment
Unless the stone is very small, when there is a possibility that it will pass spontaneously, it should be removed either by means of crushing with an endoscopic lithotrite under direct vision, by disintegration in a shockwave lithotripter (if available) or by open cystotomy through a suprapubic incision. At this operation any underlying cause, e.g. a diverticulum or urethral obstruction, must be dealt with or the stone will rapidly recur.

BLADDER TUMOURS

Pathology
Bladder tumours may be classified as follows:

Benign
Transitional cell papilloma.

Malignant
1   *Primary:*
(a) transitional cell carcinoma
(b) squamous carcinoma (arising in an area of metaplasia)
(c) adenocarcinoma (uncommon)
(d) sarcomas (rare)
2   *Secondary:* invasion from adjacent colonic, renal, ovarian, uterine or prostatic growths.

Transitional cell papillomas grade imperceptibly into malignant tumours and many pathologists regard them as low grade carcinomas, especially since they have a tendency to recur after treatment, to seed elsewhere in the bladder and to undergo frank malignant change.

Tumours are found usually in middle-aged and elderly patients. Males are far more frequently affected than females. There is a raised incidence in smokers.

Bladder tumours were extremely common among aniline dye and rubber workers because of the excretion of carcinogens such as beta naphthylamine in the urine. The manufacture of many of the more dangerous dyes and chemicals has been abolished in this country. There is a high incidence of malignant change in the exposed bladder mucosa of ectopia vesicae (page 287), in diverticula of the bladder and in the bladder infested with schistosomiasis.

Although any part of the bladder may be involved, growths are particularly common at the base, trigone and around the ureteric orifices. They are often multiple; this represents a field change throughout the transitional uroepithelium with the tendency for tumours to develop from the renal pelvis to the urethra.

Macroscopically
The well-differentiated papillomas form fine fronds which resemble seaweed floating in the urine. The more malignant tumours are sessile, solid growths which infiltrate the bladder wall, then ulcerate, often with marked surrounding cystitis.

Microscopically
The papillomas have a connective tissue core and no involvement of the stem. The carcinomas may be well or poorly-differentiated transitional cell tumours but, rarely, keratinizing squamous cell tumours or adenocarcinomas may be seen.

Spread
This may be:
1   *Local,* with infiltration of the bladder wall, the prostate, urethra, sigmoid colon

and rectum, or, in the female, the pelvic viscera. The ureteric orifices may be occluded, producing hydronephrosis and ultimately renal failure. The pelvic skeleton may be directly invaded.

2 *Lymphatic*, to the iliac and para-aortic lymph nodes.
3 *Blood-borne* spread occurs late to the liver and the lungs.
4 *Implantation* may take place into the scar if open operation is performed.

Clinical features

Bladder tumours usually present with painless haematuria. A malignant tumour which ulcerates and invades may also produce dysuria, frequency and urgency of micturition. Occasionally the patient may present with hydronephrosis due to ureteric obstruction or with retention of urine due either to clot, or to growth involving the urethra. In late cases there may be severe pain from pelvic invasion or uraemia from bilateral ureteric obstruction.

Examination is usually negative in benign papilloma, but a malignant tumour is quite frequently palpable on bimanual examination.

Bimanual palpation under a general anaesthetic enables local staging of the tumour to be performed:

T_1 confined to the mucosa: the tumour is impalpable.

T_2 penetrating the bladder wall: a localized thickening is palpated but the tumour is mobile.

T_3 penetration of the bladder wall: the tumour is mobile but the mass is larger than suggested by its cystoscopic appearance.

T_4 fixed to adjacent structures (pelvis or prostate): the mass is immobile.

Special investigations

1 *Examination of the urine* usually reveals blood, either to the naked eye or microscopically. Cytological examination may detect malignant cells.
2 *An intravenous urogram* may demonstrate a filling defect and perhaps ureteric obstruction or hydronephrosis. At the same time the presence of pelvic bony secondaries may be revealed.
3 *Cytoscopy* is the most valuable investigation since the exact nature of the tumour can be determined and a biopsy obtained.

Treatment

Papilloma

Most benign papillomas can be controlled by fulguration or resection via an operating cytoscope. Once the patient has developed a papilloma there is a high risk of further lesions occurring and he should be supervised by regular cystoscopic examinations.

Carcinoma

The management of bladder carcinoma is difficult and the results are often poor. Factors to be taken into consideration are the degree of differentiation of the tumour (information obtained by endoscopic biopsy), the extent of local spread, evidence of dissemination and the general condition of the patient.

The uncommon lesion occurring in the vault of the bladder can be removed by partial cystectomy.

Tumours which do not penetrate the bladder wall (T_1 and T_2) may be removed by endoscopic resection followed by regular cystoscopic review. Recurrences are treated either by cystoscopic coagulation or further endoscopic removal.

If the bladder wall has been breached (T_3) or the pelvic wall or prostate actually invaded (T_4) then radiotherapy is used, often preceded by a preliminary debulking of the tumour by transurethral resection.

The place of total cystectomy in the treatment of bladder cancer is still controversial. Some surgeons advise this procedure (in otherwise fit patients) in the treatment of locally advanced tumours once these have been shrunk down by radiotherapy. Others, who are more conservative, advise cystectomy only if the tumour fails to respond or recurs after radiotherapy.

Total cystectomy may also be indicated where there is extensive papillomatosis which cannot be controlled by diathermy, or to remove a seriously damaged post-irradiation bladder which is grossly fibrosed or subject to persistent haematuria as a result of postradiotherapy telangiectasia.

Total cystectomy necessitates transplantation of the ureters, either into the sigmoid colon or into an isolated loop or ileum. Transplantation of the ureters into the colon alone may give useful palliation even if the bladder growth is itself inoperable.

When such procedures are performed, there is the risk of ascending infection and *hyperchloraemic acidosis* and uraemia due to excessive reabsorption of chlorides from the urine passed into the colon. This is avoided by using a short ileal loop or by ensuring that the patient empties his rectum frequently if colonic transplantation has been employed. The blood biochemistry of the patient is checked regularly and, in addition, sodium bicarbonate by mouth is prescribed.

Chapter 38
The Prostate

There are two common conditions of the prostate that require consideration, benign enlargement and carcinoma.

BENIGN ENLARGEMENT

Pathology

Some degree of enlargement of the prostate is extremely common from the age of 45 onwards, but this enlargement often produces either no, or only minor, symptoms. The prostate, like the breast and thyroid, is composed of glandular tissue and stroma which have periods of activity and involution throughout life. Associated with these periods, the gland may become enlarged, and there may be excessive proliferation of both fibrous and epithelial tissue. The condition is therefore similar to nodular goitre and chronic mastitis.

Enlargement of the prostate may result in elongation and tortuosity of the prostatic urethra and the median lobe may become a large, rounded swelling overlying the posterior aspect of the internal urinary meatus. Here it can act like a ball valve, producing urinary obstruction.

The bladder hypertrophies in prostatic obstruction and the thickened muscle bands produce trabeculation; the areas between the bands form saccules which may distend into diverticula. Urinary infection may occur (especially after catheterization) and vesical calculi may become deposited. Back pressure on the ureters may cause a progressive hydronephrosis and eventually renal failure.

Clinical features

These anatomical changes are responsible for the symptoms of prostatic enlargement. The narrowing of the prostatic urethra and the possible median lobe enlargement cause the patient's difficulty in passing urine, with a poor and intermittent stream.

The deranged anatomy in the region of the internal meatus may allow urine into the prostatic urethra. The urine in this situation sets up a desire to micturate and this produces one of the most common symptoms of prostatism, namely frequency. This is particularly worrying to the patient at night as it interferes with his sleep. Associated with the enlargement there may be partial obstruction and congestion of the prostatic plexus of veins which may produce haematuria which usually occurs at the end of micturation when the bladder contracts around the enlarged intravesical part of the prostate.

The obstruction to the outflow of the blader may result in renal failure with drowsiness, headache and impairment of intellect due to uraemia. It is therefore always wise to examine the bladder for enlargement and to determine the blood urea on an old man with inexplicable behavioural changes.

Eventually the bladder is likely to fail to overcome the obstruction and this results in retention of urine.

This may be *acute*, with sudden onset and severe pain, or *chronic*, in which the bladder gradually becomes distended and the patient develops dribbling overflow incontinence, with little or no pain. It is in the latter group that uraemia is likely to occur. In some instances a complete obstruction then supervenes ('*acute on chronic obstruction*').

On examination the patient with an enlarged prostate, if uraemic, is likely to be pale and wasted, with a dry, furred tongue; he may be mentally confused. Examination of the abdomen may reveal a large bladder which may reach to the umbilicus or even above. The swelling has the typical globular shape of the bladder and it is dull to percussion. If there is acute obstruction the bladder will be tender to palpation.

On rectal examination the prostate will be enlarged; typically in benign enlargement the lateral lobes are enlarged and a sulcus is palpable between them in the midline posteriorly. This is in contrast to carcinoma which usually involves the posterior part of the gland and obliterates the sulcus with a craggy, hard mass. The size of the prostate may appear to be larger than it really is if the bladder is grossly enlarged and pushes the prostate down towards the examining finger. The gland should therefore be palpated again after catheterization and before operation.

Special investigations

1 *The blood urea* and the *serum acid phosphatase* should be determined; the latter is raised above 3 units in 50 per cent of malignant prostates and often denotes the presence of bone deposits.

2 *The haemoglobin* is estimated, since uraemia inhibits the bone marrow and leads to anaemia.

3 *A midstream specimen of urine* should be cultured since it is especially important to determine whether the urine is infected, as an infected renal tract severely complicates prostatic disease. Most of the patients with prostatic disease do not have an infected urine until the bladder and urethra have been instrumented.

4 *An intravenous urogram* will give useful evidence of renal function; normally contrast medium should be visible after 5 minutes. More specifically the pyelogram will show evidence of back pressure of the kidneys (namely hydronephrosis and hydro-ureter), enlargement of the bladder with chronic retention, or residual urine due to inability to empty the bladder completely. Bladder diverticula may be demonstrated. Intravesical enlargement of the prostate is shown by a globular filling defect at the base of the bladder and acute hooking of the terminations of the ureters due to the enlarged prostate pushing up the trigone of the bladder.

The films of the lumbar spine and bony pelvis should be scrutinized for evidence of secondary deposits (present in about 25 per cent of malignant prostates).

Complications of prostatic hypertrophy

These are classified into:

1   *At prostatic level:*
    (a) acute retention
    (b) chronic retention
    (c) haemorrhage
2   *At bladder level:*
    (a) diverticula
    (b) urinary infection
    (c) stone formation
3   *At kidney level:*
    (a) hydronephrosis
    (b) uraemia

Treatment

This depends on whether the patient is an elective case, with troublesome prostatic symptoms, especially marked nocturnal frequency, or whether he presents urgently with retention (see page 298). However, cure is invariably dependent on carrying out some type of prostatectomy.

Usually, this is performed endoscopically. However, if the prostate is very large or if there is some co-existent intravesical pathology, such as a large diverticulum or tumour that requires removal at the same time, an open operation may be necessary. This is performed either by the transvesical route or by the retropubic approach (Millin's prostatectomy).

Endoscopic prostatectomy — transurethral resection

The prostate can be removed endoscopically by means of an operating cystoscope, using a diathermy cutting loop. It is useful in dealing with fibrotic and malignant prostatic obstruction but it is also used routinely for benign enlargement. The mortality and morbidity in skilled hands are very low, and this technique is now the treatment of choice in all but very enlarged prostates. Removal of too little of the gland results in the recurrence of the patient's symptoms, whilst removing too much may damage the urethral sphincteric mechanism.

CARCINOMA OF THE PROSTATE

Pathology

This is a relatively common tumour in elderly males but is rare below the age of 50. Many prostates without clinical evidence of malignancy reveal a carcinomatous focus on careful histological examination.

Macroscopically

The tumour is usually situated in the posterior part of the prostate beneath its capsule and appears as an infiltrating hard, pale area.

Microscopically

An adenocarcinoma, usually well differentiated but occasionally anaplastic.

Spread

1 *Local:* there is invasion of the peri-prostatic tissues and adjacent organs, i.e., the bladder, urethra, seminal vesicles and, rarely, invasion around and ulceration into the rectum.

2 *Lymphatic:* to the iliac and para-aortic nodes.

3 *Blood-borne:* especially to the pelvis, spine and skull, usually as osteosclerotic lesions. Secondaries may also be found in the liver and lung.

Clinical features

The symptoms of carcinoma of the prostate may be identical to those of benign enlargement, but in addition the patient may present with symptoms of secondary deposits, particularly with pain in the back from involvement of the vertebrae. As with cancer anywhere, the patient's general condition is likely to be poor with weight loss and anaemia.

As the tumour enlarges locally, three stages can be recognized on clinical examination (Fig. 38.1)

1 A hard nodule in one lobe of the prostate.

2 A craggy mass replacing the prostate and abolishing the normal sulcus between the two lateral lobes.

3 The same, together with infiltration of the tissues on either side of the prostate.

Special investigations

The same initial investigations are performed as for benign enlargement. The particularly useful finding is a high serum acid phosphate (above 3 units), present in approximately 50 per cent of cancer cases. Some 25 per cent have bone scan or X-ray evidence of bony secondary deposits which, unlike most other growths, are usually osteosclerotic.

Biopsy material can be obtained either by needle puncture via the perineum or rectum, or trans-urethrally using the diathermy loop.

Treatment

Occasionally a tiny prostatic carcinoma is completely removable by prostatec-

(A)   (B)   (C)

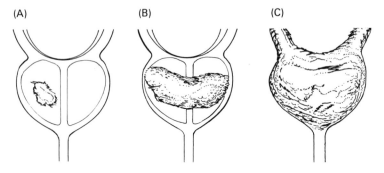

Fig. 38.1. The clinical stages of prostatic carcinoma: (A) a hard nodule in the prostate; (B) a mass obliterating the median sulcus; (C) infiltration outside the prostatic capsule.

tomy; this fortunate occurence happens most often by accident when an apparently benign prostate is removed and is found microscopically to contain a malignant focus. A carcinoma of the prostate found on incidental rectal examination and which is either symptomless or with minimal symptoms, especially in an elderly patient, can be left untreated.

Carcinoma of the prostate is more usually discovered at a stage when it has already spread beyond its capsule and may well have involved other organs, particularly the pelvic cellular tissues, bladder base and bone.

The mainstay of treatment of this disease is androgen suppression or the use of specific androgen antagonists, which will produce symptomatic relief in disseminated prostatic cancer in about 75 per cent of patients. Huggins showed that castration of patients with prostatic carcinoma very often relieved their symptoms and sometimes produced dramatic remissions in the course of the disease. It was subsequently found that similar results could be obtained by the administration of oestrogens. At present, oestrogen treatment is used primarily in the majority of cases. The usual regime is 1mg of Stilboestrol three times daily by mouth.

Stilboestrol may produce gynaecomastia, nipple and scrotal pigmentation and testicular atrophy. More importantly, it may result in fluid retention and precipitate congestive cardiac failure. Indeed, it is contra-indicated in elderly patients with cardiovascular disease. Under such circumstances, bilateral orchidectomy should be performed.

Other techniques of hormonal manipulation include:
Cyproterone acetate: a steroid androgen antagonist.
Aminoglutethimide: which prevents adrenal androgen secretion.
Leuteinising hormone releasing hormone (LHRH) agonists: which produce a fall of leuteinising hormone from the anterior pituitary, with consequent reduction of testicular secretion of testosterone.

Palliation produced by hormonal treatment of prostatic cancer has completely changed the nature of this disease for many patients, a useful and happy life being preserved in some cases for many years. However, the results are not always so satisfactory. Radiotherapy may relieve the pain of bony deposits and can also be employed for local control to supplement hormonal therapy.

Urinary obstruction due to the prostatic carcinoma may resolve on stilboestrol therapy; if not, an endoscopic prostatectomy is indicated.

PROSTATITIS

Bacterial infection of the prostate may be very difficult to diagnose as it may mimic both benign enlargement and carcinoma. However, if the patient has previously suffered from tuberculosis anywhere in the body, but particularly anywhere in the genito-urinary tract, then infection of the organ with tubercle bacilli should be suspected. The treatment is standard anti-tuberculous chemotherapy.

Non-tuberculous prostatitis is usually due to faecal organisms, particularly *Escherichia coli* and *Streptococcus faecalis*.

Clinical features

The patient will usually have symptoms of prostatism and may present with acute retention. However, unlike most cases of retention, the urine will probably have been infected before any instrumentation has been attempted. In addition the patient may be pyrexial with a leucocytosis and the prostate is acutely tender on palpation.

Treatment

If the disease is recognized early enough treatment with the appropriate antibiotics may cause resolution. Untreated, an abscess may form and rupture spontaneously into the urethra.

BLADDER NECK OBSTRUCTION

Bladder neck obstruction may be due to congenital valves in the region of the prostatic urethra and internal meatus, or fibrosis of the prostate.

Congenital valves usually produce hydronephrosis and retention of urine in childhood. They may be difficult to diagnose in that instruments may pass freely into the bladder, although the valves obstruct micturition. Early treatment by surgical removal of the valves before renal failure occurs is important.

Prostatic fibrosis produces the symptoms of prostatic hypertrophy but without enlargement of the prostate. The onset may be in childhood or early adult life.

Treatment

Comprises endoscopic incision of the bladder neck.

THE MANAGEMENT OF URINARY RETENTION

Apart from transient episodes of acute retention, for example post-operative, the definite treatment of the condition can only be decided upon after three essential steps have been carried out. These are:

1   The diagnosis of the cause.
2   The assessment of any degree of renal damage due to back pressure.
3   The assessment of the general condition of the patient — is the patient fit for any surgical procedure which may be necessary?

Diagnosis of the cause

The diagnosis can be classified into:

1   *General causes (no organic obstruction to urinary flow):*
   (a) post-operative
   (b) CNS disease, e.g. tabes, multiple sclerosis, spinal tumour
   (c) drugs, e.g. Pro-Banthine
2   *Local causes:*
   (a) in the lumen of the urethra, e.g. stone or blood clot
   (b) in the wall, e.g. stricture
   (c) outside the wall, e.g. prostatic enlargement (benign or malignant), faecal impaction, pelvic tumour, pregnant uterus

General causes of retention of urine must always be borne in mind. The commonest cause of acute retention is indeed seen post-operatively. The patient is not used to passing urine lying in bed, is weak and often in pain. Usually the condition can be overcome by giving an injection of morphia and sitting the patient with his legs over the side of the bed, but if this does not succeed, catheterization may be required; the catheter can either be removed once the bladder has been emptied or, if the patient is particularly ill, can be left *in situ* until next morning. Carbachol should not be used; it causes intense pain and there is the risk of rupture of the bladder if any obstructive element is present. A catheter is kinder, safer and more certain. Sometimes a patient with an enlarged prostate is precipitated into retention of urine following some other surgical procedure and it may then be necessary to proceed to prostatectomy.

In every case the central nervous system must be carefully examined since retention of urine may be due to interruption of the sacral nervous pathway. There is a tendency to think of retention of urine in an elderly man as being invariably due to prostatic disease, but every now and then one of these patients will be found to have a spinal tumour, tabes dorsalis or some other neurological condition.

The diagnosis of the cause of retention is made by the usual three steps.

History

This may reveal the typical progressive symptoms of prostatism, a story of urethral infection suggesting stricture, a preceding episode of ureteric colic suggesting stone, etc.

Examination

Includes a rectal examination to determine the size and nature of the prostate, palpation of the urethra for stone or stricture, inspection of the urethral meatus and examination of the CNS.

Special investigations

X-ray of the pelvis may reveal a calculus at the bladder base or bony secondaries from prostatic carcinoma.

The serum acid phosphate is estimated; a figure above 3 units suggests carcinoma.

Assessment of the degree of renal damage

The patient with retention of urine may have damaged his kidneys by back pressure; obviously this is far more likely to occur in long-standing cases of chronic retention, but the possibility must be considered in every case. This assessment again is made under three headings:

History

Renal failure is suggested by headaches, anorexia, vomiting, and mental disturbance.

Examination

Is the patient pale and drowsy with the dry, coated tongue of uraemia?

Special investigations

The blood urea is estimated — elevation above 7 mmol/l (40 mg per cent) suggests at least some degree of renal impairment.

Serum creatine is estimated — elevation above 100 mmol/l suggests renal impairment.

Assessment of the general condition of the patient

The average patient with retention of urine admitted to hospital is an elderly gentleman. Before proceeding to major surgery his general condition must obviously be carefully investigated — again the three headings:

History

Exercise tolerance, the presence of cough and sputum and a history of previous coronary episodes are enquired into.

Examination

Chest, cardiovascular system and blood pressure.

Special investigations

The chest is X-rayed and an ECG performed if necessary. The haemoglobin level is checked.

Scheme of management

The three common causes for an emergency surgical admission of a man with acute urinary retention are benign prostatic hypertrophy, malignant disease of the prostate and urethral stricture. The following scheme outlines the management of such cases (see Fig. 38.2). The patient is catheterized under full aspectic precautions:

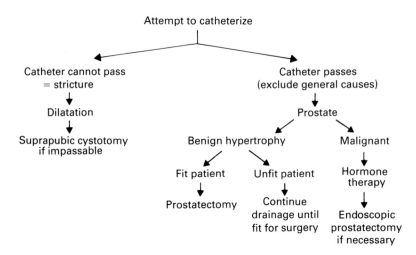

Fig. 38.2. Treatment of acute retention.

Benign prostatic enlargement

Proceed to prostatectomy as soon as convenient if the renal function and general condition of the patient are satisfactory. If renal damage or general poor condition preclude operation, drainage by catheter is continued until these can be improved. Thus a mild degree of heart failure is treated with digitalis and diuretics or a chest infection by antibiotics and physiotherapy. If the patient is in such poor health that operation will obviously never be possible, for example a bedridden cardiac cripple, then he is best managed by permanent urethral drainage, the catheter being changed regularly and urinary antiseptics used if necessary should urinary infection occur. A self-retaining Foley catheter is far kinder to the patient than a leaky and smelly permanent suprapubic cystotomy tube.

Malignant disease of the prostate

Hormone therapy is commenced; an endoscopic prostatectomy is required if symptoms persist.

Urethral stricture (see page 304)

The catheter will not pass and the urethra must be gently dilated with bougies under local or general anaesthetic. Following this, it is then possible to catheterize the patient and then to continue with regular urethral dilatations or to divide the stricture with a urethrotome. Rarely the stricture is impassible and the patient then requires a temporary suprapubic cystotomy. Once the oedema has been allowed to subside it then often becomes possible to dilate the urethra after about a week and close the suprapubic fistula. Occasionally a plastic operation on the stricture is indicated but only rarely is a permanent suprapubic drainage required.

Chapter 39
The Male Urethra

CONGENITAL ABNORMALITIES

In the course of its development the urethra may be malpositioned so that it terminates on the ventral aspect of the penis or rarely on its dorsal aspect (*hypospadias* and *epispadias* respectively). In the female the urethra may open into the anterior vaginal wall. Both epispadias and hypospadias may interfere with potency and fertility and there are a variety of plastic operations that have been designed to correct these abnormalities.

The other important congenital anomaly of the urethra is the presence of valves. These can obstruct the flow of urine, resulting in chronic retention of urine and uraemia in infants.

INJURIES OF THE URETHRA

These may be classified (Fig. 39.1) into rupture of:

1 The bulbous urethra may be damaged by a direct blow, e.g. a fall astride a bar or similar object, or during forcible dilatation or cystoscopy. The patient will complain of severe pain in the perineum and usually bright red blood will be seen dripping from the external meatus. There will be marked bruising in the region of the injury.

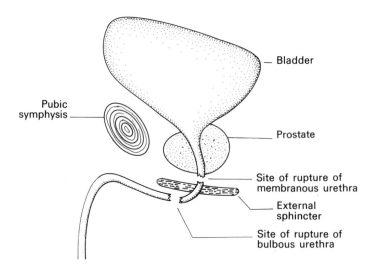

Fig. 39.1. The two commonest sites of urethral rupture.

2 *The membranous urethra* may be injured in pelvic fractures, especially those involving dislocation of a portion of the pelvis, and is torn at its junction with the prostatic urethra. As with extraperitoneal rupture of the bladder (page 288), blood and urine are extravasated in the extraperitoneal space and produce a swelling dull to percussion above the pubis. If the urethra is torn from the bladder the prostate is displaced and there will be a feeling of emptiness on rectal examination.

The attempted passage of a catheter in a patient with a pelvic fracture can be both misleading and dangerous; misleading in that the catheter may pass along a partially-ruptured posterior urethra into the bladder so that the diagnosis is missed, and dangerous in that the catheter may complete the tear in a partially ruptured urethra or produce a false passage.

Treatment

Satisfactory management depends particularly on early diagnosis since extravasation of urine is liable to lead to secondary infection, which will greatly complicate the condition. If the membranous urethra is torn then urgent surgery is indicated. If at operation the bladder is found to be in its normal position then the tear in the membranous urethra is a partial one. The bladder is drained with a suprapubic tube, the retropubic space drained and antibiotic therapy commenced. If even part of the urethra is thus preserved then subsequent stricture formation may be avoided. The diagnosis is confirmed about 10 days later by means of a urethrogram which can be safely carried out at this stage.

If the bladder is found to be 'floating' out of the pelvis, then a complete rupture is diagnosed; it is accepted that subsequent stricture formation is inevitable and so there is no point in avoiding instrumentation of the urethra. A sound is passed along the urethra as far as the tear and then the bladder is exposed extraperitoneally and opened. A second sound is passed through the internal meatus, and the two instruments are manipulated so that the urethral sound follows the path of the bladder sound, the procedure being known as 'railroading'. This should bring the urethral sound into the bladder when a rubber catheter is fastened to the end of the sound and drawn in a retrograde way from the bladder to the urethra. This is used to pull through a Foley's balloon catheter which is inflated and mild traction of 1/2 pound (0.22 kg) weight can be exerted on the catheter over a pulley, thus approximating the bladder neck to the prostatic urethra. This catheter will require to remain *in situ* for 2 weeks; at the same time a suprapubic catheter is inserted into the bladder to drain the urine.

Treatment of trauma to the bulb of the urethra will depend on the degree of damage to the urethra. If a catheter can be passed easily into the bladder, then obviously there has been only incomplete rupture of the urethra; catheter drainage will allow the damaged urethral wall to heal. However, with complete laceration of the bulbous urethra, it is necessary to perform an open operation, suture the tear and divert the urinary stream by suprapubic drainage.

Injuries to the urethra are usually followed by stricture formation due to scarring; subsequent regular dilatations by urethral bougies are necessary. Definitive plastic repair may be possible.

URETHRAL STRICTURE

Aetiology
1 Post-traumatic; rupture of urethra, previous urethral or prostatic surgery or instrumentation.
2 Post-gonococcal.
3 Carcinoma of urethra (extremely rare).

Clinical features
The patient with a urethral stricture complains of difficulty in passing urine with a poor stream and states that only by straining can he empty his bladder. This is in contrast with a patient with prostatic obstruction who usually finds straining aggravates the dysuria.

Treatment
The treatment of an established urethral stricture, whether due to infection or trauma, is primarily conservative. The patient is subjected to regular dilatations of the urethra by passage of sounds. This can be carried out in the outpatients department and may be necessary once a month, or even more frequently.

If a stricture progresses in spite of dilatation then it may be necessary to excise the stricture and perform a plastic repair of the urethra, or to carry out a urethrotomy through an operating urethroscope.

The management of acute retention due to urethral stricture is dealt with on page 301.

Chapter 40
The Penis

PHIMOSIS

Phimosis is gross narrowing of the preputial orifice. It occurs rarely as a congenital lesion, but may result from the scarring following the trauma of forcible retraction of the prepuce (see below) or as a result of chronic balanitis.

Clinical features

On micturition, the prepuce is seen to balloon and the urinary stream is reduced to a dribble.

Treatment

Circumcision is performed. In some cases of chronic balanitis with considerable inflammation of the prepuce a dorsal slit is an efficient, but less aesthetic, method of cure.

NON-RETRACTILE PREPUCE

At some time or other a large number of the male infants in this country are presented to the doctor or nurse because the parents notice that the prepuce cannot be retracted. In fact, the foreskin is normally non-retractile in the first few months of life; 50 per cent retract at the first year and the vast majority can be retracted by the third or fourth year as congenital adhesions between the glans and the prepuce gradually lyse.

Forcible attempts to retract the foreskin traumatize the tissues and the resultant scarring may lead to a true phimosis. Inability to retract the foreskin in the infant is no indication in itself for circumcision; indeed, in the 'nappy' stage the prepuce protects the delicate glans and the urethral orifice from the excoriation of ammoniacal dermatitis.

Circumcision is performed in children only on religious grounds, in the occasional case where the prepuce cannot be retracted in a child over the age of 4, or when an organic phimosis is present.

AMMONIACAL DERMATITIS

This is a common cause of inflammation of the penis in children and is due to the presence of ammonia liberated from urea by urea-splitting organisms. This is especially liable to occur if the child's nappies are not frequently changed and he is allowed to remain wet. The ammonia causes a painful, red, oedematous rash on the perineum, penis and foreskin.

Treatment

Treatment is to change the child's nappies frequently and to cover the skin with a protective barrier cream or zinc oxide and castor oil.

Circumcision should be avoided in the presence of ammoniacal dermatitis, since a meatal ulcer is likely to result.

PARAPHIMOSIS

A condition in which the foreskin becomes retracted around the corona and interferes with the venous return of the glans, resulting in swelling of the glans and extreme pain.

An important practical point: always ensure that the patient's prepuce is pulled forward again after the insertion of an indwelling catheter — if not, paraphimosis may well follow.

Treatment

Once the lesion has become established it is usually too tender to manipulate without an anaesthetic and therefore under general anaesthesia the foreskin is pulled forward into the correct position. However, the condition is likely to recur and it is best to advise the patient to have a circumcision. A dorsal slit of the foreskin may be necessary to reduce a severe paraphimosis.

BALANITIS

Balanitis is an acute inflammation of the foreskin and glans and it is usually due to the common pyogenic organisms, for instance coliform bacilli, stapylococci and streptococci. It may result in phimosis from scarring.

It is important to test the urine for sugar to exclude diabetes which may predispose to the inflammation, in which case *Candida* may be the infecting organism.

Treatment

Consists of administering the appropriate antibiotic after the organism has been cultured and its sensitivity has been determined. Local toilet with weak disinfectant solutions may give relief symptomatically.

CARCINOMA OF THE PENIS

Pathology

This tumour usually affects elderly subjects. It is uncommon in this country although relatively frequently seen in Africa and the East. It is almost invariably associated with the presence of retained smegma and is virtually unknown among Jews, who are circumcised soon after birth.

The most frequent site of the tumour is in the sulcus between the glans and the prepuce.

Macroscopically

Carcinoma of the penis may present either as a papillary growth on the glans or as an ulcerating and infiltrating tumour; the latter is more common.

Microscopically

These lesions are squamous carcinomas which are usually well differentiated.

Spread

1 *Local:* the tumour may fungate through the prepuce to present as an ulcerating lesion on the penile skin. Proximal spread along the shaft may destroy the substance of the penis.
2 *Lymphatic:* the inguinal lymph nodes are frequently involved, often bilaterally.
3 *Blood-borne* spread occurs late and is unusual.

Clinical features

The patient may report with an ulcer on the glans or because of a purulent or blood-stained discharge from below the non-retractile prepuce. He may wait until the tumour has ulcerated through the prepuce or until most of his penis has been destroyed by growth. Surprisingly enough, carcinoma of the penis never seems to occlude the urethra sufficiently to produce retention of urine.

Death from this condition usually results from haemorrhage from fungating nodes in the groins.

Treatment

In summary:
1 *Urethra intact* — radiotherapy.
2 *Urethra involved* — amputation.
3 *Lymph nodes involved* — block dissection if operable, radiotherapy as a palliative measure if matted together and fixed.

Early growths can be treated adequately by radiotherapy or by partial amputation of the penis if the urethra is encroached upon. Lesions that have spread to the regional lymph nodes are difficult to treat. Radical surgery may effect a cure, and consists of total amputation of the penis and bilateral block dissections of the inguinal lymph nodes. This operation, though mutilating, does not interfere with micturition since both the internal and external sphincters are preserved. However, the patient after a total amputation of the penis will need to micturate sitting down.

Inoperably fixed lymph nodes are treated by palliative irradiation.

Chapter 41
The Testis

ABNORMALITIES OF DESCENT

Embryology

The testis arises from the mesodermal germinal ridge in the posterior wall of the abdominal cavity. It links up with the epididymis and vas deferens which develop from the mesonephric duct. As the testis enlarges it undergoes caudal migration. By the 3rd month of fetal life it is in the iliac fossa, by the 7th month it crosses the inguinal canal, by the 8th month it has reached the external inguinal ring and by the 9th month, at birth, it has descended into the scrotum. A prolongation of peritoneum called the processus vaginalis projects into the fetal scrotum; the testis slides behind this and is thus covered in its front and sides by peritoneum. The processus vaginalis becomes obliterated at about the time of birth leaving the testis covered by the tunica vaginalis.

Pathology

When the testis cannot be found in the scrotum, three important abnormalities must be differentiated from each other:

1 Retractile testis (very common).
2 Ectopic testis (common).
3 Undescended testis (relatively uncommon).

The retractile testis is a normal testis with an excessively active cremasteric reflex resulting in the testis being drawn up to the external inguinal ring.

An ectopic testis has descended to an abnormal site. The commonest position is in the superficial inguinal pouch which lies anterior to the external oblique aponeurosis. The testis reached this site after migrating through the external inguinal ring and then leaves the normal tract of descent to pass laterally. Other situations are the goin, perineum, the root of the penis and the femoral triangle.

An undescended testis lies in the normal course of descent anywhere from the abdominal cavity, along the inguinal canal, to the top of the scrotum. The vast majority are not due to hormonal abnormalities but represent a local defect in development. The affected testis is always small and it is probable that this imperfect development impairs descent rather than the imperfect descent impairs development. The undescended testis is usually accompanied by a congenital inguinal hernia. Unilateral undescended testes are four times as common as bilateral. The condition of bilateral undescended impalpable testes is termed *cryptorchidism.*

Most, if not all, testes which *are* going to descend do so within the first few months of life. If the testis is not in its normal scrotal position at puberty then it is very unlikely that it will be capable of spermatogenesis. However, the interstitial cells are functional, so that secondary sex characteristics develop normally.

The risk of malignant change in the undescended testicle is undoubtedly greater than in the normal organ. This appears to be true even if surgical correction is carried out.

Differential diagnosis

The commonest mistake in diagnosis is to fail to differentiate a true maldescent from a retractile testis. Retractile testis, associated with an extremely active cremasteric reflux, is a common condition and often the parents think that the testes have failed to descend; indeed, when the scrotum is palpated the testes may not be felt. However, careful examination will probably reveal the testis at the external inguinal ring or at the root of the scrotum and the testis can, by downward stroking or by gentle traction, be coaxed into the scrotum. A useful trick is to examine the child in the squatting position; this often encourages a retractile testis to descend into the scrotum. It is also worth while asking the parents to examine the child when he is relaxed in a warm bath; again the retractile testis may now slip into its normal position.

If the testis is easily palpable in the groin and remain easy to feel when the child tenses his abdominal wall muscles, then it is lying in the ectopic position and not in the inguinal canal — where it is usually impalpable or, at the most, in a thin boy, detected as a vague, tender bulge.

Treatment

The child with retractile testes is normal; reassurance of the parents is all that is required.

The ectopic or undescended testis must be placed in the scrotum before puberty if it is to function as a sperm producing organ — in addition operation is indicated for cosmetic and psychological reasons. The operation is therefore carried out before the age of 7 and consists essentially of mobilizing the testis and its cord, removing the coexisting hernial sac and fixing the testis in the scrotum without tension.

Hormone treatment is only indicated in those rare cases of bilateral un-descended testes where there is definite evidence of endocrine deficiency; here a short course of injections of chorionic gonadotrophin is given.

Complications of maldescent

1 Defective spermatogenesis: sterility if bilateral.
2 Increased risk of torsion.
3 Increased risk of trauma.
4 Increased risk of malignant disease.

EXAMINATION OF SWELLINGS OF THE SCROTUM
(Fig. 41.1)

1 *Can the examiner get his fingers to meet above the swelling?* If this is not possible then the swelling arises from the abdomen and is an inguinoscrotal hernia.
2 *If it is possible to palpate clearly the upper edge of the swelling, is the swelling*

SCROTAL SWELLINGS

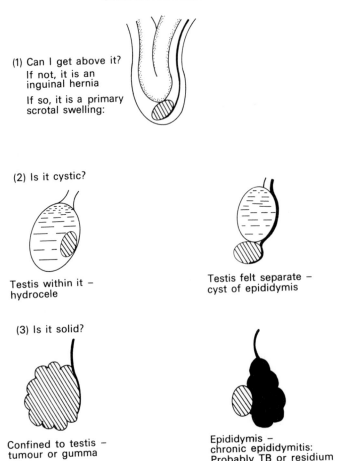

(1) Can I get above it?
If not, it is an inguinal hernia
If so, it is a primary scrotal swelling:

(2) Is it cystic?

Testis within it –
hydrocele

Testis felt separate –
cyst of epididymis

(3) Is it solid?

Confined to testis –
tumour or gumma

Epididymis –
chronic epididymitis:
Probably TB or residium
of acute infection

Fig. 41.1. The differential diagnosis of a scrotal swelling.

cystic? If it is cystic on transillumination and the testis is palpable separate from the swelling then the swelling is a cyst of the epididymis. However, if the testis is within the cyst, it is a hydrocele.

3 *If the swelling is solid* then the following must be considered:
(a) the swelling is an abnormal testis, e.g. a tumour or a gumma.
(b) the epididymis is involved; this is usually an inflammatory condition, either acute or chronic. The latter is either tuberculous or the residual chronic thickening which may persist for many months after an acute pyogenic infection which has been treated with an antibiotic.

Ultrasound examination is valuable in determining whether there is an underlying solid mass in relation to the presence of a scrotal cystic swelling.

CYSTS OF THE EPIDIDYMIS

Epididymal cysts are often multiple, may be bilateral, and produce a fluctuant and usually highly translucent swelling in the scrotum. As they arise from the epididymis, the testis is palpable separately from the cyst. This is the main differentiating point from a hydrocele. The contained fluid may be water-clear or may be milky and contain sperm, hence the old term spermatocele. Clinically there is no way of differentiating between a cyst of the epididymis and a spermatocele and the latter term is best abandoned.

Large cysts of the epididymis may trouble the patient by getting in the way of his clothes and chafing his legs. If producing symptoms, cysts of the epididymis should be removed surgically. Cysts usually develop in adult life but occasionally small congenital cysts may be found in relation to remnants of testicular and epididymal development.

HYDROCELE

A hydrocele is an excessive collection of fluid in the tunica vaginalis.

A primary or idiopathic hydrocele is usually large and tense and there is no disease of the underlying testis.

A secondary hydrocele is usually smaller and lax and the testis is diseased. It is due to the serosal sac surrounding the testis becoming filled with an exudate secondary to tumour or inflammation of the underlying testis or epididymis.

Primary hydroceles are divided into vaginal, congenital, infantile and hydrocele of the cord (Fig. 41.2):

1 *The vaginal hydrocele* is the usual type of hydrocele surrounding the testis and separated from the peritoneal cavity. The patient presents with a cystic transilluminable swelling in the scrotum. On examination the testis is difficult to feel and lies at the back of the swelling which, due to the anatomy of the tunica, encompasses the anterior and lateral portions of the organ.

2 *The congenital hydrocele* is associated with a hernial sac; it opens into the peritoneal cavity through a narrow orifice. When elevated it gradually empties.

3 *An infantile hydrocele* extends from the testis to the internal inguinal ring but does not pass into the peritoneal cavity.

4 *Hydrocele of the cord* is rare. It lies in, or just distal to, the inguinal canal,

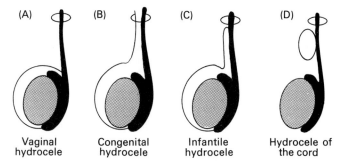

(A)	(B)	(C)	(D)
Vaginal hydrocele	Congenital hydrocele	Infantile hydrocele	Hydrocele of the cord

Fig. 41.2. The anatomical classification of hydroceles (the ring at the upper end of each diagram represents the internal inguinal ring).

separate from the testis and the peritoneum. Diagnosis is confirmed by the simple test of downward traction on the testis, which pulls the hydrocele of the cord down with it.

Treatment

Hydroceles in infants should be left alone — most disappear spontaneously. If the hydrocele persists after the first year, operative treatment is advisable. The sac is opened, the testis inspected to exclude a testicular tumour or other pathology and the patent processus vaginalis is ligated and divided.

Hydroceles in adults should be tapped to remove the fluid in order to enable the testis to be palpated to exclude primary lesions of the testicle. The position of the testis is located by transillumination and carefully avoided. A little local anaesthetic is inserted into the skin of the scrotum, a trocar and cannula are introduced into the hydrocele and fluid removed. In the primary hydrocele the fluid is pale yellow and may have flecks of cholesterol in it. If the fluid is bloodstained then this is more likely to be a secondary hydrocele, although the bleeding may be due to trauma. Once the fluid has been removed the testis is palpated to exclude malignancy or infection.

Primary hydroceles can be managed by intermittent tapping or they can be excised surgically; most patients prefer the latter form of treatment since aspiration must be repeated every few months. Secondary hydroceles require treatment for the underlying condition. Ultrasonography is of use for examination of the testis in these cases.

ACUTE INFECTIONS OF THE TESTIS

Acute infections may be due to mumps (producing an orchitis), and gonorrhoea and coliform bacilli (which infect the epididymis).

With acute orchitis due to the virus of mumps the other stigmata of mumps will probably be present (see page 132). Adults are particularly likely to be affected; there may be residual damage to the testis and if both sides are involved fertility may be impaired.

Bacterial epididymitis may follow cystitis and prostatitis, or may occur *de novo*. It can also be a complication of prostatectomy.

Clinical features

The patient will have a very painful swelling in the testis, often with a secondary hydrocele and constitutional effects (pyrexia, headache and leucocytosis). Examination of the urine may reveal the presence of organisms and pus cells, but the urine need not invariably be abnormal.

Treatment

Bed rest and the appropriate antibiotic. If frank abscesses have formed with fluctuation then drainage is required. However, with early adequate treatment resolution is more likely. The patient will often have residual swelling of the epididymis, which may be rather firm, and differentiation from the tuberculous epididymitis may be difficult unless the history of the previous acute attack is obtained.

CHRONIC INFECTIONS OF THE TESTIS

Gumma

Although once common, syphilis of the testis is now a rarity. Apart from the fact that they produce enlarged testes which makes clinical differentiation from a carcinoma difficult, but which melt away on penicillin, gummata of the testis will not be further considered.

Tuberculosis

This often occurs in association with tuberculosis in other parts of the genito-urinary tract.

Clinical features

The patient usually presents with swelling of the epididymis. The vas deferens may be thickened and feel nodular. A cold abscess may develop in relation to the epididymis and rupture through the scrotum, usually posteriorly, resulting in a chronic sinus. The seminal vesicles may be enlarged and palpable on rectal examination.

Diagnosis depends on isolating tubercle bacilli from the urine or biopsy material, or evidence of tuberculosis elsewhere.

Treatment

This is the same as for tuberculosis in other situations (see page 283). If a chronic sinus has developed, then unilateral orchidectomy is probably the best form of treatment, since the testis is unlikely to be functional, is a continued source of infection and may lead to spread of the disease elsewhere.

TORSION OF THE TESTIS

Aetiology

Usually this is a torsion of the spermatic cord in a congenitally abnormal testis, often maldescended or hanging like a bell-clapper with a completely investing tunica vaginalis. Occasionally true torsion of the testis occurs without involving the cord when there is an extensive mesorchium between the testis and epididymis. It is probably impossible for torsion to occur in an anatomically completely normal testis. Untreated, the testis undergoes irreversible infarction within a few hours and there is a typical transudation of blood-stained fluid into the tunica vaginalis.

Clinical features

Torsion of the testis is an acute surgical emergency which usually occurs in children or adolescents. There may be a history of mild trauma to the testis or of previous attacks of pain in the testis due to torsion and spontaneous untwisting.

The patient presents with an acutely swollen and painful testis and also with pain in the lower abdomen, since the nerve supply of the testis is mainly from T10 sympathetic pathway. Rarely the pain is limited to the abdomen. Patients with torsion of the right testis have been operated on for acute appendicitis because the testis has not been examined with care.

On examination the testis is swollen, painful to touch and tends to lie high in the scrotum.

Differential diagnosis

The main difficulty in differential diagnosis is from acute epididymitis. In this latter condition the testis does not lie so high in the scrotum, there is a systemic reaction with pyrexia and leucocytosis, and there is usually a history of urinary infection with pus cells and organisms in the urine. A useful factor in differential diagnosis is the age of the patient, since torsion of the testis is unusual after the age of 20, whereas epididymitis is rare before that age.

Torsion may also mimic a strangulated inguinal hernia.

Treatment

If there is any doubt as to the diagnosis it is best to explore the testis as soon after admission as possible since every hour increases the likelihood of irreversible damage to the testis. If still viable, the testis is untwisted and sutured to the tunica vaginalis. If infarcted, it is removed. In every case fixation of the other testis should be performed at the same time since any congential anomaly is likely to be bilateral and torsion of the opposite testis may therefore occur.

VARICOCELE

This is a condition of varicosities of the pampiniform plexus of veins. It is much commoner on the left than the right. Suggested causes are that the left testis is lower than the right, that the loaded sigmoid colon compresses the left testicular vein, and that the left testicular vein, entering the renal vein close to where the suprarenal vein also joins the renal, becomes constricted by release of adrenaline into the vein. None of these theories seems to explain the condition very satisfactorily. Most cases occur without other associated pathology, but very occasionally a varicocele can be secondary to a tumour or other pathological process blocking the testicular vein. The best-known example of this is a tumour of the kidney involving the renal vein and obstructing the drainage of the left testicular vein.

Clinical features

On examination in the standing position the varicose veins within the scrotum feel like a 'bag of worms'. The condition may be associated with defective spermatogenesis and patients with varicocele are often subfertile.

Treatment

Usually the condition requires no treatment apart from reassurance that the condition is not likely to give rise to any dangerous complications. If the weight of the varicocele and testis cause an ache then a suspensory bandage may help the patient. If he demands treatment, and in cases of male infertility, the varicose veins can be divided and ligated.

TUMOURS OF THE TESTIS

Testicular tumours are the commonest solid malignancy in young adult males.

Pathology

There are two main forms of malignant tumours of the testis, seminoma and teratoma.

The seminoma (60 per cent) arises from cells of the seminiferous tubules, usually occurs between 30 and 40 years of age and is relatively slow growing. The tumour is solid and the cells vary from well-differentiated spermatocytes to undifferentiated round cells. Some 10 per cent arise in undescended testes.

The teratoma (40 per cent) occurs in a younger age group, the peak incidence being 20 to 30 years. The precise origin is not known, but it is thought to arise from more primitive germinal cells. It has a markedly cystic appearance and used to be called fibrocystic disease. The cut surface may appear like a colloid goitre. Microscopically the cells are very variable and the tumour may contain cartilage, bone, muscle, fat and other tissues.

A rare form of teratoma is the *chorionepithelioma of the testicle*. This is usually a solid, haemorrhagic tumour and microscopically consists of syncytial tissue, very similar to the tumour of the same name occurring in women. It is very rapidly growing and tends to metastasize to the lungs and liver (and can do this even when the tumour in the testis is quite small.) This tumour usually produces a positive pregnancy test in the urine due to the fact that it secretes trophoblastic hormone and there may be associated gynaecomastia.

Spread

1 *Local:* the testis is progressively destroyed by the tumour. Spread through the capsule is unusual, but occasionally in an advanced case there may be ulceration of the scrotum.

2 *Lymphatic:* to the para-aortic nodes via lymphatics accompanying the testicular vein. In advanced cases there may be enlargement of the supraclavicular nodes, especially on the left side.

3 *Blood-borne:* spread from the teratoma occurs relatively early to the lungs and liver. In the seminoma this tends to be late in the disease.

Special investigations

Chest X-ray and CT scan of the abdomen for secondaries.

Blood is taken preoperatively for tumour markers (*alpha-feto protein* and human *chorionic gonadotrophin*). These are useful not only in making a diagnosis but in subsequent follow-up.

A scrotal ultrasound may reveal a solid tumour in a hydrocele but a negative finding cannot exclude malignancy.

Clinical presentations

1 As a lump in the testis.
2 As a hydrocele.
3 Rarely as a painful rapidly enlarging swelling which may be mistaken for orchitis.
4 As secondaries, usually metastatic growths in the lung, as a mass in the abdomen due to involved abdominal lymph nodes, or as a cervical lymphadenopathy.

Tumours of the testis usually present as a painless, swollen testicle which is hard and may be associated with an overlying secondary hydrocele which sometimes contains bloodstained fluid.

Treatment

If it is suspected that the testicular swelling is due to a tumour, early exploration is mandatory. The spermatic cord is exposed through an inguinal incision and occluded by an atraumatic clamp and the testis delivered. The clamp prevents dissemination of tumour cells. If the diagnosis is now obvious, immediate orchidectomy is performed. If the diagnosis is in doubt, a biopsy is taken and submitted to frozen section examination. Orchidectomy is performed if the diagnosis is now confirmed.

Seminomas are highly radio-sensitive so that, following orchidectomy, radiotherapy is given to the abdominal lymph nodes. If the tumour is a teratoma, better results are probably obtained by treating lymph node deposits (demonstrated clinically or on CT scan) by combination cytotoxic therapy. Patients with disseminated disease in either group are treated by cytotoxics.

Prognosis

Node-negative cases have an extremely good prognosis of about 100 per cent five year survival. Even with early abdominal lymph node spread there is still a 95 per cent five year survival and with disseminated disease, long term survivals are often achieved with chemotherapy.

Chapter 42
The Neck

(For thyroid, see page 320)

Differential diagnosis of a lump in the side of the neck

When considering the swellings which may arise in any anatomical region, one enumerates the anatomical structures lying therein and then the pathological swellings that may arise therefrom. The side of the neck is an excellent example of this exercise:

1   *Skin and superficial fascia:*
    (a) sebaceous cyst
    (b) lipoma
2   *lymph nodes:*
    (a) infective
    (b) malignant
    (c) the lymphomas, lymphatic leukaemia (see page 77).
3   *Lymphatics:* cystic hygroma
4   *Artery:*
    (a) carotid body tumour
    (b) carotid aneurysm
5   *Salivary glands:*
    (a) submandibular salivary tumours or sialectasis
    (b) tumours in the lower pole of the parotid gland
6   *Pharynx:* pharyngeal pouch
7   *Branchial arch remnant:* branchial cyst

BRANCHIAL CYST AND SINUS

Aetiology

The 2nd branchial arch in the embryo grows down over the 3rd and 4th arches to form the cervical sinus. This sinus usually disappears, but its persistence may lead to formation of a branchial cyst, sinus or fistula.

Clinical features

The cyst usually presents in early adult life and forms a soft swelling 'like a half-filled hot water bottle' which bulges forward from beneath the anterior border of the sternomastoid into the carotid triangle. It is lined by squamous epithelium and contains pus-like material which is in fact cholesterol. Clinical diagnosis can be clinched by aspirating a few drops of this fluid from the cyst and demonstrating cholesterol crystals under the microscope. Occasionally the cyst may become infected. Differential diagonsis is from a tuberculous gland of neck or from an acute lymphadenitis. A first branchial arch cyst may present just below the external auditory meatus with extension closely related to the VII nerve.

The branchial sinus presents as a small orifice discharging mucus which opens over the anterior border of sternomastoid in the lower part of the neck. The majority are present at birth but a secondary branchial sinus may form if an infected branchial cyst ruptures. The sinus extends upwards between the internal and external carotid arteries to the side wall of the pharynx. It may open into the tonsillar fossa (which represents the 2nd internal cleft) to form a branchial fistula.

Treatment

Surgical excision

TUBERCULOUS CERVICAL ADENITIS

With a general decline in tuberculosis, this once common lesion (mainly of children) is now relatively rarely seen in this country, except in the aged, sufferers from AIDS and in immigrants from Asia. Cervical nodes are usually secondarily involved from a tonsillar primary focus, although the adenoids or even the dental roots may occasionally be the primary source of infection. The organisms may be human or bovine and occasionally the disease is secondary to active pulmonary infection. The upper jugular chain of nodes is most commonly affected.

Clinical features

At first the nodes are small and discrete; then, as they enlarge, they become matted together, caseate, and the abscess so formed eventually bursts through the deep fascia into the subcutaneous tissues, producing a 'collar stud' abscess. Left untreated, this discharges onto the skin resulting in a chronic turberculous sinus.

Differential diagnosis

Solid nodes must be differentiated from acute lymphadenitis, one of the lymphomas or secondary deposits. The breaking-down abscess must be differentiated from a branchial cyst (see above).

Diagnosis is assisted by an X-ray of the neck; usually the chronic tuberculous nodes show flecks of calcification.

Treatment

A full course of anti-tuberculous chemotherapy is given (see page 283). Small nodes are treated conservatively and the patient is kept under observation. If the nodes enlarge, e.g. one centimetre or more in diameter, they should be excised. If the patient presents with a 'collar stud' abscess, the pus is evacuated, a search made for the hole penetrating through the deep fascia and the underlying caseating gland evacuated by curettage.

It is not usually necessary to deal with the infected tonsils or adenoids since these resolve with the chemotherapy.

CAROTID BODY TUMOUR (CHEMODECTOMA)

Pathology

A slow-growing tumour which arises in the carotid body at the carotid bifurcation. It eventually becomes locally invasive and may metastasize. To the naked eye, it is a lobulated, yellowish tumour closely adherent to the major arterial trunks. Histologically it is made up of large chromaffin polyhedral cells in a vascular fibrous stroma.

Clinical features

The tumour presents as a slowly enlarging mass in a patient over the age of 30, which transmits the carotid pulsation. The mass itself may be so highly vascular that it too demonstrates pulsation. Occasionally pressure on the carotid sinus from the tumour produces attacks of faintness.

Special investigation

Arteriography shows the carotid bifurcation to be splayed open by the mass and the rich vascularity of the tumour is demonstrated.

Treatment

it is often possible to dissect the tumour away from the carotid sheath. If the carotid vessels are firmly involved, resection can be performed with graft replacement of the artery.

In the eldery, these slowly growing tumours can be left untreated.

Chapter 43
The Thyroid

CONGENITAL THYROID ANOMALIES

The embryological line of descent of the thyroid gland, from the region of the foramen caecum of the tongue to its normal position in the neck, may be the site of fistula or cyst formation (Fig. 43.1). Rarely the thyroid fails to descend properly into the neck and such a patient may present with a lump at the foramen caecum (*lingual thyroid*) or at the front of the neck near the body of the hyoid bone. Such a swelling may not be suspected as being thyroid and if this is removed the patient may have no other functioning thyroid tissue. In all cases of unexplained nodules in the line of thyroid descent, a radio-iodine scan should be performed to ensure that there is normal thyroid tissue present in the correct place before the lump is removed. Occasionally the thyroid descends beyond its normal station into the superior mediastinum — *a retrosternal thyroid*.

THYROGLOSSAL FISTULA

This presents as an orifice in the line of the thyroid descent, in the midline of the neck. It may discharge thin, glairy fluid and attacks of infection can occur.

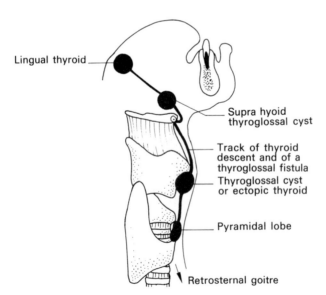

Lingual thyroid

Supra hyoid thyroglossal cyst

Track of thyroid descent and of a thyroglossal fistula

Thyroglossal cyst or ectopic thyroid

Pyramidal lobe

Retrosternal goitre

Fig. 43.1. The descent of the thyroid, showing possible sites of ectopic thyroid tissue or thyroglossal cysts, and also the course of a thyroglossal fistula. (The arrow shows the further descent of the thyroid which may take place retrosternally into the superior mediastinum).

Treatment

The treatment is to excise the fistula and this excision must be complete. The track runs in close relationship with the body of the hyoid, therefore this should be removed in addition to the fistula and the dissection is continued up to the region of the foramen caecum of the tongue.

THYROGLOSSAL CYST

Forms in the embryological remnants of the thyroid and presents as a fluctuant swelling in the midline of the neck. Clinically the cyst moves upwards when the patient protrudes the tongue because of its attachment to the tract of the thyroid descent, and moves on swallowing because of its attachment to the larynx by the pretracheal fascia.

Treatment

Such cysts should be removed surgically.

THYROID PHYSIOLOGY

The thyroid gland is concerned with the synthesis of the iodine containing hormones thyroxine (tetra-iodothyronine, T4) and tri-iodothyronine (T3) which control the metabolic rate of the body. It also secretes calcitonin from its parafollicular C cells, which reduces the level of serum calcium and is therefore antagonistic to parathormone.

Iodine in the diet is absorbed into the blood stream as iodide which is taken up avidly by the thyroid gland. After entering the follicle, the iodide is converted into organic iodine which is then bound with the tyrosine radicals of thyroglobulin to form the precursors of the thyroid hormones. The colloid within the thyroid vesicles is composed of thyroglobulin synthesized in the follicular cells. Within thyroglobulin, iodine and tyrosine combine first to form mono-iodotyrosine from which T3 and T4 are formed and stored within the thyroglobulin colloid. These hormones are released into the blood stream after being separated from thyroglobulin within the follicular cells. In the general circulation about 99 per cent of T3 and T4 is bound to protein (protein-bound iodine) and it is the minute amount of unattached thyroid hormones in the circulating blood which produces the endocrine effects of the thyroid gland.

The concentration of the thyroid hormones in the blood under normal conditions is maintained within narrow limits. The immediate control of synthesis and liberation of T3 and T4 is by the thyroid-stimulating hormone (TSH) produced by the anterior pituitary. TSH is secreted in response to the level of thyroid hormones in the blood by a negative feedback mechanism so that a drop in the level of these hormones stimulates TSH production and vice versa. The secretion of TSH is also under the influence of the hypothalamic thyrotrophin-releasing hormone (TRH).

The production of thyroid hormones can be inhibited by the thiouracils and carbimazole which block the binding of iodine but do not interfere with the uptake of iodide by the gland. Although less T3 and T4 are produced, the thyroid gland tends to become large and vascular with treatment by these drugs.

High doses of iodide given to patients with excessive thyroid hormone production result in an increase in the amount of iodine-rich colloid, and a diminished liberation of thyroid hormones; the gland also becomes less vascular. The effects of iodide treatment are maximal after two weeks of treatment and then diminish.

Lack of iodine in the diet prevents the formation of thyroid hormones and excess pituitary TSH is produced which may result in an iodine deficient goitre. Thiocyanates prevent the thyroid gland from taking up iodide.

PATHOLOGY OF GOITRE

Nodular goitre
Like the breast, ovary and the prostate, the thyroid gland undergoes periods of activity and regression at different times. There is excessive thyroid activity at puberty and during pregnancy and a fall after the menopause. The commonest cause of enlargement of the thyroid gland in Great Britain is a nodular goitre, and this has similarities with the commonest pathological conditions of the breast and prostate, namely fibroadenosis and benign hyperplasia. In a nodular goitre, the gland is enlarged, irregular and partly cystic. The pathology would appear to be an excessive degree of activity and regression resulting in a varied appearance of the gland. some vesicles are lined with hyperactive epithelium and others with flattened atrophic cells. Some contain no colloid, others an excessive amount. The thyroid interstitium is excessive with a certain amount of fibrosis and round cell infiltration. Nodular goitres may produce a normal amount of thyroxine, but sometimes excessive thyroxine production results in hyperthyroidism in this condition ('secondary thyrotoxicosis').

Complications of nodular goitre
1 Tracheal displacement or compression.
2 Haemorrhage into a cyst (which may produce urgent tracheal compression).
3 Toxic change.
4 Malignant change (rare).

Colloid goitre
All diseases of the thyroid are commoner in geographical locations in which the water and diet are low in iodine. In Great Britain the most notorious district was Derbyshire and the frequency of goitres in this region gave rise to the term 'Derbyshire neck'. Iodination of table salt has all but abolished this state of affairs. Switzerland, Nepal, Ethiopia and Peru are also areas where natural iodine is very scarce in the diet and water, and there thyroid disease is common. The commonest lesion of the thyroid gland due to iodine deficiency is the colloid goitre in which the gland as enlarged and the acini are atrophic with a large amount of colloid. As has been mentioned, this accumulation of colloid is probably due to over-secretion of TSH from the anterior pituitary, acting on the thyroid which is unable to produce thyroxine.

Hyperplasia
In primary Grave's disease the thyroid is uniformly enlarged and there is hyperac-

tivity of the acinar cells with reduplication and infolding of the epithelium. The gland is very vascular and there is little colloid to be seen. Lymphocyte infiltration is usually a pre-dominant feature.

CLINICAL CLASSIFICATION OF THYROID SWELLINGS

The clinical assessment of a patient with an enlarged thyroid falls into two phases:

1 *First,* determine the physical characteristics of the gland itself — is it smoothly enlarged, is there a single nodule present, is it nodular?

2 *Second,* determine the endocrine state of the patient; euthyroid, hyperthyroid or hypothyroid?

A synthesis of these two phases gives a simple clinical classification of the vast majority of thyroid swellings.

The common findings are:

1 A smooth, non-toxic enlargement of the thyroid gland: this is the 'physiological' goitre which tends to occur at puberty and pregnancy.

2 A nodular, non-toxic gland — there being either a solitary nodule or multiple nodules. This is the common nodular goitre.

3 A smooth toxic goitre: primary thyrotoxicosis or Graves' disease.

4 A nodular toxic enlargement: secondary thyrotoxicosis.'

The less common findings are:

5 A smooth, firm enlargement (although sometimes asymmetrical and irregular) with myxoedema, usually in a middle-aged female: Hashimoto's disease.

6 An invasive enlargement: carcinoma.

Riedel's thyroiditis and acute thyroiditis are uncommon.

Clinical features

Patients may present complaining of a lump in the neck and/or with symptoms due to excessive or diminished amounts of circulating thyroxine.

The thyroid swelling

The characteristics of an enlarged thyroid are a mass in the neck on one or both sides of the trachea, which moves on swallowing, since it is attached to the larynx by the pre-tracheal fascia. The draining lymph nodes, lying in the anterior triangle of the neck, are palpated.

Evidence of retrosternal enlargement of the thyroid should be sought by percussion over the sternum. A retrosternal thyroid can block the venous return to the superior vena cava and result in engorgement of the jugular veins and their tributaries and in oedema of the upper part of the body — a cause of the superior mediastinal syndrome. In such cases X-rays of the thoracic inlet should be taken; the enlarged thyroid will be shown as a radio-opaque mass in the retrosternal position.

The trachea should be examined to determine displacement or compression by the thyroid enlargement; the patient should be asked to take a deep breath, when stridor may become apparent.

The vocal cords should be examined by indirect laryngoscopy, as thyroid enlargement may result in damage to the recurrent laryngeal nerves and vocal cord paralysis. If surgery is contemplated it is obviously important to know whether or not the cords are functioning normally before operation.

Symptoms and signs of hyperthyroidism

Patients with hyperthyroidism (thyrotoxicosis) are usually female.

Clinical features are conveniently grouped into systems from above downwards:

1   CNS: the patient is irritable, nervous and demonstrates tremor of the out-stretched fingers, she cannot keep still.

2   The skin: is moist and hot, the patient prefers winter to summer.

3   The eyes: exophthalmos in 85 per cent (see below).

4   The thyroid: this is usually enlarged but not invariably so; it may be highly vascular and demonstrates a bruit and thrill.

5   CVS: a rapid pulse is almost invariable and typically the sleeping pulse is also raised. There may be atrial fibrillation and indeed the patient may present with heart failure.

6   Alimentary system: the patient's appetite is increased and yet she loses weight. Diarrhoea is occasionally a feature.

Exophthalmos is present in 85 per cent of patients with primary thyrotoxicosis. The extraocular muscles undergo lymphocyte infiltration and are swollen by oedema. It appears to be immunologically mediated, with the extra-ocular muscles as the main target, but no antibody has been identified to date.

The eyes have a staring appearance and when the patient is asked to follow the examiner's finger from above the head to below it, the whites of the eyes have a staring appearance and when the patient is asked to follow the examiner's finger from above the head to below it, the whites of the eyes will be visible above the pupils ('lid-lag'). If there is doubt, then the degree of protrusion of the eyes can be measured by an ophthalmologist. In extremely severe exophthalmos the extrinsic muscles of the eye may be damaged, resulting in incoordination of eye muscles (exophthalmic ophthalmoplegia).

The exophthalmos is an extremely distressing condition for the patient and, if severe, the patient is unable to close her eyelids; the eyes are then liable to corneal ulceration and eventual blindness. This condition is difficult to treat. Severe cases may respond to high dosage corticosteroids but may require surgical decompression of the orbit and also suture of the eyelids across the eyeball — tarsorrhaphy.

A rare clinical feature of hyperthyroidism is thickening of the subcutaneous tissues in front of the tibia, the so-called 'pretibial myxoedema'.

From the clinical aspect, patients with thyrotoxicosis fall into two groups, the primary and secondary (see Table 43.1).

1   *Primary thyrotoxicosis* (Graves' disease) occurs usually in young women with no preceding history of goitre. The gland is smoothly enlarged and exophthalmos is a common feature. Symptoms are primarily those of CNS disturbance, perhaps because the young and healthy are little disturbed by the high pulse rate.

2   *Secondary thyrotoxicosis* is a disease of middle-age, occurring in patients with a pre-existing non-toxic goitre. The gland is nodular and there are no eye changes.

Table 43.1. Primary and secondary toxic goitres compared.

	Primary	Secondary
Age:	Young	Middle aged
Pre-existing goitre	–	+
Thyroid	Smooth	Nodular
Exophthalmos	+	–
CNS features	+ + +	+
CVS features	+	+ + +

Symptoms fall more on the CVS than on the nervous system, the patient often presenting in heart failure with atrial fibrillation, although nervousness, irritability and tremor may also be present.

It is now considered that primary thyrotoxicosis is due to the action of 'long-acting thyroid stimulator' (LATS), a gamma-globulin produced by lymphocytes and probably an antibody to some thyroid antigen. TSH–receptor antibodies can be demonstrated in most patients with this condition. Secondary thyrotoxicosis is overactivity developing in an already diseased and hyperplastic gland.

Hypothyroidism

Congenital hypothyroidism or cretinism is a condition in which the child is born with little or no functioning thyroid. He is stunted and mentally defective, with puffy lips, a large tongue and protuberant abdomen, often surmounted by an umbilical hernia.

In adults hypothyroidism or myxoedema usually affects women, and most often occurs in the middle-aged or elderly. These patients have a slow, deep voice and are usually overweight and apathetic, with a dry, coarse skin and thin hair, especially in the lateral third of the eyebrows. In contrast with hyperthyroidism, myxoedematous patients usually feel cold in hot weather, have a bradycardia and are constipated. They are often anaemic and may suffer from heart failure due to myxoedematous infiltration of the heart.

Investigations in thyroid disease

The simplest and most reliable clinical test of hyperthyroidism is *the sleeping pulse rate:* the greatest difficulty in the clinical diagnosis of hyperthyroidism is its differentiation from an acute anxiety state. However, such patients when sleeping will have a normal pulse rate, whereas in patients with hyperthyroidism the sleeping pulse will remain elevated.

Laboratory investigations

1 *The serum thyroxine (T4) and tri-iodothyronine (T3)* can be estimated directly. Their elevation are valuable test for hyperthyroidism.

2 *Radio-iodine studies* of the thyroid gland provide very useful information. A small tracer dose of gamma ray emitting I^{131} is injected intravenously; the rate at which it is cleared from the blood stream is a measure of thyroid activity. The gland itself can be scanned with a gamma ray detector and areas of high activity mapped

out. For instance, a nodule in the thyroid gland which is hyperactive can be pinpointed by this method, a so-called 'hot nodule'. Similarly, a nodule that is not producing thyroxine will not take up the radio-iodine, for example a cyst or tumour.

3   *The serum cholesterol* is usually raised in myxoedema and may be normal or a little low in hyperthyroidism.

4   *The basal metabolic rate* is quite a useful assessment of thyroid function, provided it is done by a reliable method and the patient is under really basal conditions; because of these difficulties it is now rarely used in clinical practice. Increase in the basal metabolic rate occurs in hyperthyroidism and the reverse in myxoedema.

5   *An ECG* in myxoedematous cardiac involvement will show low electrical activity with small complexes. Atrial fibrillation complicating hyperthyroidism will be confirmed.

6   *Thyroid antibodies:* these are detected in Hashimoto's (autoimmune) thyroiditis.

7   *Ultrasound* gives valuable information as to whether the mass is solid or cystic.

8   *Fine needle aspiration* allows material to be obtained for cytological examination.

OUTLINE OF TREATMENT OF GOITRE

Non-toxic nodular enlargement

Thyroidectomy is advised in patients with an enlarged, non-toxic, nodular goitre when there are symptoms of tracheal compression. In addition, in younger patients, it is reasonable to advise operation because of the danger of haemorrhage into a thyroid cyst with acute tracheal compression, and because of the small risks of toxic or malignant change in the gland. The patient may be concerned with the cosmetic appearance of her swollen neck, which is a perfectly valid indication for surgery.

In elderly patients with a long-standing goitre which is symptomless it is good practice to leave well alone.

In the patient with a single nodule in the thyroid this may be a solitary benign adenoma, a malignant tumour, or most likely of all, a cyst in a thyroid showing the histological changes of a nodular goitre.

Just as every solitary lump in a woman's breast is best removed, it is similarly wise to advise removal of any solitary thyroid nodule.

Hyperthyroidism

The available therapy in thyrotoxicosis comprises:

1   Anti-thyroid drugs, of which carbimazole is the drug of choice.

2   Beta-adrenergic blocking drugs.

3   Anti-thyroid drugs combined with subsequent thyroidectomy.

4   Radio-active iodine.

Carbimazole

This is given in a dosage of 10 mg tds and is combined with sedation and bed rest in the acute phase of hyperthyroidism. There is rapid regression of toxic symptoms, the patient beginning to feel better and to gain weight with reduction of tachycardia within a week or two. Unfortunately, a high relapse rate occurs after ending treatment, even if this is prolonged for two or more years. Medical treatment alone is therefore usually confined to the treatment of primary hyperthyroidism in children and adolescents.

The toxic effect are drug rash, fever, arthropathy, lymphadenopathy and agranulocytosis; the last is the dangerous complication which is potentially lethal, but occurs in well under 1 per cent of patients. The first symptom is a sore throat and patients on carbimazole must be warned to discontinue treatment immediately if this occurs and to report to hospital. Antibiotic therapy is commenced, fresh blood transfusion given if necessary and the patient barrier-nursed until the bone marrow recovers.

Beta-adrenergic blocking drugs

In patients with severe hyperthyroidism propranolol induces rapid symptomatic improvement of the cardiovascular features while the hyperthyroidism comes under control with specific anti-thyroid therapy.

Drugs and surgery combined

The majority of adult patients in this country are treated by preliminary carbimazole until euthyroid and are then submitted to subtotal thyroidectomy.

Radioactive iodine

From the patient's point of view this is the most pleasant treatment since all she has to do is swallow a glass of water containing the radio-iodine. There is no need for prolonged treatment with drugs nor the risk of operation; it is particularly useful in recurrence of hyperthyroidism after thyroidectomy. It usually takes 2 or 3 months before the patient is rendered euthyroid. Antithyroid drugs, with or without a beta-blocker, may be used to control symptoms during this time.

There is a theoretical risk of malignant change in the irradiated gland although there has been no report of this occurring in humans. It is, however, current practice not to use radio-iodine in patients under the age 45 and, in addition, not to employ it in young women who may become pregnant during treatment, since there is a very real danger of affecting the infant's thyroid. Another disadvantage of this treatment is the production of a high incidence of late myxoedema which rises to near 30 per cent after 10 years and which requires replacement therapy with thyroxine.

COMPLICATIONS OF THYROIDECTOMY

In addition to the hazards of any surgical operation there are special complications to consider following thyroidectomy. These can be divided into hormonal disturbances (the thyroid itself and the adjacent parathyroid glands) and injury to closely related anatomical structures.

1 *Hormonal:*
   (a) tetany (parathyroid removal or bruising)

(b) thyroid crisis

(c) myxoedema (due to extensive removal of thyroid tissue)

(d) late recurrence of hyperthyroidism (inadequate operation in the toxic gland)

2 *Damage to related anatomical structures:*

(a) recurrent laryngeal nerve

(b) injury to trachea

(c) pneumothorax

3 *The complications of any operation*

Especially:

(a) haemorrhage

(b) sepsis

(c) post-operative chest infection

Some of these complications require further consideration here.

Hypoparathyroidism

May result from inadvertent removal of the parathyroids or their injury during operation. The patient may develop tetany (page 332) a few days post-operatively with typical carpo-pedal spasms, which may be induced by tourniquet around the arm (Trousseau's sign), and a positive Chvostek's sign; this is elicited by tapping lightly over the zygoma when the facial muscles will be seen to contract. The serum calcium falls to below 1.5 mmol/l (6 mg per cent).

Treatment

Consists of giving 10 ml of 20 per cent calcium gluconate intravenously followed by oral calcium lactate 15 g daily, together with dihydrotachysterol. Often the tetany is transient and the injured parathyroids recover; in other cases permanent treatment is required. Parathormone is not used because the patient quickly acquires resistance to it.

In addition to frank tetany, which occurs in about 1 per cent of cases, milder degrees of hypoparathyroidism may occur and may present with mental changes (depression or anxiety neurosis), skin rashes and bilateral cataracts. A low post-operative calcium is treated by the administration of calcium lactate 15 g daily by mouth.

Thyroid crisis

An acute exacerbation of thyrotoxicosis seen immediately post-operatively is now extremely rare because of the careful pre-operative preparation of these cases. It is, however, a frightening phenomenon with mania, hyperpyrexia and marked tachycardia which may lead to death from heart failure. The cause is not fully understood, but it may be due to a massive release of thyroxine from the hyperactive gland during the operation.

Treatment

Comprises heavy sedation with barbiturates, propranolol, intravenous iodine and cooling by means of ice packs.

Recurrent laryngeal nerve injury

The recurrent laryngeal nerve lies in the groove between the oesophagus and trachea in close relationship to the inferior thyroid artery. Here it is at risk of division, injury from stretching, or compression by oedema or blood clot.

If one nerve alone is damaged the patient may have little in the way of symptoms apart from slight hoarseness because the opposite vocal cord compensates by passing across the midline during phonation. However, if both recurrent nerves are damaged there is almost complete loss of voice and serious narrowing of the airway; a permanent tracheostomy may be required, although an incomplete injury may recover in time. It is estimated that the nerve is injured in about 2 to 3 per cent of thryroidectomies.

Haemorrhage

This occurring shortly after thyroidectomy is a dangerous condition as bleeding into the thyroid bed may compress the trachea already softened by pressure from the thyroid swelling. The neck becomes distended with blood; there is acute dyspnoea and stridor, as well as shock from blood loss.

Treatment

This may be an extreme emergency and must be dealt with at once by decompressing the neck in the ward. The skin and the subcutaneous sutures are removed, the wound is opened and the blood clot expressed. The patient can then be transferred to theatre, anaesthetized, and bleeding points secured and the wound resutured.

THYROID TUMOURS

Classification

Benign

Adenoma

Malignant

1 *Primary:*
   (a) adenocarcinoma (papillary of follicular)
   (b) anaplastic
   (c) medullary carcinoma (arises from the parafollicular cells, secretes calcitonin)
   (d) lymphoma (rare)
2 *Secondary:*
   (a) invasion from adjacent structures, e.g. oesophagus
   (b) very rare site for blood-borne deposits

BENIGN ADENOMA

Although benign encapsulated nodules in the thyroid gland are common, the majority are part of a nodular colloid goitre. A small percentage represent true benign adenomas.

THYROID CARCINOMA

Pathology

Affect females twice as often as males, often arise in pre-existing goitres and have been reported following radiation of the neck in childhood. There are two main groups:

1 The well-differentiated adenocarcinomas (papillary, follicular and medullary).
2 Anaplastic spheroidal cell carcinoma.

Such important differences occur between these two groups that they might almost be considered separate disease entities.

The well-differentiated tumours comprise:

1 *Papillary:* the commonest type of thyroid cancer. It occurs in young adults, adolescents or even children. It is a slow-growing tumour and lymphatic spread occurs late. Deposits in the regional lymph nodes may be solitary and in the past have been mistakenly regarded as lateral aberrant thyroid tissue. However, a careful search of the thyroid gland will reveal a well differentiated tumour in the homolateral lobe.

2 *Follicular:* occurs in young and middle-aged adults. It has a greater tendency to blood stream spread and therefore a worsened prognosis.

3 *Medullary:* arises from the parafollicular C cells and may secrete calcitonin. It may occur at any age and, unlike other thyroid tumours, has a roughly equal sex distribution. It may be familial and may be associated with phaeochromocytoma, and with adenomas in other endocrine glands The characteristic finding is deposits of amyloid between the nests of tumour cells.

The anaplastic carcinomas occur in the elderly; there is thus a reversal of the usual state of affairs in that the more malignant tumours of the thyroid occur in the older age group. Rapid local spread takes place with compression and invasion of the trachea; there is early dissemination to the regional lymphatics and blood stream spread to the lungs, skeleton and brain.

Treatment

The well-differentiated carcinoma presenting with a localized mass in the thyroid should be treated, after histological confirmation of the diagnosis, by total removal of the affected lobe of the thyroid together with block dissection of the lymph nodes if these are involved.

Many of these well-differentiated tumours take up radioactive iodine and it is possible to treat recurrences or metastases by I^{131} therapy. A tracer dose of radioactive iodine will give evidence of the suitability of isotope therapy by confirming uptake of the radio-iodine in the secondary deposits.

The anaplastic carcinomas may be treated by radical thyroidectomy but frequently these patients present with an already inoperable mass in the neck. Palliative radiotherapy may give temporary relief and tracheostomy may be required for the obstructed airway.

The thyroid cells are under the control of the anterior pituitary and this applies even to the well-differentiated tumours. It has been shown that giving thyroxine will suppress the thyrotrophic hormone of the pituitary and there have been remarkable examples of regression of well differentiated thyroid cancer when large doses of thyroxine have been given.

Prognosis

This is very different in the two groups of cases; the well-differentiated tumours are often associated with long survival, even in the presence of lymph node deposits, whereas patients with anaplastic tumours are usually dead within a year or two either from local invasion or widespread dissemination.

HASHIMOTO'S DISEASE

This is an uncommon thyroid disease which has received considerable attention since it was the first of the auto-immune diseases to be elucidated. The patient is usually a middle-aged female with clinical evidence of hypothyroidism. The gland is uniformly enlarged and firm, although it may occasionally be asymmetrical and irregular. Its cut surface is lobulated and greyish yellow.

Histologically there is diffuse infiltration with lymphocytes, increased fibrous tissue and diminished colloid. It is considered to be an autoimmune disease in which the patient has developed circulating antibodies to her own thyroid. Such antibodies, which react against thyroglobulin, can be demonstrated in about 90 per cent of cases.

It is important to diagnose the condition correctly by demonstrating the presence of thyroid antibodies and, if necessary, by biopsy since thyroidectomy will precipitate severe hypothyroidism in the cases.

Treatment

Thyroxine 0.3 mg is given daily; on this regime the gland shrinks and symptoms of myxoedema disappear.

RIEDEL'S THYROIDITIS

An extremely rare disease of the thyroid in which the gland may be only slightly enlarged but is woody hard with infiltration of adjacent tissues. The cause of this condition is not known, but it may represent a late stage of Hashimoto's disease or possibly be inflammatory in origin.

It is mistaken clinically for a thyroid carcinoma, but histologically the gland is replaced by fibrous tissue containing chronic inflammatory cells.

A wedge resection of a portion of the gland may be required if symptoms of tracheal compression develop.

Chapter 44
The Parathyroids

Anatomy and development

The parathyroid glands are four organs (sometimes three or five) about the size of split peas which usually lie in two pairs behind the lateral lobes of the thyroid gland. The superior parathyroids arise from the *fourth* branchial pouch and the inferior glands from the *third* pouch, in association with the developing thymus. The inferior parathyroids may lie almost anywhere in the neck and also in the superior mediastinum in relationship to the thymus gland.

Physiology

The parathyroids produce parathormone which has profound influence on calcium and phosphate metabolism. The exact mechanisms of its action are not known, but there appear to be two main effects:

1   It produces excessive excretion of phosphorus from the kidney by inhibiting the tubular reabsorption of phosphate.

2   It stimulates osteoclastic activity in the bones resulting in the decalcification and liberation of excessive amounts of calcium and phosphorus in the blood.

Thus, an increased production of parathormone produces:

1   A raised serum calcium and a lowered serum phosphate, as these substances are related reciprocally.

2   An increased excretion of both calcium and phosphate in the urine.

3   Raised serum alkaline phosphatase associated with decalcification of the bones.

Tetany

Lack of parathormone results in a low serum calcium and hyper-irritability of skeletal muscle with carpopedal spasms, the syndrome being called tetany. The most common cause of this is removal or bruising of the parathyroids in thyroidectomy (see page 328). Tetany is liable to occur if the serum calcium falls below 1.5 mmol/l (6 mg/100 ml). Spasms may affect any part of the body, but typically the hands and feet. The wrist flexes and the fingers are drawn together, the so called 'main d'accoucheur'. This spasm may be induced by a tourniquet around the arm — Trousseau's sign. The hyper-irritability of the facial muscles may be demonstrated by tapping over the facial nerve which results in spasm — Chvostek's sign.

Note that clinical tetany may occur with a normal level of serum calcium in alkalosis (e.g. overbreathing, excessive prolonged vomiting) because of a compensatory shift of ionized calcium to the unionized form in the serum.

PARATHYROID TUMOURS

Pathology

These are usually single. The lower glands are affected more commonly than the upper ones. The tumours are soft, encapsulated and a brown-grey colour — most are benign adenomas; carcinoma of the parathyroid is rare.

The tumour may coexist with other endocrine tumours (multiple endocrine adenoma syndrome) — pancreatic islet cell tumour, anterior pituitary adenoma, thyroid medullary carcinoma and phaeochromocytoma.

Clinical features

These depend on the results of excessive production of parathormone by the tumour (see above). In some 10 per cent of hyperparathyroidism the condition is found to be due to a hyperplasia of all four parathyroid glands. This occurs in patients with renal failure maintained by dialysis. Presenting symptoms may be one or more of the following:

Bone changes

Spontaneous fractures or pain in the bones. X-rays will show decalcification of the bones with cyst formation. The weakened bones may be deformed; this condition is known as osteitis fibrosa cystica or Von Recklinghausen's disease of bone. There may be metastatic calcification in soft tissues, arterial walls and the kidneys.

Renal effects

Renal stones (see page 277), infection associated with renal calculi, calcification in the renal substance or uraemia. It is important to remember that chronic renal disease with impaired excretion of phosphate may result in secondary hyperplasia of the parathyroid glands with features similar to those of a primary adenoma of the parathyroid.

Vague ill health associated with high serum calcium

The patient very often complains of lassitude, weakness, anorexia and loss of weight.

Peptic ulceration

Dyspepsia or frank duodenal ulceration is sometimes associated with parathyroid adenoma.

The main effects are summarized as: 'Stones, bones, abdominal groans'.

Special investigations

1   *Serum calcium* is usually raised to above 2.75 mmol/l (11 mg per cent). Other causes of raised serum calcium include metastatic cancer, multiple myeloma, sarcoidosis and the milk alkali syndrome; in all these the serum calcium falls if a 10-day course of cortisone is given, but no significant change takes place in true hyperparathyroidism (*the cortisone suppression test*).

2   *Serum parathormone level* is raised.

3 *Excretion of calcium by the kidneys:* the urinary excretion of a standard calcium intake is increased.

4 *Serum phosphate* is low.

5 *Serum alkaline phosphatase* is raised.

6 *X-rays of the bones* may show subperiosteal decalcification and cyst formation.

7 *Abdominal X-rays and IVU* may show renal stones or nephrocalcinosis.

8 *Subtraction scanning:* a technetium scan is taken up by the thyroid; this is followed by a thallium scan, taken up by both the thyroid and parathyroid. Subtraction of the first from the second reveals a 'hot spot' denoting a functioning parathyroid tumour.

Treatment

Removal of the parathyroid adenoma. This may be rather difficult to find as often quite small tumours can produce gross metabolic disturbances. The neck is very carefully explored, first of all in the usual sites of the parathyroid glands and if no tumour is found then more extensive dissection is made into the neck and into the superior mediastinum.

HYPOPARATHYROIDISM

This is usually secondary to surgery in the neck, especially thyroidectomy and is considered on page 328.

Chapter 45
The Adrenal Medulla

ADRENAL MEDULLARY TUMOURS

Classification
1 Ganglioneuroma.
2 Neuroblastoma.
3 Phaeochromocytoma.
4 Secondaries (a common site, especially from breast and bronchus).

Ganglioneuroma
A benign slowly growing tumour of sympathetic ganglion cells which only becomes clinically manifest if it reaches a large size. Only about 15 per cent arise in the adrenal; the rest elsewhere along the sympathetic chain.

Neuroblastoma
A highly malignant tumour of sympathetic cells occurring in children under the age of 5. It may be bilateral with early spread to adjacent tissues, the regional nodes and by the blood to bones and the liver.

Treatment
The tumour is usually inoperable but radio-sensitive and may respond well to cytoxic therapy.

Phaeochromocytoma
A physiologically active tumour of chromaffin cells which secretes noradrenaline and adrenaline in varying proportions. Ten per cent are malignant and 10 per cent are multiple; 10 per cent occur outside the adrenal in the sympathetic chain or the organ of Zuckerkandl (the '10 per cent tumour').

Any age may be affected, but the tumour is particularly found in young adults.

Clinical features
These are produced by excess of circulating adrenaline and noradrenaline. There is hypertension, which is paroxysmal or sustained, and which may be accompanied by palpitation, headache, blurred vision, fits, papilloedema and episodes of pallor and sweating. There may be hyperglycaemia with glycosuria.

Occasionally the tumour may coexist with a medullary carcinoma of the thyroid or a parathyroid adenoma (multiple endocrine adenoma syndrome).

Special investigations
1 *Phentolamine*, which is a noradrenaline antagonist, brings the blood pressure down to normal levels.

2 *The urinary catecholamines* are usually raised, particularly during an acute hypertensive attack.

3 *CT scanning or ultrasonography* may demonstrate the site and size of the tumour.

4 *X-rays:* a variety of techniques are available. A plain X-ray of the abdomen may occasionally outline a large tumour. Selective angiography of the adrenal arteries enables the tumour to be delineated. Blood samples from the adrenal veins may be obtained under X-ray control for catecholamine estimation; a raised value in the blood obtained from the IVC at this level is useful confirmatory evidence of the presence of a tumour.

Treatment

Surgical excision. Manipulation of the tumour during the operation may cause gross hypertension which is countered by an intravenous phentolamine drip. Immediately following removal of the tumour the blood pressure may fall to unrecordable levels and this is countered by blood transfusion and by a noradrenaline drip, which may have to be continued for a day or two following the operation.

Chapter 46
The Adrenal Cortex

Physiology

The adrenal cortex secretes three groups of steroids:

1 *Glucocorticoids,* which regulate carbohydrate metabolism (diabetogenic), protein break-down and fat mobilization.

2 *Androgenic corticoids,* which are virilizing.

3 *Mineral corticoids,* which regulate mineral and water metabolism. Aldosterone acts to retain sodium and water and to excrete potassium.

Representatives of these groups overlap in their action; thus cortisone, a glucocorticoid, also affects salt and water metabolism and has sex steroid effects (acne, hirsutism) if given in large amounts.

Hyperadrenocorticism

Hyperfunction of the adrenal cortex may be due to hyperplasia of the gland, a functioning cortical adenoma or carcinoma, or occasionally may be secondary to a basophil adenoma of the pituitary which produces an excess of adrenocortical stimulating hormone.

The syndromes produced by hyperfunction of the adrenal cortex can be attributed to excess of each of its three groups of hormones:

1 Glucocorticoids: Cushing's syndrome.

2 Androgenic corticoids: virilism (the adrenogenital syndrome).

3 Mineral corticoids: primary aldosteronism (Conn's syndrome).

CUSHING'S SYNDROME

A syndrome produced by the over-secretion of adrenal corticosteroids. The majority of cases result from pituitary dependent hyperplasia of the adrenal cortex, but about 10 per cent are due to benign or malignant cortical tumours or, rarely, a basophil adenoma of the pituitary.

Clinical features

The syndrome usually affects young adults (occasionally children); females more often than males. The appearance is characteristic; adiposity with central distribution, abdominal striae, a red moonface and diabetes. There may be osteoporosis, leading to vertebral collapse. Associated mineral and androgenic corticoid over-secretion produce varying degrees of hypertension, hirsutism and acne, with amenorrhoea in the female or impotence in the male.

Special investigations

The urinary and plasma cortisol level is raised. This level rises still further in cases of adrenal hyperplasia following the additional stimulation of ACTH. Failure of the level to rise on this therapy suggests an adrenal autonomous tumour rather than a simple hyperplasia which is still under pituitary control and is a useful investigation in differentiating between these two conditions.

An X-ray of the skull may reveal an enlarged pituitary fossa suggesting basophil adenoma.

CT scanning of the abdomen often demonstrates the tumour and is a valuable non-invasive investigation.

Treatment

If due to bilateral hyperplasia, bilateral adrenalectomy is performed and the patient placed on a maintenance dose of cortisone. Removal of the affected adrenal is carried out in cases of adenoma or carcinoma.

Cases due to basophil adenoma of the pituitary respond to hypophysectomy.

THE ADRENOGENITAL SYNDROME

This syndrome results from the hypersecretion of adrenal cortical androgens. It can be divided into a congenital and an acquired variety.

1 *The congenital form* appears to be due to an inborn defect of normal steroid synthesis (especially hydrocortisone) by the adrenal cortex. Excessive ACTH production by the pituitary then occurs with resulting hyperplasia of the cortex and hypersecretion of cortical androgens.

2 *The acquired variety* in children is always due to an adrenal cortical tumour which is usually malignant. In young adults the condition may be due either to a tumour or to cortical hyperplasia in cases of Cushing's syndrome where androgen production is excessive.

Clinical features

These are conveniently divided into three varieties depending on age of onset.

Infancy

In the congenital variety of the adrenogenital syndrome the new-born female has a large clitoris and is often mistaken for male (female pseudohermaphrodite). Growth is initially rapid, but the epiphyses fuse early so that the final result is a stunted child. There may be episodes of acute adrenocortical insufficiency, especially with stress or infection.

Childhood

Virilization occurs in the female and precocious sexual development, particularly of the penis, in the male. This can be well summarized as 'little girls become little boys and little boys become little men'.

Adults

Amenorrhoea, hirsutism and breast atrophy in the female, often associated with other features of Cushing's syndrome. In the male feminization is seen, but this is extremely rare.

Differential diagnosis

Differentiation must be made from the masculinizing tumour of ovary, in which the 17 ketosteroid urinary excretion is normal, and also the common condition of simple hirsutism in the female.

Treatment

Bilateral cortical hyperplasia in infancy is treated by suppressing the excess ACTH secretion with cortisone; on this regime the virilizing features clear and growth progresses normally. In the acquired variety, the tumour is treated by removal and hyperplasia by bilateral adrenalectomy with cortisone maintenance.

PRIMARY HYPERALDOSTERONISM (CONN'S SYNDROME)

This is a rare syndrome produced by an aldosterone-secreting adenoma of the adrenal cortex.

Characteristically there is a low serum potassium (which results in episodes of muscle weakness or paralysis), raised serum sodium and alkalosis with hypertension. There may be polyuria and polydipsia.

The diagnosis is confirmed by demonstration of excess aldosterone in the plasma.

The tumour, which is often small, may be demonstrated by an abdominal CT scan although selective angiography may be needed to delinerate the lesion.

Treatment

The involved adrenal is explored and the tumour (which is usually small) removed.

The condition is interesting because, although rare, it represents a curable cause of hypertension.

NON-FUNCTIONING TUMOURS OF THE ADRENAL CORTEX

Small non-secreting adenomas of the adrenal cortex are common post-mortem findings which are of no significance. Non-functioning carcinomas of the adrenal cortex are rare; they resemble renal carcinoma in appearance (hence the original hypothesis that the hypernephroma was of adrenal origin). They are highly malignant and frequently invade the subjacent kidney.

Chapter 47
The Thymus

The thymus gland controls the development of immunologically competent cells (T lymphocytes) in the embryo and neonate.

In adult life the thymus atrophies to a vestigial remnant, but to the surgeon it is of importance in having an ill-understood connection with myasthenia gravis and of being a rather rare site of mediastinal tumour.

MYASTHENIA GRAVIS

A condition of muscle weakness apparently due to a defect at the neuromuscular junction in which the motor end plate becomes refractory to the action of acetylcholine. About 10 per cent of cases are associated with a tumour of the thymus and it was this observation which led to thymectomy being performed in cases of myasthenia with cure in a proportion of patients. It has been suggested that myasthenia may be an auto-immune response to the protein of muscle or motor end plate.

Clinical features

Women are twice as commonly affected as men and the disease usually commences in early adult life. The extrinsic ocular muscles are most often affected and may indeed be the only ones involved, with ptosis, diplopia and squint. The affected muscles become weak with use and recover, partially or completely, after rest. The voice is weak and death may eventually occur from respiratory muscle failure.

Treatment

The majority of cases are controlled by choline esterase inhibitors, e.g. Prostigmin (neostigmine).

Thymectomy is indicated if the disease is progressive and the prognosis is best in young females (under the age of 40) with a history of 5 years or less. The results are less good in those cases associated with a thymic tumour.

THYMIC TUMOURS

Tumours of the thymus are of complex pathology; they may arise from either the epithelium (Hassall's corpuscles) or lymphoid tissue, or from a mixture of both. They may be benign (occasionally cystic) or malignant and rapidly invasive.

Clinical features

There are three modes of presentation:

1 A mediastinal mass.

2 Associated with myasthenia gravis.
3 Associated with immune deficiency states

Treatment

Thymectomy — combined with radiotherapy if malignant.

Chapter 48
The Breast

Lymphatic drainage

The lymphatic drainage of the breast is important, but there is no mystique about it; as with any other organ, its lymph drainage follows the pathway of its blood supply and therefore travels:

1 Along the tributaries of the axillary vessels to the axillary lymph nodes.

2 Along the perforating branches of the internal thoracic vessels, which pierce each intercostal space, to the lymph nodes along the internal thoracic chain. These lymph nodes also receive lymphatics which accompany the lateral perforating branches of the intercostal vessels.

Although the lymph vessels lying between the lobules of the breast communicate freely, there is a tendency for the lateral part of the breast to drain towards the axilla, and the medial part to be served by the internal thoracic chain.

A subareolar plexus of lymphatics below the nipple (the plexus of Sappey) and another deep plexus on the pectoral fascia have, in the past, been considered to be the central points to which the superficial and deep parts of the breast drain before passing to the main efferent lymphatics. These plexuses are, however, relatively unimportant, the main drainage proceeding directly to the regional lymph nodes.

The axillary lymph nodes drain the pectoral region, upper abdominal wall and the upper limb in addition to the lymphatics of the breast, and are arranged in five groups:

1 Anterior: lying deep to pectoralis major.

2 Posterior: along the subscapular vessels.

3 Lateral: along the axillary vein.

4 Central: within the axillary vein.

5 Apical: immediately behind the clavicle at the apex of the axilla-receiving lymph from all the other axillary nodes.

The subclavian lymph trunk emerges from the apical nodes. On the left this trunk usually drains directly into the thoracic duct; on the right it either empties directly into the subclavian vein or else joins the right jugular trunk.

Lymphatic spread of a growth in the breast may occur further afield when these normal pathways have become interrupted by malignant infiltration, surgical ablation or radiotherapy. Deposits may then be found in the lymphatics of the opposite breast or opposite axilla, the groin lymph nodes (via lymph vessels in the trunk wall), the cervical nodes (as a result of retrograde extension from the blocked thoracic duct or jugular trunk) or intraperitoneal lymphatics as retrograde spread from the lower internal thoracic nodes.

Symptoms of breast disease

There are three common symptoms of breast disease; a lump, bleeding or discharge from the nipple, and pain.

A lump in the breast

Ninety-five per cent of all lumps in the breast will be one of the four following:
1   Carcinoma of the breast.
2   Cyst.
3   Fibroadenoma.
4   A localized area of fibroadenosis

In addition, the following possible causes need to be considered:
1   Traumatic: fat necrosis.
2   Other cysts:
    (a) galactocele
    (b) chronic abscess
    (c) cystadenoma
    (d) retention cyst of the glands of Montgomery
3   Other tumours:
    (a) sarcoma (extremely rare)
    (b) duct papilloma
4   Swellings arising from the chest wall:
    (a) tuberculosis or tumour of a rib
    (b) lipoma
    (c) eroding aortic aneurysm
    (d) cold abscess (empyema necessitatis)
    (f) thrombosis of superficial veins of breast or chest wall (Mondor's disease)

Although useful information can be derived about a lump in the breast by careful examination, it is a good clinical rule that any discrete lump in the breast must be excised for histological examination or aspirated for cytological examination: 'No lady should have a lump in the breast.'

If the lump is considered likely to be a cyst, it is safe practice to aspirate it to confirm the diagnosis. If it disappears, no further treatment is required. However, if no fluid is obtained, the lump should be surgically removed or submitted to fine needle aspiration and cytological examination of the material obtained (see page 347).

Discharge from the nipple

This may be:
1   *Bloodstained:*
    (a) duct papilloma
    (b) intraduct carcinoma
    (c) Paget's disease
    (d) invasive carcinoma (unusual)
2   *Serous:* Early pregnancy.
3   *Yellowish, brown or green:* fibroadenosis.
4   *Milky:* following lactation

5 *Purulent:* breast abscess.

It is the first, the bloodstained discharge, which alarms the patient. Its management is as follows:

The patient is carefully examined; there may be one of the following possibilities:

1 A mass is discovered, pressure on which produces the discharge; the mass is excised and further treatment is based on the result of histological examination.

2 If a mass is not discovered, it may be possible by pressing on one spot adjacent to the nipple to obtain a discharge. This segment of the breast is surgically explored and submitted to histological examination; again a limited or more extensive operation may be required, depending on the results of pathological examination. It is, however, very rare for a malignant condition to be present without a lump having been detected.

3 If no mass can be felt and no duct can be incriminated, a conservative approach is adopted; the patient is kept under supervision either until the site of discharge is located and excised, or the bleeding ceases; again, this is most unlikely to be the presentation of malignant disease of the breast.

Special investigations which may help are a *mammogram* and a '*ductogram*', performed by injecting contrast into the discharging duct.

Pain in the breast

The possible causes to be considered are:

1 *Breast abscess.*

2 *Fibroadenosis:* typically the pain is present immediately before each period.

3 *Carcinoma of the breast:* this occasionally gives rise to a 'pricking' pain.

4 *Lesions, not of the breast, but of the chest wall,* e.g. chondritis of the coastal cartilage. This syndrome (Tietze's disease) is of unknown aetiology, affects one or more of the 2nd, 3rd or 4th costo-chondral junctions and, left alone, resolves over a number of months.

TRAUMATIC FAT NECROSIS

Pathology

Disrupted fat cells released by trauma produce a foreign body giant cell reaction with subsequent fibrosis and perhaps calcification.

Clinical features

Many women presenting with a lump in the breast attribute this to injury. A clinical diagnosis of fat necrosis should only be made when the trauma was sufficient to cause bruising of the breast and when the patient is obese. The lump itself may have become smaller in size and this again would suggest a non-malignant condition, in spite of the fact that clinically the lump may be tethered to the skin and accompanied by large axillary lymph nodes.

Treatment

This is excision since it is impossible to be quite certain of the diagnosis without biopsy; a section through the lump reveals a pale, fibrous mass which may contain central fluid fat or chalky material.

ACUTE INFLAMMATIONS OF THE BREAST

Classification

1 *Mastitis of the newborn* } probably hormonal but may
2 *Mastitis of puberty*   } proceed to suppuration.
3 *Mumps mastitis:* rare complication.
4 *Traumatic* (due to the chafing of braces, etc.)
5 *Subareolar:* from infection of one of the glands of Montgomery which are sebaceous-like glands around the areola.
6 Acute bacterial mastitis and acute mammary abscess.

The last cause is the commonest and most important. The majority occur during lactation, caused either by invasion by *Stapyhylococcus aureus* through an abrasion of the nipple resulting in a circumareolar abscess, or along the milk ducts themselves, producing a deep intramammary infection. Typically it affects mothers in the first month after their first pregnancy. Breast abscess may also occur in non-lactating women, but it is a rarity after the menopause.

Clinical features

The infection commences as a cellulitis which localizes into an abscess after several days.

Treatment

Milk engorgement is relieved by manual expression or a breast pump. It is best to stop lactation with stilboestrol 10 mg daily for 1 week. If the patient is seen within the first 24 hours of the onset, when the condition is still a spreading cellulitis of the breast, infection may be aborted by antibiotic therapy. If the infection has been present for more than a day or two it is almost certain that a localized abscess will have commenced to form. In these circumstances it is best to be old-fashioned and to apply poultices which comfort the patient until a localized fluctuant mass forms which can then be drained. If chemotherapy is persisted with in these later cases, an unpleasant condition may result of chronic and recurrent abscesses burrowing through the breast.

CHRONIC ABSCESS OF THE BREAST

Tuberculosis, gumma and actinomycosis of the breast are all very rare. The most likely chronic abscess of the breast is one following prolonged and misguided chemotherapy in the treatment of acute breast abscess ('antibioticoma' or 'penicillinoma').

FIBROADENOSIS, 'CHRONIC MASTITIS', OR CHRONIC DYSPLASTIC MASTITIS

This is the commonest of all breast conditions. Indeed, some degree of fibroadenosis is probably present in most women.

Aetiology

Any organ in the body which undergoes cyclical changes of proliferation and regression is prone to abnormalities of this process; these are the prostate, thyroid and ovary as well as the breast. Fibroadenosis is found in women from puberty to menopause, after which it only occurs occasionally in the form of large cysts within the breast. It is frequently bilateral.

Pathology

Macroscopically

The affected breast tissue is tough, yellowish white and of india-rubber consistency. It is not encapsulated. Cysts are usually present and vary from numerous tiny ones to solitary, large, blue domed cysts (of Bloodgood). The cyst fluid may be yellow, green or brown in colour. Sometimes the ducts contain toothpaste-like material.

Microscopically

The main features are:
1 Glandular hyperplasia.
2 Connective tissue hyperplasia.
3 Cyst formation.
4 Papillary formation within cysts.
5 Lymphocytic infiltration.
(It is this lymphocytic infiltration which induced the early microscopists to label this condition 'chronic mastitis'.)

It is probable that duct papilloma is in essence a localized form of the papillary formation seen in chronic mastitis, and that fibroadenoma is a localized glandular and connective tissue hyperplasia (see below).

Clinical features

The patient, who may be of any age from teens to the menopause, may present with one or more of the following: a lump in the breast, pain in the breast, particularly before the periods, or discharge from the nipple, which may be bloodstained, yellow, green or brown.

Examination may reveal diffuse lumpiness of both breasts or a mass confined to one sector of the breast, particularly the upper, outer quadrant. It is characteristic that this lumpiness is best defined by palpation between the index finger and the thumb, and it is more difficult to feel with the flat of the hand (in contrast to a carcinoma). This is because the segment of fibroadenosis has almost the same consistency as the surrounding breast tissue.

Less commonly the patient presents with a local, smooth, spherical lump in the breast which may be of considerable size. It may be possible to elicit fluctuation or transillumination in such a lump, and then to be tolerably certain that the diagnosis is a cyst. Quite commonly shotty nodes are palpable in the axilla.

Differential diagnosis

The differential diagnosis from an early carcinoma of the breast may be very difficult, indeed impossible; moreover, it is far from rare to find both conditions present within the same breast, although there is no definite evidence that fibroadenosis is premalignant. It is sound practice therefore *to submit every localized mass in the breast to biopsy, either by needle aspiration or excision*.

Special investigation

A soft tissue X-ray of the breast (*mammography*) may be helpful in revealing a small malignant lesion which typically shows an area of speckled calcification. It may also be helpful in reassuring the patient that a lesion is benign. It must be stressed, however, that errors may occur even in the most expert interpretation of these X-rays so that biopsy is the safest policy in any doubtful case.

Treatment

The golden rule is that 'no lady is allowed to have a lump in her breast'. A discrete lump which may be a cyst is subjected to immediate aspiration under local anaesthetic in the out-patient clinic. If clear fluid is obtained and the lump completely disappears, we can be certain that it is a simple cyst. The rare condition of a carcinoma in the wall of a cyst (cystadenocarcinoma) will yield blood-stained fluid on aspiration and a persistent lump can still be felt; urgent excision biopsy is then necessary.

If no fluid is obtained, a tissue diagnosis must be made. This is performed either by excision biopsy or by fine needle aspiration and cytological examination. Should this prove to be an area of benign fibroadenosis, the patient is reassured and suitable follow-up arranged. If a fibroadenoma is confirmed, local excision is all that is necessary. If the biopsy proves to be a carcinoma, further treatment is discussed on page 352.

The patients who are not submitted to surgery are the large group of women with diffuse granularity of one or, more usually, both breasts with no localized mass. A mammogram is helpful (see above), particularly in post-menopausal women, but usually the patient can be reassured that there is no evidence of malignant disease and kept under supervision in the out-patient clinic. Monthly self-examination can also be taught and the patient advised to report if she find any discrete lump.

Many patients with fibroadenosis complain of pain in the breasts, which may or may not be cyclical. Most can be managed by reassurance and analgesics. Severe cyclical breast pain may require treatment with the prolactin inhibitor bromocriptine or with danazol, which inhibites gonadotrophin release. Both, however, may have quite unpleasant side effects.

TUMOURS OF THE BREAST

Classification

Benign

1   fibroadenoma
2   intraduct papilloma

Malignant
> 1 *Primary:*
>   (a) carcinoma
>   (b) intraduct carcinoma
>   (c) Paget's disease of the nipple
>   (d) fibrosarcoma
> 2 *Secondary:*
>   (a) direct invasion from tumours of the chest wall
>   (b) metastatic deposits from melanoma

FIBROADENOMA

Pathology

This is a firm, encapsulated, benign tumour with a whorled appearance on cut surface.

Microscopically it comprises fibrous tissue surrounding epithelial duct proliferation.

Clinical features

Fibroadenomas occur after the age of puberty, commonly in young women; they are highly mobile 'breast mice' which are not attached to the skin. Rarely in middle-aged or elderly women a very large lobular fibroadenoma may be found which may even ulcerate the overlying skin by pressure necrosis (serocystic disease of Brodie). The majority of these remain benign, but a few may undergo sarcomatous change.

Treatment

Excision and histological confirmation of the diagnosis.

DUCT PAPILLOMA

This maybe part of a generalized papillomatosis or may occur as a solitary entity.

The duct papilloma is usually situated in one of the 15 to 20 ducts near the nipple in a young woman. The patient complains of bleeding from the nipple and the examiner may either find a small elliptical swelling adjacent to the nipple, pressure on which produces this discharge, or he may merely find that pressure on one spot causes blood to emerge from the mouth of the duct.

An X-ray 'ductogram' may define the lesion.

Treatment

Excision of the lump with, of course, histological examination of the specimen, or, if no lump can be felt, excision of the small segment of breast tissue from which the discharge can be expressed.

CARCINOMA

Pathology

This is an immensely important subject — the commonest malignant disease of females in the United Kingdom, accounting for about 13 000 deaths annually in England and Wales; less than 1 per cent occur in men. Any age may be affected, but it is rare below the age of 30.

There is no definite evidence of any predisposing factors in humans, but there is a familial tendency; it is rare in orientals and less likely to affect women who have had pregnancies in their teens. There is no proved association with the contraceptive pill.

Clinical and macroscopic types

1 *Scirrhous:* hard and encapsulated; the cut surface is grey, concave, gritty and with white spots resembling an unripe pear.

2 *Atrophic scirrhous:* scar-like tumour occurring in the shrivelled breast of the elderly.

3 *Encephaloid:* large, soft and 'brain-like'.

4 *Papillary:* intraduct or intracystic.

5 *Lactational:* a fulminating form occurring in or after pregnancy ('mastitis carcinomatosa').

6 *Paget's disease of the nipple* (see page 354).

Microscopic classification

Carcinomas of the breast are all derived from ductal or alveolar epithelium. They may be classified as follows:

1 *Adenocarcinoma:* well-differentiated acini in a fibrous stroma.

2 *Spheroidal cell:* clumps of spheroidal cells in a fibrous stroma.

3 *Carcinoma simplex:* (anaplastic carcinoma) undifferentiated cells arranged in solid masses.

4 *Colloid or mucoid carcinoma:* where excessive mucus production is a feature.

5 *Intraduct carcinoma:* arising in a duct and invading its wall.

6 *Papillary cystadenocarcinoma:* arising in a cyst wall.

7 *Squamous cell:* arising in squamous metaplasia, usually in a cyst wall.

8 *Paget's disease.*

9 *Lobular carcinoma in situ:* a premalignant condition, often present in both breasts.

Spread

1 *Direct extension:* involvement of skin and subcutaneous tissues leads to skin dimpling, retraction of the nipple and eventually ulceration. Extension deeply involves pectoralis major, serratus anterior and eventually the chest wall.

2 *Lymphatic:* blockage of dermal lymphatics leads to cutaneous oedema pitted by the orifices of the sweat ducts, giving the appearance of *peau d'orange*. Dermal lymphatic invasion produces daughter skin nodules and eventually *'cancer en cuirasse'*, the whole chest wall becoming a firm mass of tumour tissue. The main lymph channels pass directly to the axillary and internal thoracic lymph nodes. Later spread occurs to the supraclavicular, abdominal, mediastinal, groin, and opposite axillary nodes.

3 *Blood spread:* especially to lungs, liver and bones (at the sites of red bone marrow, i.e. skull, vertebrae, pelvis, ribs, sternum, upper end of femur and upper end of humerus). The brain, ovaries and adrenals are also frequent foci of deposits.

4 *Trans-coelomic:* pleural and peritoneal seeding occurs commonly in advanced disease, accompanied by pleural effusion and ascites respectively.

Staging

The following clinical staging is in common use (Fig. 48.1)

I The lump is confined to the breast, with or without some degree of skin fixation to it or with indrawing of the nipple.

II As above, but in addition, the axillary lymph nodes are enlarged and quite mobile.

III The tumour and/or the nodes are fixed superficially or deeply.

IV Distant metastases are present.

There is a high degree of clinical error, about 25 per cent in fact, in estimating whether a tumour is stage I or II; axillary lymph nodes may be involved although they cannot be felt, conversely axillary nodes which are palpable may prove free

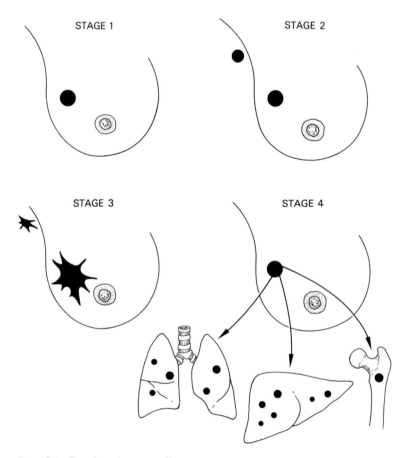

Fig. 48.1. The clinical staging of breast cancer.

from tumour. However, the classification is of great practical importance since patients with stage I and II lesions are usually submitted to 'curative' surgery, whereas those in stages III and IV are only suitable for palliative treatment (*see* section on treatment below).

TNM classification

There are considerable variations in the classification of malignant tumours which makes exchange of information between centres difficult. The International Union against Cancer has devised a clinical system for staging tumours which has already been applied to most sites. The initial letters TNM stand for: T — the tumour, N — the regional lymph nodes and M — distant metastases. The addition of numbers of the three components indicates different degrees of extent of the malignant process.

The classification applied to the breast is as follows:

T — Primary tumour

T.0: no evidence of primary tumour.

T.1: the tumour is 2 cm or less in diameter, skin not involved, except in the case of the Paget's disease where confined to the nipple; no nipple retraction or fixation to underlying tissues.

T.2: tumour more than 2 cm but not more than 5 cm in diameter, or incomplete skin fixation with tethering or dimpling of the overlying skin, or nipple retraction, but no fixation to underlying tissues.

T.3: tumour more than 5 cm but not more than 10 cm in diameter, nor infiltration nor ulceration of the skin or *peau d'orange* or fixation to the pectoral muscles.

T.4: tumour of more than 10 cm diameter or skin involvement or *peau d'orange* wide of the tumour or fixation to the chest wall.

N — Regional lymph nodes

N.0: no palpable homolateral axillary nodes.

N.1: palpable, mobile homolateral axillary nodes.

N.2: homolateral axillary nodes fixed to one another or to other structures.

N.3: homolateral supra- or infra-clavicular nodes movable or fixed, or oedema of the arm.

M — Distant metastases

M.0: no evidence of distant metastases. (This includes X-rays of the chest and skeleton, bone scan and liver ultrasound).

M.1: distant metastases present, including skin involvement wide of the breast, involvement of contralateral nodes or breast, and clinical, scanning or X-ray evidence of spread to lungs, pleural cavity, skeleton, liver etc.

Clinical features

The patient may present with local symptoms, usually a painless lump in the breast (although occasionally a pricking discomfort is complained of). Sometimes the principal complaint is of recent indrawing of the nipple or of bloodstained discharge. In addition, a small percentage of patients present with symptoms produced by secondaries, for example backache, pathological fracture, or dyspnoea from lung and pleural involvement.

Examination of a patient with a lump in the breast must be carried out in an orderly manner:

The breasts are inspected for evidence of nipple elevation or retraction, or of skin fixation to the underlying tumour; the latter is then checked by gently moving the lump within the breast. Recent nipple retraction is very suggestive of malignant disease, but the nipple may have been indrawn since birth or following a previous acute infection. Skin fixation is also strong supporting evidence of carcinoma, although it may be seen rarely over an area of chronic mastitis and may accompany fat necrosis or follow chronic abscess.

Palpation commences first with the normal breast. The diseased breast is then examined, the clinical features of the lump being determined with especial reference to skin attachment and deep fixation. The axillary nodes and then all the other lymph node areas are palpated. A search is made of the other foci of possible distant spread; examine the chest, palpate the liver, test for the presence of ascites and examine the pelvis.

Investigations

The chest is X-rayed and a radiological and bone scan skeletal survey of skull, spine and pelvis is performed for secondary deposits.

A full blood count is performed, since anaemia and leucopenia suggest widespread bone marrow involvement.

Diagnosis is confirmed by fine needle aspiration or biopsy.

Treatment

Stages I and II

When the disease is clinically confined to the breast tissue alone or has only involved the axillary lymph nodes with no evidence of either spread into adjacent tissues, or of widespread dissemination, the surgeon hopes to be able to eradicate the disease and achieve a 'cure'. Unfortunately, in a proportion of these patients, microscopic metastases will already have occurred and so evidence of dissemination may become manifest months or years after the primary tumour has been removed. There is wide variation in the treatment of these cases in different centres. Surgery ranges from, at one end of the spectrum, removal of the lump only, through simple mastectomy, mastectomy with clearance of the axillary nodes, radical mastectomy in which the pectoral muscles are removed, to, at the other extreme, radical mastectomy combined with excision of the internal thoracic chain. There is no uniformity of opinion as to whether any of these methods should be combined with either pre- or post-operative irradiation or whether or not the ovaries should be either ablated or irradiated in pre-menopausal patients. The reason for this controversy is the rarity, to date, of carefully controlled clinical trials comparing the results of these various combinations of therapy. Such trials have now shown that no form of local treatment has any advantage over the other as regards patient survival.

Current opinion favours a relatively conservative approach. Most surgeons perform either simple mastectomy with clearance of the axilla, or else local removal of the tumour ('lumpectomy') combined with radiotherapy; the latter has the great advantage of an excellent cosmetic result and long-term studies indicate that life expectation and local tumour control are as good for this technique as for more radical mutilating surgery.

Because of the relatively poor prognosis in advanced stage II disease (those with extensive lymph node involvement), suggesting that in 60 per cent of these patients occult dissemination of tumour has already occurred at the time of presentation, there is particular interest in the trials in progress on the value of adjuvant cytotoxic or hormonal therapy in this group.

Stage III cases

Surgical clearance of the disease is now impossible. Local radiotherapy often produces useful palliative results although a 'toilet' operation may later be required to remove a fungating and ulcerating local lesion.

Stage IV and recurrences after previous mastectomy

A solitary distant deposit, for example in one bone, or local recurrence in the scar following mastectomy, is best treated by local radiotherapy.

Topical injection of a cytotoxic may be used in the treatment of malignant ascites or pleural effusion after preliminary aspiration of the fluid.

Where dissemination is widespread, sex hormones or 'hormone surgery' are used. About 30 per cent of all breast tumours are hormone dependent. The tumour oestrogen receptor assay, at present only performed at special referral centres, is helpful in predicting the likelihood of response. ER positive tumours respond to hormone therapy in 60 per cent of cases, whereas ER negative tumours are rarely hormone dependent (10 per cent). Hopefully refinement of this type of assay will enable more accurate assessment to be made in the future.

There are several methods of hormone therapy available Tamoxifen, a potent anti-oestrogen, has a low incidence of side-effects and should be the first line of treatment in both pre- and post-menopausal patients.

Patients who do not respond to Tamoxifen are managed:

1 If the pre-menopausal or early post-menopausal: ovarian ablation, either by oöphorectomy or radiotherapy.
2 Post-menopausal women: either stilboestrol or ethinyl-oestradiol.
3 Bilateral adrenalectomy.
4 Hypophysectomy.

These last two major surgical procedures are now rarely employed and have been replaced by:

5 'Pharmacological adrenalectomy', which may be effected by means of Amino-glutethimide, which inhibits synthesis of cortisol and adrenal androgen and oestrogen.

In patients with widespread disease not responding to hormone therapy temporary regression may be effected by means of cytotoxic drugs, particularly in the form of combination therapy.

Pregnancy and breast cancer

Fortunately carcinoma of the breast occurs rarely during pregnancy and lactation. The disease process, presumably because of hormonal effects, may be considerably accelerated with the appearance of an inflammatory type of lesion, the so-called mastitis carcinomatosa. In most cases, however, the tumour behaves like a cancer of the same stage in a non-pregnant woman.

Although the prognosis is serious it is not necessarily hopeless. Treatment is carried out along the lines already indicated according to the stage at which the disease presents. Most surgeons advise termination of the pregnancy.

Carcinoma of the male breast

This accounts for less than 1 per cent of all cases of breast cancer. The prognosis is worse than in the female, probably because of the sparse amount of breast tissue present, which allows rapid dissemination of the growth into the regional lymphatics.

Treatment consists of radical mastectomy, but since so little skin is available it is often necessary to carry out a skin graft to the cover the resulting cutaneous defect.

Orchidetomy and cytotoxic therapy may be employed in advanced cases with disseminated disease.

Prognosis

The 5-year survival rate in stage I tumours is approximately 80 per cent; stage II lesions approximately 40 per cent. A small number of stage III and IV growths may also have prolonged survival, especially if slow growing or hormonally dependent.

In addition to the staging of the tumour, histological grading is also of great importance; the less differentiated the tumour, the worse the prognosis.

PAGET'S DISEASE OF THE NIPPLE

Paget described diseases of bone, penis and nipple, all of which bear his name.

Pathology

The nipple lesion occurs in middle-aged and elderly women. It presents as a unilateral red, bleeding, eczematous lesion of the nipple which is eventually destroyed. It is associated with a carcinoma of the underlying breast which may or may not form a palpable mass.

Microscopic appearance

The epithelium of the nipple is thickened with prolongations of the rete pegs. The deeper layers of the epithelium contain multiple clear Paget cells with small dark-staining nuclei; these are hydropic malignant cells. The underlying dermis contains an inflammatory cellular infiltration.

Careful search of the breast after mastectomy usually reveals the presence of an associated intraduct carcinoma, even if this was clinically impalpable and some distance from the nipple.

Aetiology
　　Paget's disease probably represents the invasion of the nipple by malignant cells arising in a duct which also gave origin to the associated breast tumour.

Treatment
　　Mastectomy or local excision with post-operative radiotherapy. In the absence of a palpable mass the prognosis is excellent. When a mass is present the prognosis resembles carcinoma of the breast in general and depends on the stage of the tumour and its histological grade.

BREAST SCREENING

　　Since micrometastases are frequently present when only a small lump can be detected by palpation, much effort has been devoted to discover breast cancer before there is a lump. A nationwide mammography breast screening is now in progress in the UK. All women between 50 and 65 are offered mammography every three years. A suspicious lesion on X-ray that cannot be felt has to be localized by 3 dimensional radiography and a wire inserted into the radiological abnormal tissue so that the surgeon can remove the area by local excision and confirm that the specimen is the correct portion of breast by X-ray. Then histological examination will establish the diagnosis. If carcinoma is found, management is as for Stage I tumours outlined above. Early data from screen trials indicate a pickup of 1 suspicious mammogram in 1000 and of these selected cases, 50 per cent are malignant. It is hoped that this early detection will be rewarded by a significant improvement in survival and that the expensive screening process does not in itself cause harm from the radiation exposure.

Chapter 49
The Skin and its Adnexae

SEBACEOUS CYST (EPIDERMOID CYST OR WEN)

A sebaceous cyst is a retention cyst produced by obstruction to the mouth of a sebaceous gland: sebaceous cysts may therefore occur wherever sebaceous glands exist and are not found on the gland-free palms and soles. They are especially common on the scalp, face, scrotum and vulva and on the lobule of the ear. The cyst is fluctuant and cannot be moved separately from the overlying skin. There may be a typical central punctum and the contents are cheesy with an unpleasant smell. The lining membrane consists of squamous epithelium.

Complications

1 Infection
2 Ulceration, which may then resemble a fungating carcinoma — ('Cock's peculiar tumour').
3 Calcification, producing a hard subcutaneous tumour misnamed a 'benign calcifying epithelioma'.
4 Horn formation.
5 Malignant change — very rare.

Treatment

The uninfected sebaceous cyst should be removed to prevent possible complications. A small incision is made over the cyst under local anaesthetic, the capsule incised, the contents evacuated and then the capsule avulsed with artery forceps. If acutely inflamed, drainage will be required, followed later by excision of the capsule wall.

Rhinophyma is the name applied to the red bulbous nose produced in the elderly subject by hypertrophy of the sebaceous tissues. If treatment is demanded for cosmetic reasons the excess tissue is pared down with a scalpel; rapid regeneration of skin occurs from the deep remnants of the sebaceous glands.

IMPLANTATION DERMOID

This is a subcutaneous cystic swelling commonly found on the fingers. It usually follows a puncture injury with consequent implantation of epithelial cells into the subcutaneous tissues; the typical, white, greasy material of the cyst content results from, degeneration of the desquamated cells. In some examples there is a tell-tale old healed scar over the cyst, confirming a preceding injury and clinching the diagnosis.

VERRUCA VULGARIS (WART)

This is the familiar well-localized horny projection which is common on the fingers, hands, feet and knees, particularly of children and young adults. Crops of warts may occur on the genitalia and perianal region, in many cases spread by sexual contact. The lesion is often multiple and is due to a virus infection.

Microscopically, there is a local hyperplasia of the prickle cell layer of the skin (acanthosis) with marked surface cornification.

Treatment

Untreated, warts usually vanish spontaneously over a number of months, hence the apparent efficacy of folk-lore 'wart-cures'. Often reassurance that these lesions will disappear is all that is required, but if treatment is demanded they can be burnt down by the application of a silver nitrate stick or podophyllin or curetted with a sharp spoon under local or general anaesthesia.

Plantar warts are verrucas which occur on the weight-bearing areas of the foot. Pressure forces the wart into the deeper tissues, producing intense local pain on walking. They may occur in epidemics in schools, etc., where the hygiene of the communal bath or changing room is not of a high standard.

They should be treated by silver nitrate or curettage.

MOLLUSCUM SEBACEUM (KERATOACANTHOMA)

A lesion which occurs most commonly on the face and nose (75 per cent) but may also be found on the fingers, hands and elsewhere on the skin in patients of the 50 to 60 age group. It appears as a rapidly-growing nodule which may reach an inch or more in diameter in a few weeks and which closely resembles an epithelioma or rodent ulcer in appearance; indeed, it is only this story of very rapid growth which helps differentiate it from the latter.

Histologically it consists of a central crater filled with keratin surrounded by hypertrophied squamous stratified epithelium. There is no invasion of the surrounding tissues.

If left untreated, the natural history of lesion is its disappearance over a period of 4 or 5 months, leaving a faint white scar. Its aetiology is unknown, but it does not appear to be a virus infection; attempts to transfer it by means of tissue extract have failed; moreover, its solitary situation and occurrence in mainly elderly patients are both against a viral origin.

Treatment

It is safest to remove the lesion, if only to establish histological proof of the diagnosis with confidence.

GANGLION

Although ganglia are amongst the commonest of surgical lumps, their origin is uncertain. They may represent a benign myxoma of joint capsule or tendon sheath, a hamartoma or a myxomatous degeneration due to trauma.

Ganglia occur especially around the wrist and the dorsum of the foot (joint capsule origin), or along the flexor aspect of the fingers and on the peroneal tendons (tendon sheath origin). They are unilocular thin-walled cysts with a synovial lining which contain mucoid fluid having the microscopic appearances of

Wharton's jelly. Histologically, they are indistinguishable from cysts of the lateral cartilage of the knee and semimembranosus bursae.

Treatment

The patient may complain of discomfort or of the cosmetic appearance; if so the cyst should be excised under a general anaesthetic and in a bloodless field produced by a tourniquet. The old-fashioned treatment of hitting the ganglion with the family Bible ruptures the cyst, but recurrence usually occurs after some time. Recurrence is unfortunately quite common after surgical excision if even a fragment of the ganglion wall is left behind.

PILONIDAL SINUS

The majority of pilonidal sinuses occur in the skin of the natal cleft. They may be solitary or appear as a row in the midline. Frequently tufts of hair are found lying free within the sinus (pilonidal = nest of hair).

Usually young adults are affected, males more than females, and more often in dark-haired individuals; the sinuses are rarely seen in children. They may also occur in the clefts between the fingers as an occupational disease of barbers and are found rarely in the axilla, at the umbilicus, the perineum and the sole of the foot as well as on amputation stumps.

Aetiology

Complicated embryological theories of failed fusion and of tail-bud retraction are invoked, but although post-anal pits are seen in the new-born, pilonidal sinuses rarely present until adolescence. Moreover, a congenital theory of origin does not explain the occurrence of pilonidal sinuses elsewhere and the occurrence of such sinuses on the hands and feet of men working with cattle, where the contained hair is clearly of animal origin, all seem to be in favour of the hypothesis that these sinuses occur by implantations of hair into the skin; these set up a foreign body reaction and produce a chronic infected sinus. It may be that in some cases the post-anal pits act as traps for loose hairs, thus combining both the congenital and acquired theories of origin. The hair enters the skin follicles from its distal end and works its way in due to tapered lateral hair extensions angled proximally.

Clinical features

The pilonidal sinus is symptomless until it becomes infected; there is then a typical history of recurrent abscesses which have either required drainage or have discharged spontaneously.

Treatment

If an acute abscess is present, this must be drained in the usual way. In the quiescent phase the track is excised or simply laid open and allowed to heal by granulation. Recurrence is diminished by keeping the surrounding skin free from hair by rubbing with fine sandpaper, shaving or the use of depilatory creams.

THE NAILS

These are the site of some common and important surgical conditions:

PARONYCHIA

Paronychia denotes infection of the nail fold, usually of the finger, but it may complicate an ingrowing toe-nail (see below).

Diagnosis of acute paronychia is obvious; the nail fold is red, swollen and tender, and pus may be visible beneath the skin.

Treatment

If seen before pus has formed, at the cellulitic stage, infection may be aborted by a course of penicillin or other appropriate antibiotic together with immobilization by a splint to the finger and a sling to the arm. If pus is present, drainage is performed through an incision carried proximally through the nail fold, combined with removal of the base of the nail if pus has tracked beneath it.

Chronic paronychia is seen in those whose occupation requires constant soaking of the hands in water, but it may also occur as a result of fungus infection of the nails and where the peripheral circulation is deficient, e.g. Raynaud's phenomenon.

Ingrowing toe-nail

This is nearly always confined to the hallux and is usually due to a combination of tight shoes and the habit of paring the nail downwards into the nail fold, rather than transversely; the sharp edge of the nail then grows into the side of the nail bed, producing ulceration and infection.

Treatment

If seen before infection has occurred, advice is given on correct cutting of the nails, 'winkle-picker' shoes are vetoed, and a pledget of cotton wool tucked daily into the side of the nail bed after preliminary soaking of the feet in hot water to soften the nails to enable the nail to grow up out of the fold.

If an acute paronychia is present, drainage will be required by means of removal of the side of the nail or avulsion of the whole nail. For recurrent cases when the infection has settled, the nail should be obliterated, either by excision of the nail root (Zadek's operation) or by treating the nail bed with phenol.

Onychogryphosis

This condition of an intensely coiled 'ram's horn' deformity of the nail may affect any of the toes, although the hallux is the commonest site. It may follow trauma to the nail bed and is usually found in elderly subjects.

Treatment

Relatively mild examples can be kept under control by trimming the nail with bone cutting forceps. Merely avulsing the nail is invariably followed by recurrence and the only adequate treatment is excision of the nail root.

Lesions of the nail bed

It is here convenient to list a number of relatively common conditions which affect the nail bed:

1. Haematoma

As a result of crush injury to the terminal phalanx, with or without fracture of the underlying bone, a tense, painful haematoma may develop beneath the nail. Relief is afforded by evacuating the clot through a hole made either by a dental drill or by a red hot needle; both procedures are painless. Occasionally a small haematoma may develop after a trivial or forgotten injury and clinically may closely simulate a subungual melanoma.

2. Subungual exostosis

This is nearly always confined to the hallux and is especially found in adolescents and young adults. The exostosis may actually ulcerate through the overlying nail, producing an infected granulating mass. The diagnosis is confirmed by X-raying the toe and treatment is to remove the nail and excise the underlying bone nodule.

3. Melanoma

The nail bed is a common site for malignant melanoma (see page 363). The lesion should be confirmed by excisional biopsy followed by amputation of the digit. If the regional lymph nodes are involved, block dissection is performed.

4. Glomus tumour

The nail bed of the fingers and toes is a common site of this extremely painful lesion which is a benign tumour arising in a subcutaneous glomus body (highly innervated arterio-venous anastomosis). It is considered on page 368.

TUMOURS OF THE SKIN AND SUBCUTANEOUS TISSUES

Classification

1. Epidermal

    (a) *Benign:*
        (i) Papilloma.
        (ii) Senile keratosis.
        (iii) Seborrhoeic keratosis.
    (b) *Malignant:*
        (i) Bowen's disease.
        (ii) Squamous cell carcinoma.
        (iii) Basal cell carcinoma.
        (iv) Secondary deposits (e.g. from carcinoma of breast and lung, leukaemia, Hodgkin's disease).

2. Benign and malignant melanomas

3. Tumours of sebaceous and sweat glands

4. Dermal tumours

From blood vessels, lymphatics, nerves, fibrous tissue or fat.

EPIDERMAL TUMOURS

Papilloma

A common, benign, pedunculated tumour, often pigmented with melanin. Microscopically it comprises a keratinized papillary tumour of squamous epithelium.

Senile (solar) keratosis

A small, hard, brown, scaly tumour on exposed surfaces, e.g. the face and hands of the elderly.

Microscopically hyperkeratosis is present, often with atypical dividing cells in the prickle layer.

The importance of this lesion is that it may undergo change into a squamous cell carcinoma.

Seborrhoeic keratosis

A common tumour of the elderly. It appears as a yellowish or brown raised lesion on the face, arms or trunk and is often multiple.

Microscopically, there is hyperkeratosis, proliferation of the basal cell layer and melanin pigmentation.

The lesion is quite benign, but differential diagnosis from a melanoma can only be made with certainty by excising the lump and submitting it to histological examination.

Bowen's disease

This is a 'carcinoma *in situ*'. It appears as a very slowly growing, thickened, brown lesion with well-defined margins.

Microscopically, there is marked mitotic activity in the prickle cell layer with the presence of giant cells and large, clear Paget cells.

Treatment is adequate excision; if left untreated eventually a squamous cell carcinoma will supervene.

Squamous cell carcinoma (epithelioma)

Occurs usually in the elderly male, especially in skin areas exposed to sunshine, i.e. face and back of the hands. It is relatively common in white subjects who live in the tropics.

Predisposing factors

Include:
1 Senile keratosis.
2 Bowen's disease.
3 Lupus vulgaris.
4 Exposure to sunshine or irradiation.
5 Carcinogens — e.g. pitch, tar, soot.
6 Chronic ulceration (Marjolin's ulcer — see below).
7 Immunosuppressive drugs.

Pathology

Macroscopically it presents as a typical carcinomatous ulcer with raised everted edges and a central scab. *Microscopically* there are solid columns of epithelial cells growing into the dermis with epithelial pearls of central keratin surrounded by prickle cells. Occasionally anaplastic tumours are seen in which these pearls are absent.

Spread occurs by local infiltration and then by lymphatics. Blood spread occurs only in very advanced cases.

Treatment

Consists of either wide excision or radiotherapy, depending on the site of the lesion.

If the regional lymph nodes are involved, block dissection is indicated.

Marjolin's ulcer

The name applied to malignant change in a scar, ulcer or sinus, e.g. a chronic varicose ulcer, an unhealed burn, or the sinus of chronic osteomyelitis. It has the following characteristics:

1 Slow growth, because the lesion is relatively avascular.
2 Painless, because the scar tissue does not contain cutaneous nerve fibres.
3 Lymphatic spread is late, because the scar tissue produces lymphatic obliteration.

Once the tumour reaches the normal tissues beyond the diseased area, then rapid growth, pain and lymphatic involvement take place.

Basal cell carcinoma (rodent ulcer)

Occurs usually in elderly subjects, males twice as commonly as females. Ninety per cent are found on the face above a line joining the angle of the mouth to the external auditory meatus, particularly around the eye, the naso-labial folds and the hair line of the scalp. The tumour may, however, arise on any part of the skin and this includes the anal margin. Predisposing factors are exposure to sunlight or irradiation. The tumour is particularly common in white-skinned subjects in tropical regions.

Pathology

Macroscopically the tumour has raised, rolled, but not everted edges. It consists of pearly nodules over which fine blood vessels can be seen to course. Starting as a small nodule, the tumour very slowly grows over the years with central ulceration and scabbing.

Microscopically solid sheets of uniform, darkly staining cells arising from the basal layer of the skin are seen. Prickle cells and epithelial pearls are both absent.

Spread is by infiltration with slow but steady destruction of surrounding tissues; in advanced cases the underlying skull may be eroded or the face, nose and eye may be destroyed, hence the name 'rodent'.

Lymphatic and blood spread occur with extreme rarity.

Treatment

By excision where this can be done with an adequate margin and without cosmetic deformity. It is also indicated in late cases where the tumour has recurred after irradiation or has invaded underlying bone or cartilage. In the majority of cases, however, superficial radiotherapy gives excellent results. Where the tumour occurs on or near the eyelid, the conjunctiva must be protected by means of a lead shield during irradiation therapy.

MELANOMA

Aetiology

Melanomas develop from melanoblasts which are situated in the basal layer of the epidermis and which are now considered to be derived from dermal nerve end organs and to originate from the neuro-ectoderm of the embryonic neural crest. Some melanoblasts contain no visible pigment, but all are characterized by a positive DOPA reaction; they can all convert dihydroxyphenylalanine (DOPA) into melanin.

Classification

The melanomas may be classified into:
1 Intradermal melanoma or naevus (the common mole).
2 Compound melanoma or naevus.
3 Juvenile melanoma.
4 Junctional melanoma or naevus.
5 Malignant melanoma.

Nearly everyone possesses one or more moles; some have hundreds although they may not become apparent until after puberty. Those moles which are entirely within the dermis remain benign, but a small percentage of the junctional naevi, so called because they are seen in the basal layer of the epidermis at its junction with the dermis, may undergo malignant change (Fig. 49.1).

Intradermal melanoma or naevus

This is the commonest variety of mole. The naevus may be light or dark in colour and may be flat or warty. A hairy mole is nearly always intradermal. They may be found in every situation except the palm of the hand, the sole of the foot or the scrotal skin.

Histologically they are situated entirely in the dermis where naevus cells form non-encapsulated masses. They never undergo malignant change.

Compound melanoma or naevus

Clinically this is indistinguishable from the intradermal naevus, but histologically it has junctional elements which make it potentially malignant.

Juvenile melanoma

Melanomas before puberty are relatively unusual. Microscopically they may be

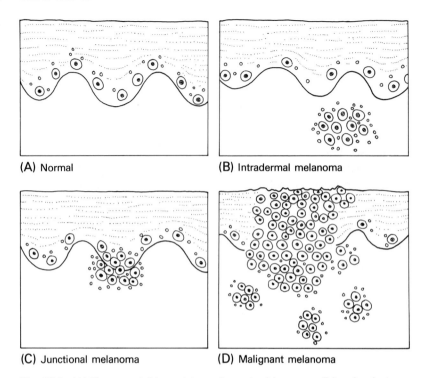

(A) Normal

(B) Intradermal melanoma

(C) Junctional melanoma

(D) Malignant melanoma

Fig. 49.1. (A) The normal skin contains melanocytes (shown as cells) and melanin pigment shown as dots. The pigment increases in sunburn and freckles. (B) A benign intradermal naevus; the melanocytes are clumped together in the dermis to form a localized benign tumour, (C) a junctional naevus with melanocytes clumping together in the basal layer of the epidermis. These are usually benign but may occasionally give rise (D) to an invasive malignant melanoma.

indistinguishable from malignant melanoma; yet fortunately and surprisingly these usually pursue a completely benign course. Melanomas in children should therefore always be dealt with by conservative surgery in spite of their frightening histological appearance.

Junctional melanoma or naevus

The junctional naevus is pigmented to a variable shade from light brown to almost black. It is nearly always flat, smooth and hairless. It may occur anywhere in the body and, unlike the intradermal naevus, may be found on the palm of the hand, sole of the foot and the genitalia. Histologically, naevus cells are seen in the basal layers of the epidermis from which the cells may spread to the surface.

Only a small percentage of junctional naevi undergo malignant change, but it is from this group that the vast majority of malignant melanomas arise.

Malignant melanoma

About 3000 cases of malignant melanoma occur annually in the UK.

The majority are cutaneous, but malignant melanoma may also be found on the mucous membrane of the nose, mouth, anus and intestine. Another important group arise from the conjunctiva, the choroid and the pigmented layer of the retina.

The tumour may be found on any part of the skin, but especially on the lower limb, the sole of the foot, the nail beds and the head and neck. Recent figures show an increasing tendency for malignant melanoma to occur on the lower limbs of young women, and increasing exposure to sunlight has been blamed for this. It is, surprisingly, rare in the pigmented skin of coloured races where, for practical purposes, it is only found in the non-pigmented skin on the sole of the foot. The prognosis of malignant melanomas of the face is rather better than elsewhere.

The majority probably arise in pre-existent junctional naevi.

Immunology

A number of observations suggest that there may be an immunological mechanism concerned in the growth of malignant melanoma. It is well known, for example, that a melanoma may cease to grow or even undergo, very rarely, a spontaneous regression. In some patients antibodies specific to melanoma antigens can be demonstrated at an early stage of the disease but these disappear when secondary deposits occur, which suggests that spread of the tumour has resulted from loss of this immunological barrier.

Signs of malignant change in a naevus

1 Increase or irregularity in size
2 Increase or irregularity in pigmentation
3 Bleeding or ulceration.
4 Spread of pigment from the edge of the tumour.
5 Itching or pain.
6 Formation of daughter nodules.
7 Lymph node or distant spread.

Microscopically pleomorphic cells are seen which spread through the layers of the epidermis and which are usually pigmented. Occasionally the cells are amelanotic, in which case they are still DOPA positive.

Spread

As well as local growth and ulceration, malignant melanomas seed by lymphatic permeation, which produces cutaneous nodules by progressive proximal spread, and by lymphatic emboli to the regional lymph nodes. There is also widespread dissemination by the blood stream to any and every organ in the body. Free melanin in the blood may produce generalized skin pigmentation and melanuria in late cases.

Treatment of pigmented lesions

The following is a general guide to the management of pigmented lesions of the skin:

Any pigmented tumour on the hand, sole or genitalia, or any which, in other situations, are subjected to trauma should be excised; these are the commonest among the small percentage of naevi to undergo malignant change. In addition, pigmented lesions should be removed for cosmetic reasons or if the patient is acutely anxious about their presence — this is a particularly common phenomenon among doctors, nurses and medical students. Such lesions are sent for careful histological examination and should always be removed in their entirety.

If the pigmented lesions show any of the features already listed which suggest that malignant change has taken place the tumour is first removed for urgent histological examination. If malignant melanoma is confirmed, then a wide local excision of the area is performed with primary skin grafting.

If the regional nodes are involved, these are treated by block dissection. If impalpable, they are kept under careful surveillance and block dissection performed if subsequent enlargement takes place.

Where the condition is locally irremovable some palliation may be produced by radiotherapy or by using cytotoxic agents systemically or by regional perfusion.

Prognosis

Prognosis depends on large number of factors:

1   The thickness of the primary lesion. Prognosis is good when this is less than 1.5 mm in depth. The deeper the lesion, the greater the risk of lymph node metastasis.

2   A superficial spreading melanoma has a better prognosis than a penetrating and ulcerating lesion.

3   The anatomical site — tumours on the trunk and scalp have a poor prognosis.

4   The presence of lymph node metastases are of grave prognostic significance and more so if there are cutaneous deposits.

Five-year survival in patients treated adequately before lymph node dissemination has occurred is about 75 per cent but recurrences may develop after many years, especially with melanoma of the eye which may produce liver secondaries more than 20 years after the removal of the original tumour. Hence the aphorism 'beware the patient with the large liver and the glass eye'.

Once the regional lymph nodes are involved the 5-year survival drops to 20 per cent. survival after the appearance of disseminated metastases is usually short.

TUMOURS OF SWEAT AND SEBACEOUS GLANDS

Benign and malignant tumours of these glandular adnexae of the skin are rare.

Sebaceous adenomas

These are more in the nature of a hyperplasia of the glands than true tumours. They occur as pink of yellow nodes on the nose, cheek and forehead. Microscopically they are merely overgrowths of sebaceous glands.

Sebaceous carcinoma

Found rarely on the face and scalp in elderly subjects. Carcinomatous change may occur in sebaceous cysts.

Sweat gland adenomas or carcinomas

May occur on the face and scalp and in the apocrine sweat glands of the axilla, vulva and scrotum. They are composed of columns or cylinders of clear cells and the descriptive term 'cylindroma' is applied to these tumours for this reason. On the scalp they may form masses of large nodules ('turban tumour'), but tumours of similar appearance may also be of basal cell origin.

DERMAL TUMOURS

Tumours of blood vessels usually lie in the dermis, although the underlying muscles and soft tissues may be involved. The abdominal viscera, central nervous system and bone may also be the sites of these lesions. The terminology of blood vessel tumours is confusing and is bedevilled with picturesque descriptive terms. Most benign blood vessel 'tumours' are indeed congenital malformations or hamartomas.

Classification:

1　Capillary haemangioma.
2　Cavernous haemangioma.
3　Sclerosing angioma (Fibrous histiocytoma).
4　Glomus tumour.
5　Haemangiosarcoma.
6　Kaposi's sarcoma.

Capillary haemangioma

A variety of types of congenital capillary malformation may be found in the skin, usually at birth. The 'salmon pink patch' is a common blemish on the head or neck of a new-born child and rapidly disappears spontaneously. The 'strawberry naevus' is bright red, raised, and usually disappears during the first few years of life, although there may at first be a rapid alarming enlargement, even with ulceration, before involution occurs. The 'port-wine stain', flush with the skin, usually on the face, lips and buccal mucosa, produces an extensive area of dark red, blue or purple discoloration. It shows no tendency to regress with increasing age. Campbell de Morgan spots are found on the trunk of middle age and elderly subjects. They are bright red aggregates of dilated capillaries which can be emptied by pressing on them with the tip of a pencil and are of no significance.

Note that port-wine stain of the face may have a segmental distribution corresponding to the cutaneous branches of the trigeminal nerve and may be associated with angiomas of the cerebral pia-arachnoid which may manifest themselves by focal epileptic attacks (the Sturge–Weber syndrome).

The 'spider naevus' of chronic liver disease is another example of a capillary haemangioma. Touching the middle with a pinhead causes the lesion to disappear whilst the pressure continues.

Treatment

Most strawberry naevi disappear spontaneously, but diathermy coagulation, application of CO_2 snow or excision and grafting may be required. The port-wine stain is best left alone. It may be disguised with cosmetics and occasionally excision with skin graft replacement or laser coagulation is undertaken.

Cavernous haemangioma

These are made up of large blood spaces lined with endothelium; they occur on the skin, lip, and quite commonly, as multiple nodules in the liver.

The lesions are blue, may be raised and may partly empty on pressure. They may infiltrate the underlying tissues and may be associated with unsightly overlying cutaneous thickening.

Treatment

This is often difficult. The condition may be disguised by the use of cosmetics or thrombosis can be encourage by injection of 33 per cent saline. Very unsightly lesions may be excised and skin grafted.

Sclerosing angioma (fibrous histiocytoma)

This is a pigmented tumour of the skin which may easily be confused with a malignant melanoma with which it has a close macroscopic resemblance. Palpation, however, reveals a typically hard consistency due to the dense fibrous stroma. It is probably produced as a result of fibrosis of a capillary haemangioma. The pigment is due to iron and not to melanin: this is easily shown with specific histological staining.

Glomus tumour

Glomus bodies are found in the subcutaneous tissues of the limbs, particularly the fingers, the toes, and their nail beds. They are convoluted arteriovenous anastomoses with a cellular wall comprising a thick layer of cuboidal 'glomus' cells which are modified plain muscle; between these cells are abundant nerve fibres. These structures are perhaps concerned with cutaneous heat regulation. Glomus tumours are blue or reddish small raised lesions which occur in young adults at the common sites of glomus bodies. Their characteristic is exquisite tenderness which makes their slightest touch agonizing.

Treatment

Treatment is excision of the lesion, which is rewarded by the heartfelt gratitude of the patient.

Haemangiosarcoma

Malignant tumours of the vascular endothelium are extremely rare, although they do occur at any site where haemangiomas are found. In the past the term has been applied to many highly-vascular sarcomas simply because they contained large vascular spaces.

Haemangiosarcoma of the liver has been reported in workers in the plastics industry exposed to vinyl chloride.

Kaposi's sarcoma

This tumour has a multi-centric origin. It presents as a number of bluish red or dark blue nodules scattered over the extremities of one or more of the limbs. It is usually found in elderly patients, particularly Russians and Africans. Ninety per cent are in male subjects. It is the commonest tumour to develop in patients with AIDS. The nodules spread centrally along the limb, may ulcerate and may metastasize to the liver and lungs.

Histologically there are two components, blood vessels and fibroblasts; the latter show the malignant features, thus distinguishing this tumour from a heamangiosarcoma. The tumour can be kept under control for long periods by local radiotherapy of cytotoxic drugs.

Telangiectasis

Telangiectases, althought not truly tumours, are conveniently mentioned in this section. They are dilatation of normal capillaries and are seen in a number of circumstances; in the weatherbeaten faces of countrymen, on the legs of young women, who may complain of their cosmetic appearance.

Multiple congenital telangiectases (Osler's disease) is an inherited Mendelian dominant disease with tiny capillary angiomas of the skin, lips and mucous membranes; they may give rise to repeated nose-bleeds and gastro-intestinal haemorrhage.

LYMPH VESSEL TUMOURS

Lymphangiomas are congenital in origin and similar to haemangiomas; they are lined by endothelium but contain lymph. They ar relatively uncommon, but occur mainly on the lips, tongue and cheek, resulting in macrocheilia or macroglossia.

Cystic hygroma

Arises from the jugular lymph sac in the neck, the embryonic precursor of the jugular part of the thoracic duct. It consists of a multilocular cystic mass which is often present at birth or noticed in early infancy. Characteristically it is supremely transilluminable. It may respond to injection of hypertonic saline as a sclerosant. Surgical treatment consists of excision, but this is a difficult procedure since the cysts ramify throughout the structures of the neck.

NERVE TUMOURS

Tumours of the peripheral nerves arise from the neurilemmal sheath of Schwann, hence the terms neurilemmoma, neurofibroma or Schwannoma. They push the fibres of the nerve to one side or actually grow within the substance of the nerve. The tumours may be solitary or multiple and may involve any peripheral nerve in the body. Of the cranial nerves the VIIIth is most commonly involved, often as a solitary tumour (the acoustic tumour, see page 83). Tumours may arise within the spinal canal, particularly from the dorsal nerve roots, resulting in an extramedullary, intrathecal, slow growing spinal tumour (see page 108). A part of this tumour may protrude through the intervertebral foramen, producing a dumb-bell tumour which projects either into the thoracic or abdominal cavity.

In the skin and subcutaneous tissues there is a wide range of presentations from a solitary tumour arising from a peripheral nerve to uncountable numbers involving the whole of the body (*Von Recklinghausen's disease*; his name is also applied to the osteitis fibrosa cystica of hyperparathyroidism).

Clinical features

The tumours may appear in childhood and there is often a family history, Von Recklinghausen's disease being an autosomal dominant condition. The cutaneous lesions are soft and often pedunculated. They are usually painless, although pressure may produce pain along the line of the nerve, particularly when larger nerve trunks are involved. The tumour is mobile from side to side but not longitudinally, in the line of the nerve to which is it attached. There may be associated café au lait patches of pigmentation. In some cases there are disfiguring masses of neurofibromatous tissue over which the thickened skin hangs in ugly folds. The 'Elephant Man' of the London Hospital was a gross example of the disease.

Treatment

Where the neurofibromas are solitary or few in number removal can be performed, either by enucleation, if the nerve fibres are pushed to one side, or resection with suture of the divided nerve. Incomplete removal must not be performed since sarcomatous change may follow. Where the whole body is covered by these lesions some cosmetic improvement can be effected by excising the more noticeable lesions from the face and hands.

Neurofibrosarcoma is uncommon. It may arise *de novo* or as malignant change in a neurofibroma. Clinical features are pain, rapid growth and peripheral anaesthesia or paralysis. Treatment is wide excision.

FATTY TUMOURS

Lipoma

Lipomas are the commonest of benign tumours. They usually occur in adults and the sex distribution is equal, although females are more likely to present to the surgeon for cosmetic removal of these lesions. Lipomas may arise in any connective tissue but especially in the subcutaneous fat, particularly around the shoulder and over the trunk. They do not occur in the palm, sole of the foot or in the scalp, because in these areas the fat is contained within dense fibrous septa. Occasionally lipomas appear in large numbers subcutaneously and it is sometimes quite difficult to differentiate them from neurofibromas. Elsewhere it is useful to remember 'lipomas occur beneath everything'; thus, in addition to being subcutaneous, they may be sub-fascial, sub-periosteal, sub-peritoneal, sub-mucosal and sub-pleural.

The diagnosis is rarely in doubt with this soft lobulated fluctuant tumour. The fluctuation is interesting; it is often said to be due to the fat being liquid at body temperature, but anyone observing an operation will notice that fat within the body certainly does not flow out in liquid form over the surgeon's boots when the skin is incised. The fluctuation can be explained by the histological structure of the lipoma, which consists of aggregates of typical fat cells; each cell itself forms a microscopical cyst. This is very much like the fluctuation which can be elicited in a colloid goitre made up of thyroid vesicles distended with colloid material.

Treatment

Consists of excision if the lipoma is cosmetically troublesome.

Liposarcoma

A rare tumour which probably arises as an unusual event in a pre-existing benign lipoma. The retroperitoneal site is commonest, but it may also occur around the thigh region and should be suspected if the tumour is very large, firmer than usual, vascular or rapidly growing.

Treatment

Comprises wide excision if this is possible.

Chapter 50
Transplantation Surgery

Classification of grafts
1   Allograft — viable transplant between members of the same species.
2   Isograft — viable transplant between identical twins.
3   Xenograft — transplant between members of different species.
4   Structural grafts — act as a non-living scaffold. Can be of biological origin, e.g. arterial and heart valve grafts, or synthetic, e.g. Dacron vascular prosthesis.

Responses to transplantation

The behaviour of organs and tissues transplanted within a species depend initially on surgical technique and subsequently on biological factors. The function, however, of certain transplanted tissues depends on their structure and viability is not necessary; arterial grafts and cardiac valves are examples. Corneal and cartilage grafts suffer little from biological damage due to the separation of the living cells from direct contact with the blood stream. The cornea and anterior chamber of the eye are known as privileged sites for grafting. The fate of most other tissues following successful surgical transplantation depends on the relationship of donor to recipient. Transplants of tissue between identical twins (isografts) behave the same as transplants within the same individual, they take permanently, although with the kidneys there is a danger of the original disease of the recipient affecting the transplanted organ.

The biological destruction of grafts between unrelated members of the same species (allografts) is an immune process. The graft behaves as an antigen, which specifically sensitizes the lymphoid tissues of the recipient. Antibodies and cellular immune mechanisms destroy the grafts. Should another transplant be performed from the same donor to the same recipient (second set graft) it will be destroyed more quickly than the first due to the immunity resulting from the previous graft.

Tissue typing

Some prediction of the behaviour of tissue grafted from a given donor to a given recipient can be provided by serological typing analogous to red blood cell grouping. Instead of red blood cells, lymphocytes are tested against antisera to transplantation (histo-compatibility) factors. As with red cell groups, compatibility requires that there are no antigens present in the donor which are absent in the recipient.

The most well-defined transplantation antigens are inherited in a similar way to red cell groups. These antigens belong to the HLA system which is determined by 2 linked genes on the sixth human chromosome, so that a normal diploid individual possesses 4 HLA antigens. A cytotoxicity test is used with antisera which kill lymphocytes containing the specific antigen. More accurate typing by

DNA analysis is now used for certain purposes where speed is not essential e.g. paternity testing. Nomenclature is standardized so that the typing results in one laboratory are comparable to those in all others. This is of great importance in the logistics of transplantation, since in order to obtain a good match it is necessary for there to be a large pool of recipients awaiting organ transplantation and also access to a large number of donor organs. Rapid interchange of information and transport of organs to the appropriate recipient requires an organization structure that is efficient and can operate at any time of the day or night. The data are stored in a computer in the main reference centre for each large population area, e.g. one for the United Kingdom in Bristol.

Unfortunately as more is known of transplantation antigens, so that pattern becomes increasingly complicated; there are additional antigens of the major histocompatibility locus complex (MHC) on the same chromosome as the 4HLA antigens and other antigens on different chromosomes. Any of these can be of biological importance in clinical transplantation. Within a family the HLA antigens act as markers for the other minor antigens. Thus tissue typing of two siblings will result in 25 per cent chance of a 2 chromosome match, 25 per cent chance of a 2 chromosome mismatch and 50 per cent chance of a single chromosome match. Kidney grafts between siblings of identical MHC antigens do outstandingly well. Results of grafts between blood relatives in general correlate well with HLA matching. When a kidney is grafted from an unrelated donor, the relevance of HLA matching is far weaker, since even perfect HLA matching does not imply matching of the minor antigens. The chief value of HLA typing in such cases is to prevent grafting across a positive cross-match in sensitized patients (where recipient serum kills donor lymphocytes, antibodies having resulted from a previous graft, blood transfusions or pregnancy) and avoiding HLA antigens in second grafts that were present in the first graft that had been rejected. Nevertheless an attempt is always made in organ grafting to obtain as good as match as possible, and always to match for RBC compatibility. The red cell antigens are of great importance in organ grafting and a B kidney grafted into an A recipient is unlikely to function more than an hour due to cytotoxic anti B antibodies in the recipient's circulation.

Immunosuppression

With the exception of kidney grafts between identical twins, some method of inhibiting the immune system of the recipient is always necessary. Unfortunately it has not so far been possible clinically to produce specific immunosuppression by use of donor antigen.

The most valuable immunosuppressive agents are azathioprine (Imuran, a derivation of 6-mercaptopurine), cyclosporin and corticosteroids. These agents are potentially toxic and their dosage has to be very carefully regulated. The serum antibodies of animals injected with human lymphocytes — anti-lymphocyte globulin, ALG — has been used as an additional immunosuppressive agent, but products vary in efficacy and toxicity. Monoclonal antibodies directed against human lymphocytes, T cells or lymphocyte subsets are rapidly displacing the older multivalent products. Recently it has been possible to remove the animal antigenic material from monoclonal antibodies so in future we will be able to give treatment for longer periods with 'Humanized' monoclonal antibodies.

The best form of immunosuppression for clinical organ transplantation is a triple therapy regimen of Imuran, cyclosporin and corticosteroids, each given in low relatively non-toxic doses, so that good immunosuppression is achieved without the side effects of bone marrow depression for azathioprine, nephrotoxicity for cyclosporin and Cushing's syndrome for corticosteroids. Mono- and polyclonal antibodies have been shown to be effective in the treatment of acute rejection crises. Unfortunately, after a week to 10 days, antibodies are produced against the antilymphocyte antibodies, which cause them to lose their activity.

CLINICAL ORGAN TRANSPLANTATION

Kidney transplantation has been practised for more than 30 years and in the last 10 years, liver, heart and combined heart and lung transplants have been performed on a routine basis in North America and Western Europe. A kidney donor may be a live, related volunteer; unrelated donors are not accepted as donors in the United Kingdom. Cadaveric donors have to be used for heart, lungs and liver transplantation and also for most kidney and pancreas grafts. Exceptions are lung and liver lobe grafts to children from parents and the 'Domino' heart donated from a recipient of a combined heart–lung transplant. There is a serious shortage of donor organs, which is likely to become more worrying as the results of transplantation improve, since a life-saving organ that can transform a moribund patient back to full rehabilitation is more precious than any material treasure for the patient in question. Due to prejudice, lack of information and the extra work involved, many organs are lost that could be transplanted to help the sick.

Cadaver donors

An organ must be removed from a body that is not contaminated by bacterial or viral infection or a metastasizing tumour. Most suitable donors are victims of road traffic accidents and subarachnoid haemorrhage. It is obviously futile to transplant necrotic organs; the cells of the tissue to be grafted must be alive. Therefore, organs to be used for transplantation are taken from individuals with brain stem death with the circulation still intact or just after the circulation has ceased. Criteria accepted in the UK for establishing brain death have never been seriously challenged by professional neurologists or neurosurgeons; the only concern is that the tests are performed correctly by skilled doctors. Despite attempts by certain television programmes to undermine the public's confidence in the medical profession, in general the lay population trust doctors to make the correct decision as to when to stop ventilation of a patient with brain stem death, and most people have a charitable attitude toward organ donation after death.

Organ preservation

As soon as circulation to the organ to be transplanted stops, the organ is plunged into cold physiological solution and the vasculature is perfused with cold electrolyte solution of ionic composition and osmotic pressure similar to that of intracellular fluid. The organ is then kept in a sterile environment surrounded by ice. The kidney will keep satisfactorily for more than 36 hours, the liver for 20 hours, the heart and heart lungs for 5 to 6 hours and the pancreas probably also for 20 hours.

Kidney transplantation

More than 400 000 kidneys transplants have been performed throughout the world, the results have been very carefully assessed and there are now a number of survivors with functioning grafts after more than 20 years. The kidney has an advantage over other organs for transplantation in that patients with renal failure can be maintained in reasonably good physical condition by regular twice or thrice weekly dialysis, whereas there is no equivalent luxury for patients with heart, lung and liver failure. The principles of the technique are shown in Fig. 50.1. The blood supply, venous and ureteric drainage are re-established as expeditiously as possible. Anti-rejection immunosuppressive treatment is started immediately after operation, usually with low doses of azathioprine, cyclosporin A and steroids. Daily assessment of kidney function enables rejection to be diagnosed at an early stage, usually confirmed by a transcutaneous needle biopsy of the kidney.

Cellular rejection can usually be reversed by large doses of steroids or mono-clonal antibodies. One and 5-year functional survival is approximately 90 per cent and 85 per cent if the donor was an HLA identical sibling, 85 per cent and 70 per

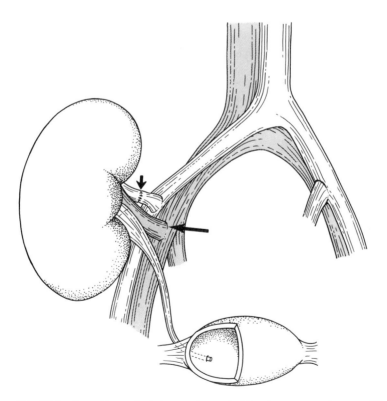

Fig. 50.1. A renal transplant. Arrows show arterial and venous anastomoses. The kidney is inserted extraperitoneally into the iliac fossa. (By courtesy of *Discovery*).

cent for a parent and 80 and 60 per cent for a cadaver donor. Most complications occur in the first 6 months after transplantation.

Liver transplantation

Liver transplantation has now been accepted as the treatment of choice for many forms of fatal liver disease. Patients should be offered the operation before they become too sick for what is the most formidable of surgical assaults. The four main categories of patients are those with primary tumours of the liver, cirrhotic processes, acute hepatic necrosis and metabolic diseases, e.g. oxalosis. Alcoholics are unreliable concerning follow-up and the taking of immunosuppression and they are liable to resume alcohol consumption after operation. However, selected cases, who have given up drinking, do well. Approximately 80 per cent of liver transplant recipients survive a year and the 5-year figure is approaching 60 per cent. The longest survivor is now alive and well 23 years after operation.

Heart, lung and combined heart lung transplants

Heart transplantation is a relatively straightforward operative procedure in a unit where open heart surgery is performed. The indications are atherosclerotic coronary artery disease and cardiomyopathy. Lung transplantation without the heart is now well established, either one or both lungs or grafted. Both lungs with the heart can be grafted en bloc, three anastomoses being required, namely aortic, trachael and right atrial. The indications for lung transplantation are primary pulmonary hypertension and chronic obstructive airways disease. The survival of recipients of both heart and combined heart and lung grafts is approximately 80 per cent at one year. The longest period of survival after heart grafting is 20 years and after combined heart and lung transplantation 10 years.

Pancreas grafting

It is likely that transplantation for the treatment of diabetes will eventually involve beta cells or islets, possibly with the help of genetic engineering, but although more than 150 islets grafts have so far been attempted in man, they have nearly all failed. The only successful results have been with transplantation of the vascular-ized pancreas or a pancreatic segment. One of the dangers of pancreas grafting is leakage of pancreatic digestive juice, which can lead to severe surgical complica-tions. A variety of techniques have been used to overcome this, namely injection of the pancreatic duct with occlusive material such as Neoprene, drainage of pancre-atic juice into the gastro-intestinal tract and drainage into the bladder. These three techniques have all produced some good long-term results.

Pancreas transplantation is still in a developmental stage, the longest survivor with a functioning graft has lived more than 12 years. Approximately 70% of grafts are functioning after one year. It remains to be proved whether a pancreas graft will prevent the development and progression of the microangiopathy, which causes retinal and renal damage. Diabetic nephropathy has been the main indica-tion of pancreas grafting and usually a kidney from the same donor has been transplanted.

With all organ transplants, not only must the surgery be performed with great care, the organs suffer no severe ischaemic damage, and rejection be controlled, but in addition the patient must be followed up in the long term. In some cases there is danger of recurrence of the original disease in the transplanted organ, for example, glomerular nephritis and diabetic nephropathy in the kidney, hepatic malignancy, hepatitis and auto-immune disease in the liver, coronary artery disease in the heart and islet cell destruction in patients who have an active auto-immune process which caused the original diabetes. Other diseases are cured, for example, polycystic kidney treated by kidney grafting and biliary atresia, inborn errors of metabolism such as Wilson's disease and alpha-1-antitrypsin deficiency treated by liver grafting. It is clear that organ grafting is now an important part of surgery, with results overall much better than those obtained with many common cancers.

Index